THE WOMAN'S GUIDE TO PEAK PERFORMANCE

THE WOMAN'S GUIDE TO

PEAK PERFORMANCE

The Ultimate Reference for All Levels of Fitness

SUSAN L. PURETZ, ED.D.

ADELAIDE HAAS, PH.D.

DONNA I. MELTZER, M.D.

CELESTIAL ARTS
Berkeley, California

Note to the Reader
The information presented in this book is designed to help you improve your health and fitness and to assist you in making informed health decisions. It is not intended to be a substitute for professional medical care or the advice of a physician. We recommend that you seek the guidance of a licensed health care provider before beginning an exercise program.

 Celestial Arts • P.O. Box 7123 • Berkeley, California 94707

Distributed in Canada by Publishers Group West, in the United Kingdom and Europe by Airlift Books, in New Zealand by Tandem Press, in Australia by Simon & Schuster Australia, in Singapore and Malaysia by Berkeley Books, and in South Africa by Real Books.

Interior design by Star Type, Berkeley
Cover design by Brad Greene
Interior illustrations by Akiko Aoyagi Shurtleff

Library of Congress Cataloging-in-Publication Data

Puretz, Susan L.
      The woman's guide to peak performance / Susan L. Puretz, Adelaide
Haas, Donna I. Meltzer.
            p.   cm.
      Includes index.
      ISBN 0-89087-841-2 (pbk.)
      1. Exercise for women. 2. Physical fitness for women.   I. Haas,
Adelaide.   II. Meltzer, Donna I.   III. Title.
RA781.P84   1997
613.7′045—dc21   97-42142
                                                         CIP

First printing, 1998
Printed in Canada

1 2 3 4 5 6 - 03 02 01 00 99 98

Contents

Acknowledgments

We are appreciative of the assistance we received from the many persons who made the writing of this book possible. They were all wonderful and generous with their time and energy. We are especially indebted to the women who openly shared their exercise stories with us.

Our editors Veronica Randall and Heather Garnos were instrumental in turning manuscript pages into a finished book. We appreciate their support, helpful advice, patience, and encouragement through some very challenging times. The research and writing of this book were sometimes collaborative efforts and sometimes individual ones. Each author's chapters were critiqued by the others, with the understanding that the named author was ultimately responsible for the final content.

From Adelaide and Susan:

Our research survey was given direction, design, and analytic help from Steve Scanfianza. Marianne Jaffee's layout design and Pat Arnst's diverse secretarial skills were invaluable. Assistance in distributing the questionnaire was provided by Ruth Haas, Ira & Sieglinde Luskin, Robert & Virgnia Nacamu, the organizers of the Kingston Classic, and many others; we appreciate their efforts.

Dedicated colleagues in the Sojourner Truth Library at SUNY New Paltz, particularly Gerlinde Barley, Corrinne Nyquist, and Gary Oliver, helped us establish a solid research foundation.

To our readers we owe our deep thanks for thoroughly and thoughtfully reviewing our manuscript: Yvonne Allenson, Brenda Bass, Hollise Carr, Ely Cohen, Beth Glace, Deana Groves, Joseph Haas, Gretchen Madoff, Mary Phillips, and Louise Tricard. For their special information and contributions we thank Anthony Dos Reis, Daniel Honig, Rhonda O'Conner, Robert Owens, and Louise Tricard.

Finally, we thank Phillip McDonald and Kurt Haas, without whose understanding and help this book would not have been written.

From Donna:

Many thanks to my colleagues, O. Jones, Cathy Alexander, and Lily B. Lepre, for their detailed and careful review of the manuscript. I appreciate the technical advice offered by Helen and Rich Gibbons and Barbara Krauss Auguston. Michael Egnor, M.D., from the Department of Neurosurgery at University Medical Center at Stony Brook, made helpful suggestions. A very special thanks should go to Bobbi Stek for her patience in modeling.

The resources available at the Health Sciences Center Library at SUNY Stony Brook, and the Oyster Bay Public Library were invaluable in helping me research articles in order to establish facts and dispel myths surrounding exercising women.

I am grateful to Daniel, Julie Nicole, and Emily Egnor, and Justin Alexander for constantly reminding me about the truly important things in life. They deserve special recognition for helping me keep everything in proper perspective.

I am indebted beyond words to my sisters, Laurie J. Meltzer and Shelley Egnor, for their unfailing advice, support, humor, and friendship. Lastly, I cherish the encouragement offered by my mother, Julie W. Meltzer, who as a septuagenarian is living proof of the virtues of staying active and fit.

Introduction

In recent years, exercise has become more and more important for women of all ages and fitness levels. Female athletes are garnering more acclaim and respect, and nearly one-half of the participants in the most recent Olympics were women. But most of us are not Olympic contenders or professional competitors: you may be an amateur athlete, a member of a fitness program, or someone who's just starting to think about embarking on a fitness regime. Maybe you used to exercise and want to regain your previous level of fitness. Regardless of your current exercise level, this book is for and about you—the female with an interest in fitness and peak performance.

The health and quality of life benefits of exercise are enormous. Despite all that is known about these benefits, reports from the Surgeon General[1] indicate that 60 percent of Americans do not engage in regular exercise, and 25 percent of adults do not exercise at all. From the teen years onward, females are more likely than males to be sedentary, and unfortunately, this situation worsens with advancing years.

Despite these depressing statistics, women of all ages can and do enjoy a full range of physical opportunities. The types of activity that we can incorporate into our lives are endless and range from the exotic, like rock climbing, to the familiar, like walking. Each has its attractions, benefits, and liabilities. Each contributes to our health and physical fitness.

We, the authors of this book, are all physically active. Throughout our lives we have managed to continue to exercise despite the obligations of home, education, and career. While some may view exercise as an indulgence, we see it as a necessity—and feel better for having been active.

As we've exercised over the years, we have been repeatedly impressed with the special needs of women. Our bodies are shaped differently than our male counterparts, hence some of the distinctions in our physical performance. In this book, we address the unique and special needs that women have when training or simply exercising. We also consider nutrition, our monthly periods, pregnancy, and the impact of children. We have come to realize that properly fitting clothing and equipment are key, and that "unisex" gear may not always be appropriate for women, and so we offer advice on finding the best gear and clothing.

When we decided to collaborate on this book, we made a unanimous decision that we wanted to contribute something important and lasting to the betterment of women's health care and fitness. We also realized the need to provide accurate, authoritative, and contemporary information on women's issues in sports. It is our hope that with this book's help you will stay fit and attain peak performance at whatever endeavor you pursue. Above all, we hope you remember that the "f" in fitness should stand for fun, not frustration, fear, or failure.

1. U.S. Department of Health and Human Services. *Physical Activity and Health: A Report of the Surgeon General.* Atlanta, GA: U.S. Department of Health and Human Services, Centers for Disease Control and Prevention, National Center for Chronic Disease Prevention and Health Promotion, 1996.

Why We Exercise

ADELAIDE HAAS, PH.D.

A day without exercise is like a day without sunshine. I'm irritable, depressed, and out-of-sorts if I don't get my daily workout fix. I sometimes settle for a brisk half-hour walk, but I usually crave and get much more. —Kim, age 31, works out at a local health club, takes aerobics classes, plays tennis, and skis.

Some women, like Kim, are strongly motivated to exercise, while many others try to avoid physical exertion and prefer to relax. Whether you are already physically active, or simply know it is good for you and want to get started, you will find much of interest in this chapter.

WHAT IS EXERCISE?

My mother doesn't understand why I belong to a health club and work out. She says that her generation got plenty of exercise cleaning the house and running after children. She thinks that if I want to do more I should spend the time helping her with her housework and volunteering to assist other older people.

—Sally, age 55, bookkeeper

Is housework exercise? Certainly you stretch, use your muscles, and get your heart pumping faster. While dedicated exercisers may believe there is a difference between work and exercise, the Surgeon General's report on physical activity and health indicates that routine chores such as washing windows, pushing a baby stroller, and shoveling snow produce the same benefits as more formal exercise.[1] We checked with the Centers for Disease Control and Prevention and the American College of Sports Medicine to help us sort this out, and gleaned the definitions that follow.[2]

Physical activity is "any bodily movement produced by skeletal muscles that results in energy expenditure." Moderate physical activity is defined as any activity that is done at the intensity level of walking three to four miles per hour, a brisk pace.

Exercise is a form of physical activity. It is a "planned, structured, and repetitive bodily movement done to improve or maintain one or more components of physical fitness."[2] According to the Consensus Symposium on Physical Activity, Fitness, and Health, held in Toronto in 1992, exercise is also a "leisure-time" activity.[3]

So, here lies the difference. Housework is clearly physical activity and may be moderate or even intense, but its purpose is home maintenance, not bodily fitness. Because of its goal, housework is generally not considered to be something one does during leisure. Nonetheless, a by-product of housework may be a degree of physical fitness. The same would apply to physical activity that is part of one's job.

Sports, since the nineteenth century, has come to refer to "highly structured, rule-laden games."[4] Before that time, activities such as hunting and fishing were considered "sport," but bowling and cricket were thought of as games.[4] Sports sociologists acknowledge difficulty in arriving at clear definitions, as do the participants in our study (see page 7). The Consensus Symposium we cited earlier notes a geographic difference in concept. In North America, sports connote physical activities that involve competition. In Europe, "sport" is used to include other forms of exercise and recreation such as recreational hiking, biking, and swimming.[5]

Physical fitness describes the body's condition. To be fit means the person possesses "a set of attributes that . . . relates to the ability to perform physical activity."[6] The term is sometimes used in a sports-related sense. In this case physical fitness focuses on the speed, power, balance, coordination, agility, and reaction time needed to play the game well. A broader health-related definition emphasizes cardiovascular endurance, muscular strength and endurance, flexibility, and body composition. (See Chapter 4, Focus on Fitness, for more information.)

Basic Vocabulary

These often confusing terms can be summarized.

- Physical activity: any bodily movement.
- Exercise: activity that has as its goal the development or maintenance of physical fitness.
- Physical fitness: the body's condition relative to its ability to perform activities, including sports.
- Sports: recreational or professional (usually competitive) activities that typically result in improved physical condition.

A LOOK BACKWARD

We may believe that our generation discovered exercise for women. After all, many of our grandmothers were raised to believe that sports and leisure time physical activity were just for males. Ladies did not sweat, and a female involved in athletics was either a cheerleader or a companion to her husband, who enjoyed attending sporting events. But even while out of the spotlight, women have been physically active in work and play for centuries. Although we can't provide a world view, we highlight some aspects of women's activities in days gone by.

Ancient Times

From primitive times onward, both women and men have engaged in physical activity, although it was likely not exercise just for its own sake. Wall hangings from the Paleolithic era, 10,000 or more years ago, are reported to show women dancing.[7] Frescoes from Crete, dated about 4000 B.C., show young people of both sexes engaged in bull vaulting—a dangerous sport, possibly of religious significance, in which participants attempted to do a handspring off the back of a bull.

About 3,000 years ago, in Sparta, Greek girls participated in sports such as running races, wrestling, discus, and javelin. Young women were encouraged to become strong, it was believed, so that they would produce powerful sons. But whatever the motivation, these ancient females reaped the benefits of vigorous exercise.

In the early Middle Ages, the fifth-century bishop of Clermont, Sidonius, described women and men playing ball games for sport and recreation. In contrast, some scholars report that in twelfth-century England, for example, women's roles in athletics were primarily as scorekeepers and award presenters. Other researchers dispute this, and suggest that, in addition to providing support for male athletes, women also participated in certain activities, such as swimming, boating, hunting, ice skating, horseback riding, and archery.[7]

The 16th, 17th, and 18th Centuries

Europe.   Dancing was apparently the most common form of exercise during this period for women of all classes in England. Additionally, some women played cricket and trapball (an early form of baseball). Paintings and literature reveal that skating, sledding, foot racing, swinging, and seesawing were prevalent in Germany, France, and other parts of continental Europe.

Despite these activities, the opportunities for females to engage in recreational exercise were limited. English feminist Mary Wollstonecraft encouraged women to develop both minds and bodies, arguing that girls should be permitted to partake in the same exercises as boys. She advocated playgrounds where all children, regardless of gender or social background, could engage in gymnastic play in the fresh air.[8]

North America.   Native American women are reported to have engaged in various forms of dancing. In addition, ball games and foot races were part of the lives of American Indians of both sexes. European immigrants commented on the strength, agility, and endurance of these native women.[9]

When daily life is filled with hard physical work, little energy remains for recreational exercise. Therefore, the early European-American settlers, especially the women, tended to engage in little physical recreation.

As life became easier for the colonists, dancing emerged as a major recreation for both women and men. African-American women, slaves in those days, also sought out dancing for pleasure.[9]

The 19th and 20th Centuries

Frontier women and those who lived on farms were generally in better physical shape than those in cities. Country life required much strenuous work but often permitted time for horseback riding, dancing, and ice skating. However, women in the cities often led restricted lives. The clothing of the day, such as tight corsets and narrow shoes, combined with prevailing concepts of female gentility to keep many women in marginal health.

The early nineteenth century saw a concern for women's physical fitness. Feminists of the day, including Catharine Beecher, Emma Hart Willard, Almira Phelps, and Mary Lyon, argued and worked for exercise programs as part of women's education. Calisthenics, dancing, walking, and horseback riding were taught in the schools with which these women were associated: Hartford Female Seminary, Troy Female Seminary, and Mount Holyoke.

Toward the end of the nineteenth century, bicycles were introduced throughout Europe and America. Cycling provided women with excellent exercise as well as transportation. This was not without repercussions, as some male physicians raised ill-founded fears of women's overexertion and erroneously asserted that bicycling caused reproductive health problems.[10] In 1895, Vassar College, then an all-women's college, introduced the first field day. Activities included running races as well as other track and field events.[11]

Finally, by the beginning of the twentieth century, physical education for women gradually and partially became an aspect of European and American school programs. It was not until the end of this century, however, that females gained almost full access to sports and athletics.[12] But we're not there yet—some gaps remain. For example, two California girls were turned away from football practice at the beginning of the 1996 school year. They had prepared for the team all summer, but when they showed up for practice, they were told that their school district did not permit girls to play contact sports, for "safety reasons."[13]

PRESENT-DAY VIEW

Who Are These Female Exercisers?

To better understand female participation in exercise, and to gather information helpful in improving our physical pursuits, we conducted a survey. We distributed 1,500 questionnaires at running races, fitness and dance centers, educational institutions, and a union meeting. About one-third (497) of the forms were completed and returned to us. The questionnaire had 54 questions, with space for explanations. (You might like to take a few minutes to think about how you would answer the questions. A copy is in the Appendix.) The discussion that follows is based on our results and also on information provided by other researchers and writers.

Some Vital Statistics

One in Four. The United States Public Health Service reports that only about one in four adults (24 percent) in the U.S. today exercises on a regular basis. This is scant improvement over the 22 percent reported in 1985. Interestingly, and regrettably, about 25 percent of American adults are not physically active *at all*.[14] Which group do you belong to?

Does Age Affect Our Exercise Habits? According to recent data, age *is* a factor. For example, a 1995 study by the Centers for Disease Control reported that women in the 18-to-34 age range are almost twice as likely to exercise regularly, compared to those 65 and older.[15]

The women who participated in our project are between 14 and 81 years of age. About 16 percent are under age 30, 26 percent are between 30 and 39, 32 percent are between 40 and 49, 18 percent are between 50 and 59, 6 percent are between 60 and 69, and 2 percent are over 70 years of age. However, as we'll see in Chapter 14, you are never too old to benefit from exercise.

Education. The women in our survey tend to be quite well educated. Two-thirds are college graduates, and half of these also hold advanced degrees. Those who have not completed college generally either have some higher education, for example a two-year degree (12 percent), or are younger and likely have not yet completed their formal training.

More About Our Respondents.   About 60 percent of the participants in our project are currently married and a similar percentage have children. They are engaged in a wide assortment of jobs. Teacher, health care professional (nurse, therapist), homemaker, and office worker are the most frequently listed occupations. Also noted are salesperson, artist, farmer, veterinarian, student, retired, and unemployed.

Almost 90 percent of the women in our survey rate their health as good or excellent. While 76 percent rank their level of fitness as good or excellent; 20 percent consider it to be only fair. How do your rate your health and fitness?

What Do Women Exercisers Do?

The World Is Our Oyster.   The women who completed our survey are active in many ways. Most do more than one form of exercise. The most popular activity is walking; 75 percent report they do this for exercise. We were surprised to find that almost half the women (49 percent) in our project report that they engage in weight training on a regular basis. This is certainly a departure from previous generations, when weights were regarded as being just for men. Other commonly reported activities are biking (47 percent), hiking (39 percent), swimming (40 percent), running (38 percent), and dancing (28 percent). Skiing (alpine and nordic), soccer, softball, volleyball, golf, tennis, and badminton also are mentioned by a fair number of our respondents. A few women engage in more unusual pursuits such as sailing, aqua jogging, jet skiing, in-line skating, rock climbing, and windsurfing. What is your pleasure?

The respondents exercise in many different places, with 36 percent using more than one location. About 15 percent exercise primarily at home; a similar percentage belong to a health club or a "Y." Public parks, roads, trails, bike paths, dance studios, beaches, and high school/college tracks and other facilities also are reported as places to exercise.

A Serious Commitment.   More than 90 percent of our survey participants exercise more than three days per week, with 11 percent exercising daily. Almost all the women (98 percent) reported that they spend a minimum of 30 minutes exercising, and almost 25 percent of our participants said that their exercise lasts longer than an hour. When asked about intensity, 65 percent termed their exercise moderate, while 20 percent noted that it was intense. Almost one in three (31 percent) reported that they compete in some activities. Are you committed or are you an armchair enthusiast?

Exercise vs. Sports

When I was in high school, a casual game of tennis was considered exercise. Nowadays, I view tennis as a healthy activity, but certainly not a major form of exercise.
—Darlene, age 45, plays tennis and belongs to a health club where she engages in weight training and aerobics

Curious as to whether today's women view exercise and sports as equivalent, we asked our respondents, "Do you make a distinction between your sports activity(ies) and the things you do for exercise?" The vast majority (72 percent) of the women noted that they made no distinction between the two. The consensus was that as long as you are moving, getting your pulse rate up, and using muscles it does not matter what the activity is. What do you think?

Those survey respondents who did distinguish between exercise and sports made some interesting observations:

"Exercise = discipline; sports = fun."
"It's the difference between work and play."
"Exercise is done routinely. I do sports just once in a while."
"Sports are a luxury; exercise is my daily bread."

In general, women who compete in their physical endeavors are more likely to view their regular exercise as a preparation for their sports activities. They reported that running and weight training help to keep them in shape for tennis and soccer. But even some non-competitors noted that regular exercise is essential if they are to be fit for seasonal treats such as skiing and mountain climbing.

Focus on Fitness.　The last couple of decades have witnessed a change in attitudes toward physical activity. Prior to the 1970s, sports were valued for their own sake (pleasure, competition, team spirit) and for the exercise that they provided. Tennis courts and playing fields were filled with people who were enjoying themselves in healthful ways.

Since that time, a not-so-subtle shift in philosophy has been apparent throughout the United States and perhaps the world. Women and men are engaging in exercise to enhance their physical fitness and they often are substituting activities that are specifically directed at improving their bodies for the games and sports of old.

Aerobics classes, jogging, and weight training have been recognized as efficient ways of developing fitness. Softball and bowling are fun and afford some healthful benefits, but if time is limited, many people now prefer to be more directed in their exercise.

Aerobics classes almost killed my business. I taught African and Jazz dance in my community for about ten years before the fitness craze changed my life. I used to be the only game in town. Women and men wanted some exercise; they took my classes. Now, only those who already have an interest in dance register with me. It is sad. I used to cast out a net and land exercisers, some of whom found they really wanted and appreciated an aesthetic experience. One thing I know. I will not teach aerobics! —Brenda, age 58, dance instructor and performer

BEGINNINGS

About 25 percent of the women in our survey started exercising regularly as children. We wanted to know how they got started.

Parents and Schools

When I was six years old, my mother enrolled me in dancing school. Every Wednesday afternoon and Saturday morning I did tap, ballet, and acrobatics. It was fun. I remember this as a regular part of my life all through elementary school. I dropped out for about 30 years (ages 12 to 45), but I'm now back to dancing about twice a week. This time it's square, line, folk, and social. —Sally, age 72, retired teacher, dances with her husband and belongs to several dance clubs

When regular exercise is introduced in childhood, it is usually the parents who are the major influence. Just as Sally was given dance lessons, other respondents reported that their parents had exposed them to tennis, swimming, or ice skating. Some women reported that competitive swimming was part of their local public pool's program. Others indicated that their parents obtained memberships at a "Y."

Among the younger women, high school was sometimes an influence. Softball, track, and soccer teams encouraged these respondents to be active. Interestingly, women over 50 reported that they did not have these opportunities in their educational settings.

When I was in high school, sports were for boys. Some girls were cheerleaders, but none of my female friends was athletic. —Darlene, age 64

It is likely that Title IX, the Education Amendment of 1972, is most responsible for the change in athletic opportunity for women in schools. (See Chapter 7, The Competitive Edge.) Title IX mandated that physical education classes throughout the United States had to contain both boys and girls, and that athletics and sports had to be equally available to members of both sexes.[16] Prior to this time, physical training for girls was largely in the hands of parents and therefore considerably dependent on financial status, social factors, and programs outside the school.

Independent Choices

Most women in our survey (75 percent) started to exercise as adults. They pursued physical activity because they wanted it. Table 1.1 shows the percentage of respondents who gave specific reasons for beginning to exercise. As you can see, weight control and health were ranked as reasons one, two, or three by the majority of women. Pleasure and personal appearance were the next most frequently given reasons for starting to exercise. Relief of tension was ranked in the top three by more than one-third of the respondents. Parents, competition, and social factors were noted by less than 15 percent of the women answering our survey.

EXERCISE TODAY

What Motivates Women to Continue to Exercise?

The majority of women (51 percent) who completed our survey have been exercising regularly for more than five years. An additional 26 percent have been exercising regularly for one to five years. We asked the regular exercisers why they continue to exercise. Table 1.2 shows the reasons women gave for exercising today. Health has emerged as the primary motivation. But weight control (which may also be considered a health factor), pleasure, and personal appearance are still important. Overlooked by many women when they began to exercise, but considered significant today, is that exercise is valuable in reducing tension.

Research Reports the Benefits of Exercise

Open almost any issue of most magazines and newspapers, and you'll see articles touting the value of exercise. They report, usually quite accurately, the research showing that exercise yields both physical and psychological advantages.

Exercise Is Good for the Body

Watching Your Weight.   Exercise is a good way to control one's weight. As we reported earlier, more than half the women in our survey indicated that this was a major reason why they worked out. Almost every diet plan includes the caveat that exercise is important in weight loss.

Exercise contributes to obtaining and maintaining a lean, healthy look in several ways. The calories we consume permit the body to do its work. (The word "calorie" refers

TABLE 1.1

....

Reasons Women Began to Exercise (N = 497)

Percentage of Respondents Ranking

Reason	#1	#2	#3	Not Ranked
Weight	27.4	17.5	10.9	34.0
Health	26.8	14.5	12.1	29.2
Pleasure	20.0	10.7	13.3	35.5
Looks	12.5	17.9	13.1	37.6
Tension	8.7	14.7	14.1	42.1
Parents	5.6	1.2	1.0	85.3
Competition	5.2	4.0	3.6	74.8
Social	3.0	6.4	5.2	63.0
Other	6.0	2.4	1.2	88.7
	115.2*	89.3	74.5	

....

* Some respondents gave more than one primary reason for beginning to exercise.

to the "energy producing property of food."[17]) Unfortunately, most of us ingest more calories than our bodies require for normal functions, including breathing, building new cells, maintaining warmth, and so on. These extra calories are converted in our bodies to fat, unless we do something about it. If you exercise, you must eat more to maintain your weight. If you do not increase your caloric intake when you exercise, you will lose fat and your weight will slowly decrease. For more about food, see Chapter 10.

Do you know people who seem to be able to eat as much as they like and not gain weight, regardless of whether they exercise? These folks probably have relatively high metabolisms; they require a larger-than-average caloric intake just to maintain their weight. A naturally high metabolism may be due to factors beyond our control, but it may also be prompted by exercise, which we do control. Exercise speeds up metabolism, which means that in addition to using many calories during physical activity, the exercising person burns more while at rest.

Despite all we've learned about exercise, many Americans are overweight. The 1996 Surgeon General's report on physical activity and health states that 33 percent of American adults are overweight. The report is clear in its message that excess weight is harmful

TABLE 1.2

....

Reasons Women Continue to Exercise (N = 497)

Percentage of Respondents Ranking

Reason	#1	#2	#3	Not Ranked
Weight	23.5	19.4	13.0	28.5
Health	35.2	17.3	12.1	20.1
Pleasure	20.1	12.9	12.7	31.6
Looks	11.1	14.9	15.9	33.4
Tension	15.3	19.5	16.1	30.4
Parents	.2	.2	.2	92.2
Competition	2.4	3.0	2.8	76.9
Social	2.4	2.8	5.8	66.0
Other	6.3	1.4	1.0	89.7
	116.5*	91.4	79.6	

....

* Some respondents gave more than one primary reason for beginning to exercise.

to health. As weight goes up, the likelihood increases that a person will suffer from health problems such as high blood pressure, diabetes, increased LDL cholesterol (the bad kind), and decreased HDL cholesterol (the good kind). All of these problems are associated with disability and premature death.[18]

Strong Bones in a Strong Body.   It's known that exercise helps to build strong bones. A study by Dr. G. A. Greendale and colleagues at the University of California at Los Angeles was designed to determine the relationship between leisure time physical activity and bone mineral density. They asked 1,014 women and 689 men, with an average age of 73, to recall their level of exercise currently, at age 50, at age 30, and during their teen years. The researchers controlled for current age, body mass, arthritis, calcium and estrogen intake, cigarette smoking, and alcohol use. They concluded that both current and lifelong exercise appear to contribute to stronger hip bone mineral density.[19] (This is discussed further in Chapter 14, Keeping it Going: The Older Athlete.)

Regardless of your past activity levels, exercising today can benefit your bones. Dr. Illka Vuori summarized the work of many scientific researchers in the *Research Quarterly for*

Exercise and Sport, reporting that physical activity can improve bone mineral density at any age. She noted that some activities that utilize particular bones (for example, tennis stresses the forearm) result in increased bone strength primarily to those bones which are involved. However, moderate weight-bearing activity, such as brisk, regular, long-term walking, appears to be most effective in preventing age-related bone loss.[20] For a further discussion of exercise and osteoporosis (weakening of the bones) see Chapter 14, Keeping it Going: The Older Athlete.

Chronic Disease.   Can exercise actually keep you from getting some serious long-term diseases? The answer is "yes," according to the Centers for Disease Control and Prevention and the American College of Sports Medicine. Exercise, just like weight control, reduces the likelihood of many disorders. Of course, as we noted earlier, exercise and weight control often go hand-in-hand, so it may be hard to say which is actually conferring the benefits.

Nevertheless, epidemiological research has shown that exercise may offer reasonable protection from coronary heart disease, high blood pressure, non-insulin-dependent diabetes mellitus, osteoporosis, and colon cancer. Cancers of the female reproductive system (the uterus, cervix, ovaries, and vagina) and breast have been reported to occur less often among women who had been athletes during college, compared to their non-athletic classmates.[21] Generally it is agreed that exercise tends to improve the lipid-cholesterol composition of the blood, the muscle-to-fat ratio, bone density, tolerance for glucose, and the general ability of the body to ward off disease.[22]

Additional evidence of the value of exercise in preventing breast cancer is found in a 1997 study of more than 25,000 women. Women who exercised for at least four hours per week were 37 percent less likely than those who were sedentary to develop breast cancer. This research comes on the heels of other work which suggested similar benefits of exercise for women.[23]

Heart Problems.   The most convincing scientific evidence of the merits of exercise relates to cardiovascular function. Individuals who are least active have twice the risk of coronary heart disease compared to those who are most active.[24] High blood pressure, obesity, and a poor lipid-cholesterol blood profile associated with lack of exercise contribute to more frequent coronary heart disease. In addition, we must caution: smoking is also a major factor in coronary heart disease.

JoAnn E. Manson, M.D. reported the results of a large-scale study of the relationship of exercise to coronary heart disease and stroke. Dr. Manson and her colleagues at the Brigham and Women's Hospital in Boston examined the health and exercise patterns of more than 70,000 female nurses for four years. Those who were most active had 44 percent fewer strokes and 42 percent fewer heart attacks than those who were least active.[25]

Exercise Is Good for the Mind and Spirit

Can Working Out Make You Smarter?   It may seem like a stretch, but some evidence suggests that exercise improves mental as well as physical function. A study of adults between the ages of 65 and 72 found that those who participated in a 16-week walking program scored higher on tests of mental ability compared to a control group.[26]

> *If I don't go to the "Y" before work, I feel sluggish and unable to function effectively. My routine is to swim a mile Monday, Wednesday, and Friday mornings, and use the exercise bike Tuesdays and Thursdays. Quick shower follows, and I'm set for the day.* —Anne, age 65, advertising copywriter

Improve Your Reaction Time.   The ability to respond quickly tends to decrease with advancing age. A study by psychologist Arthur Kramer of the University of Illinois found that when previously sedentary adults between the ages of 63 and 82 participated in ten weeks of water aerobics classes, they were quicker at pushing buttons in response to different pitched tones compared to those who remained sedentary.[27] This kind of effectiveness might translate into improved ability to word process, enter data accurately, or drive a car more safely.

Handle Stress.   No life is stress-free. Home, work, and personal problems contribute to making us feel pressured. Exercise can enable us to deal more effectively with whatever life serves us. For example, a study of 5,000 college students revealed that those who exercised regularly had less anxiety and were better able to cope with the rigors of academic life.[28]

Chase Away the Blues.   Many studies have reached the same conclusion regarding the power of exercise to alter moods. Most kinds of exercise at nearly any age are helpful in warding off and curing even significant depression. Several studies found that exercise is as effective as psychotherapy, and a lot less expensive! However, exercise combined with psychotherapy is more helpful than either one alone.[28]

Exercise can help you over those minor "down" periods. You do not need to be pathologically depressed to benefit from a mood enhancer. Exercise tends to improve self-esteem. If you feel better about yourself, you are more likely to have a positive outlook on the world.[29]

That Exercise High.   Runners speak of the "high" they get—usually in their second mile. Some say the first mile is work, but then they develop a satisfying rhythm. Others report that the good feeling of exercise doesn't occur until the activity is over. One of our respondents called it an exercise "afterglow." Almost all the women in our survey reported that exercise was enjoyable.

> *Exercise is the most positive thing I do for myself right now. People think I'm nuts for getting up at 5 A.M. to do it, but it's the only time I can be reasonably certain I won't be interrupted. It's what refuels me and gets me through a day of chasing the kids around.* —Gail, age 34, mother of two young children

How Much Exercise Is Enough?

Now that you are convinced that exercise really is good for you, the question remains: How much do you need to reap the benefits? The answer is not simple. Stanford University researcher Dr. Ralph Paffenbarger observed, "Everyone is confused. . . . Even the scientists are confused." [30]

The reason for the confusion is that the findings of recent studies contradict some earlier research conclusions. Dr. I-Min Lee and her colleagues at the Harvard School of Public Health studied more than 17,000 Harvard alumni for a period of more than 20 years. They reported that an increase in life expectancy was found among those men who engaged in regular vigorous workouts, such as running, but not among men whose exercise was more moderate, such as walking and tennis doubles. Overall, the more active the men were, the longer they were likely to live.[31]

Researcher Dr. Paul Williams, of the University of California at Berkeley, studied women as well as men, and agrees with Dr. Lee. He reported that those factors that confer cardiovascular protection, such as lower body weight, lower blood pressure, and improved levels of blood cholesterol and lipids, were significantly more apparent in those whose exercise was intense.[32]

These findings stand in contrast to the 1991 "Guidelines" from the American College of Sports Medicine. Based on multiple studies, the recommendation was that just 30 minutes a day of moderate exercise, such as walking, is enough to prevent chronic diseases and promote longer life.

So, is a half-hour daily stroll enough to make you live longer and avoid serious diseases? Probably not. But it *is* better than sitting around and doing nothing. Dr. Arthur Leon, professor of health promotion and exercise at the University of Minnesota, and his colleague, Jane Norstrom, health communication specialist with the Park Nicollet Medical Foundation in Minneapolis, Minnesota, suggest an exercise pyramid.[33]

The Exercise Pyramid

running
mountain
climbing
racquetball
weight training
Level 3

social / folk dancing
relaxed swimming
wash floor • shovel snow
softball • golf • bowling
Level 2

walk to store • knead bread • clean house
walk up stairs • rake leaves • yoga • T'ai Chi
Level 1

The activities listed are examples of exercise you should be getting on a regular basis. You should try to engage in Level 1 every day, Level 2 three to five times a week, and Level 3 when and if you can. All levels are important; new activities at higher levels can be added if you are able.

Concept adapted from Leon, A. S., & Norstrom, J. Evidence of the role of physical activity and cardiorespiratory fitness in the prevention of coronary heart disease. *QUEST*, 1995, 47, 311–319.

The Exercise Pyramid. Not everyone can exercise vigorously. Advancing age, ill health, and physical problems can impose limitations. But just about everyone can do something, and that forms the base of the pyramid.

• **Level 1.** The bottom of the pyramid consists of those activities most of us took for granted a generation or two ago. We walked to mail a letter and buy a quart of milk. We climbed stairs, swept the steps, and sometimes kneaded bread. Everyone should try to take advantage of daily chores to keep active. Instead of riding the elevator, use the stairs. Don't drive right to your destination; park a block away and walk the difference.

• **Level 2.** Active recreation comprises the middle level of the pyramid. Examples are relaxed dancing, swimming, or playing softball for at least 30 minutes several times a week.

• **Level 3.** At the peak of the pyramid is intense physical activity. Not everyone is capable of pursuing this. But if you are able, engaging in intense activity for 30 minutes or more three or four times a week, combined with the other two levels of activity, is reported to yield the greatest health benefits. Recognize, however, that this can be carried to excess. If you stop menstruating prematurely, or if your weight drops below recommended limits, you risk estrogen depletion and osteoporosis now and in your later years. Increasing your food intake is often an effective solution.[34] (See Chapter 18, Beware of the Danger Zones, for more information on these problems.)

Are You Addicted to Exercise? Scientists describe addictions as habits that persist despite rational and reasonable efforts to end them. We normally think of alcohol, narcotic, and nicotine addictions, but more benign substances such as caffeine and sugar are also addicting. Behaviors may also be addictive. Think how habitual gambling, theft, lying, and violence may become. But is an apparently harmless, even beneficial, activity like exercise addictive?[35]

If you crave exercise, and don't feel well when you can't work out, you may have developed a habit that is hard to break. Dr. William P. Morgan of the University of Wisconsin believes that some runners and other athletes exhibit an addiction. He notes that these individuals "will do almost anything to get a running 'fix.' They may have withdrawal symptoms, such as depression, irritability, and insomnia, if they can't run."[36]

But exercise addiction is only harmful if it interferes with other aspects of your life. For example, it would be unhealthy for an injured person to persist in activities that hurt. Fortunately, the old slogan "no pain, no gain" is no longer popular. You can't work through pain. You need to listen to your body. So being addicted to exercise may be a good thing, if it encourages you to persist in this worthwhile activity. But it can be harmful if you refuse to modify your routine to compensate for illness, injury, or personal considerations. (See Chapter 5, Routines: The Stars Are the Limit, for more information.)

> *I was a totally compulsive exercise addict from age 20 to 32. Then I had to quit competitive running due to chronic injuries. I had to undergo a profound spiritual conversion in order to find a new way of living. Now I exercise with care because I love to feel and look good and the comradeship. I only compete with myself or informally with others along the trail.* —Diana, age 44

Why Not Work Out?

If exercise is so great, why don't more people do it? Approximately three out of four American adults do *not* exercise regularly. Bess H. Marcus, a professor of behavioral and preventive medicine at Brown University School of Medicine, examined some of the reasons why people do not engage in physical activity.[37]

Psychological Barriers.   Adherence to an exercise program requires first recognizing the importance of this commitment. Although public health messages abound, people with higher levels of education are more likely to appreciate the value of exercise. As noted earlier, respondents to our survey generally had more than a high school education.

Secondly, to be successful, you must set realistic goals and have the perseverance to stay with your plan. Some health clubs and exercise tapes set too high an expectation for participants. Would-be exercisers get discouraged.

> *When I first decided to join our local gym to lose weight and get in shape I got totally turned off. The place was filled with younger people who already looked great. I took one look around, and then simply walked out. I decided to try an exercise video in the privacy of my home. Unfortunately, the same thing happened. The workout was led by three trim, beautiful instructors, and in the background was a group of skinny dancers. It took a long time for me to find my proper niche.*
> —Gertrude, age 48, high school English teacher

Social and psychological support for exercise is helpful. If your friends are active, you are more likely to want to join in and participate too. Compliments you receive about looking good following a workout encourage continued activity.

No Place to Exercise.   Women, especially, may find it hard to find a place to work out. We may feel shy about how we look, and we may be unwilling to exercise in public.

Private clubs tend to be expensive and often do not feel welcoming to novice exercisers. It is not surprising that many women prefer to work out at home.[37] But even at home, lack of adequate floor space and concern or embarrassment regarding others with whom you live may interfere with your commitment to exercise.

• **Safety**. While jogging or bicycling may sound attractive, safety issues hold many women back. In a city, car traffic may be hazardous and automotive exhaust unhealthy. In rural areas, dogs may present a real danger. Sometimes a not-unwarranted fear of muggers keeps would-be exercisers inside out of harm's way.

Fortunately, some businesses recognize the importance of exercise for their employees and have provided facilities. Those women who have a secure place to exercise at their job site are more likely to maintain an exercise routine than those who do not.[37]

Too Much to Do, Too Little Time.   Lack of time is probably the primary reason that more women do not exercise. Married women may have multiple demands on them from their husbands, and possibly children and jobs. Single mothers find their hours and minutes largely accounted for. Time limitations were given as the primary deterrent to exercise by 65 percent of the respondents to our survey.

Given the importance of exercise, many women do overcome time limitations.[38]

WORKING IT OUT

Make exercise a priority

1. Put your workout on your schedule. It is an important part of your day. You find time to eat, sleep, and brush your teeth. Even a short regular exercise period will serve you well.
2. Let other things go. Are there extra chores you take on that could be eliminated? Remember, organize and prioritize!

Seize the moment

1. Walk up the stairs; don't use the elevator.
2. Park your car so that you must walk a little further to your destination.
3. Keep exercise clothing handy. You may be able to do some exercise during lunch or immediately after work.

Get equipped

1. Free weights and a jump rope are not expensive and may be used anywhere. (See Chapter 9, Gearing Up.)

Involve others

1. Get your partner or a friend to exercise with you. Together it is easier to find the time because you have a commitment to one another.
2. If you have children, bring them with you when you go to a track to run. They can play in the center area or ride bikes. Babies can come along in a baby-jogger. You get twice the workout and when baby is ready, he or she can toddle around. Most health clubs have child care facilities.
3. Plan your social life around active events. Instead of meeting friends for dinner, consider taking a hike. Walking and talking is a great way to relax, get exercise, and cement a relationship, all at the same time.

The rewards of regular physical activity are many. The reasons to exercise far outweigh the drawbacks. If you are not currently active and know you should be, follow the suggestions above to put fitness into your life.

1. Burros, M. It's not just weeding. It's a full-body workout. *New York Times*, July 14, 1996, Section 4, p. 2.

2. Pate, R. R., Pratt, M., Blair, S. N., et al. Physical activity and public health. A recommendation from the Centers for Disease Control and Prevention and the American College of Sports Medicine. *Journal of the American Medical Association*, 1995, *273* (5), 402–407.

3. Blair, S. N., & Hardman, A. Physical activity, health, and well-being. An International Scientific Consensus Conference, Quebec City, May 19–21, 1995. In *Research Quarterly for Exercise and Sport*, December 1995.

4. Park, R. J. From "genteel diversions" to "bruising peg": Active pastimes, exercise, and sports for females in late 17th- and 18th-century Europe. In Costa, D. M., & Guthrie, S. R. (Eds.). *Women and sport: Interdisciplinary perspectives*. Champaign, IL: Human Kinetics, 1994.

5. Bouchard, C., & Despres, J. P. Physical activity and health: Atherosclerotic, metabolic, and hypertensive diseases. *Research Quarterly for Exercise and Sport*, 1995, *66* (4), 268–275.

6. Pate, R. R., Pratt, M., Blair, S. N., et al. Physical activity and public health. A recommendation from the Centers for Disease Control and Prevention and the American College of Sports Medicine. *Journal of the American Medical Association*, 1995, *273* (5), 402–407.

7. Kennard, J. & Carter, J. M. In the beginning: The ancient and medieval worlds. In Costa, D. M., & Guthrie, S. R. (Eds.). *Women and sport: Interdisciplinary perspectives*. Champaign, IL: Human Kinetics, 1994.

8. Park, R. J. From "genteel diversions" to "bruising peg": Active pastimes, exercise, and sports for females in late 17th- and 18th-century Europe. In Costa, D. M., & Guthrie, S. R. (Eds.). *Women and sport: Interdisciplinary perspectives*. Champaign, IL: Human Kinetics, 1994.

9. Struna, N. L. The recreational experiences of early American women. In Costa, D. M., & Guthrie, S. R. (Eds.). *Women and sport: Interdisciplinary perspectives*. Champaign, IL: Human Kinetics, 1994.

10. Vertinsky, P. Women, sport, and exercise in the 19th Century. In Costa, D. M., & Guthrie, S. R. (Eds.). *Women and sport: Interdisciplinary perspectives*. Champaign, IL: Human Kinetics, 1994.

11. Tricard, L. M. *American women's track and field: A history*. Jefferson, NC: McFarland & Co., 1996.

12. Hult, J. S. The story of women's athletics: Manipulating a dream 1890–1985. In Costa, D. M., & Guthrie, S. R. (Eds.). *Women and sport: Interdisciplinary perspectives*. Champaign, IL: Human Kinetics, 1994.

13. *Florida Today* wire service. Girls declined chance to play football. August 30, 1996.

14. Brody, J. E. Why bad health habits drive out good ones. *The New York Times*, February 1, 1995.

    U.S. Department of Health and Human Services. Physical Activity and Health: *A Report of the Surgeon General*. Atlanta, GA: U.S. Department of Health and Human Services, Centers for Disease Control and Prevention, National Center for Chronic Disease Prevention and Health Promotion, 1996.

15. *New York Times*. Lack of exercise cited in U.S. women. *The New York Times*, February 19, 1995, 29.

16. Hult, J. S. The story of women's athletics: Manipulating a dream 1890–1985. In Costa, D. M., & Guthrie, S. R. (Eds.). *Women and sport: Interdisciplinary perspectives*. Champaign, IL: Human Kinetics, 1994.

17. Morehead, A. & Morehead, L. (Eds.). *The New American Webster Handy College Dictionary*. New York: New American Library, 1981.

18. U.S. Department of Health and Human Services. Physical Activity and Health: *A Report of the Surgeon General*. Atlanta, GA: U.S. Department of Health and Human Services, Centers for Disease Control and Prevention, National Center for Chronic Disease Prevention and Health Promotion, 1996.

19. Greendale, G. A., Barrett-Connor, E., Edelstein, S. et al. Lifetime leisure exercise and osteoporosis: The Rancho Bernardo study. *American Journal of Epidemiology*, 1995, *141* (10), 951–959.

20. Vuori, I. Exercise and physical health: musculoskeletal health and functional capabilities. *Research Quarterly for Exercise and Sport*, 1995, *66* (4), 276–285.

21. Lee, I. Exercise and physical health: Cancer and immune function. *Research Quarterly for Exercise and Sport*, 1995, *66* (4), 286–291.

22. Pate, R. R., Pratt, M., Blair, S. N., et al. Physical activity and public health. A recommendation from the Centers

for Disease Control and Prevention and the American College of Sports Medicine. *Journal of the American Medical Association*, 1995, *273* (5), 402–407.

23. McTiernan, A. Exercise and breast cancer—Time to get moving? *New England Journal of Medicine*, 1997, 336 (18), 1311–1312.

    Thune, I. et al., Physical activity and the risk of breast cancer. *New England Journal of Medicine*, 1997, 336 (18), 1269–1275.

24. Elrick, H. Exercise is medicine. *The Physician and Sportsmedicine*, 1996, *24* (2), 72–76.

    Blair, S. N., & Hardman, A. Physical activity, health, and well-being. An International Scientific Consensus Conference, Quebec City, May 19–21, 1995. In *Research Quarterly for Exercise and Sport*, December 1995.

25. Bronner, L. L., Kanter, D. S., & Manson, J. E. Primary prevention of stroke. *New England Journal of Medicine*, November 23, 1995, *333* (21), 1392–1400.

26. Moul, J. L., Goldman, B., & Warren, B. Physical activity and cognitive performance in the older population. *Journal of Aging and Physical Activity*, 1995, *3*, 135–145.

27. Brink, S. Smart moves. *U.S. News & World Report*, May 15, 1995, 76–84.

28. Nicoloff, G., & Schwenk, T. L. Using exercise to ward off depression. *The Physician and Sportsmedicine*, 1995, *23*, 44–58.

29. Biddle, S. Exercise and psychosocial health. *Research Quarterly for Exercise and Sport*, 1995, *66* (4), 292–297.

30. Brody, J. E. Trying to reconcile exercise findings. *The New York Times*, April 23, 1995, 22.

31. Brody, J. E. Study says exercise must be strenuous to stretch lifetime. *The New York Times*, April 19, 1995, A1 & C10.

    Brody, J. E. Trying to reconcile exercise findings. *The New York Times*, April 23, 1995, 22.

32. Brody, J. E. Trying to reconcile exercise findings. *The New York Times*, April 23, 1995, 22.

33. Leon, A. S., & Norstrom, J. Evidence of the role of physical activity and cardiorespiratory fitness in the prevention of coronary heart disease. *QUEST*, 1995, *47*, 311-319.

34. Baar, K. Time for a fitness pyramid. *The New York Times*, March 29, 1995, C1 & C6.

35. Rodgers, J. E. Addiction: A whole new view. *Psychology Today*, 1994, *27* (5), 32-38, 72, 74, 76, 79.

36. Solomon, H. A. *The exercise myth*. San Diego: Harcourt Brace Jovanovich, 1984, 101.

37. Marcus, B. H. Exercise behavior and strategies for intervention. *Research Quarterly for Exercise and Sport*, 1995, *I* (4), 319–323.

38. Fick, D. S., & Goff, S. G. Blending exercise into family life. *The Physician and Sportsmedicine*, 1996, *24* (2), 83–84.

2

A Woman Is Not a Man

DONNA I. MELTZER, M.D.

It is September 1973, and one of the first televised Battles of the Sexes is about to take place. Twenty-nine-year-old Billie Jean King, trying to promote women's professional tennis, is about to play opposite 55-year-old self-proclaimed male chauvinist Bobby Riggs. Ms. King triumphs in three straight sets, 6–4, 6–3, 6–3, and rejects taunts from courtside fans such as: "Come on, Billie Jean, start acting feminine—miss a few."[1]

Over the last few decades, there has been a dramatic increase in the number of women participating in sporting activities. More and more women of all ages are exercising—some for health and fitness, others for fun and recreation, and many because it makes them feel good. (See Chapter 1: Why We Exercise.) The growth in women's physical activity, at both the recreational and competitive levels, has prompted interest in health issues pertaining to the female athlete. In order to better understand some of these concerns, it is important to acknowledge that there are anatomical and physiological differences between women and men—a woman is not a man!

GROWING PAINS

I have an 8-year-old son and a 6-year-old daughter. They both play soccer during the school year. If they were the same size, I do not think I could honestly say that my son is more athletic than my daughter. —Pat, age 40

A Common Blunder

An individual's sex is determined at the time the sperm fertilizes the egg; however, it is not until puberty that sexual differentiation really becomes pronounced.[2] At birth, a quick glance at the genitalia helps your birth attendant announce the ecstatic lines of "It's a boy!" or "It's a girl!" Aside from the fact that males have penises and females have vaginas, it is very difficult to differentiate between unclothed baby boys and girls.

How many times have you made eye contact with an infant or toddler and complimented the parents on their beautiful child? Naturally, half the time your adulation evolves into an insult after you innocently ask "How old is he?" only to be corrected by the parent that "SHE" is whatever. Perhaps you have also been on the receiving end of this conversation. Of course, there is a reason for this common mix-up—young children look alike above and below the diaper area.

Measuring Up

Boys and girls have a similar body size and shape until puberty, when marked biological and anatomical differences begin to appear. Females usually reach puberty between the ages of nine and thirteen, approximately one to two years earlier than males, who develop pubescent changes between the ages of ten and fourteen.

Since girls have a shorter growth period than boys, it is not surprising that the average adult female is shorter and weighs less than her male counterpart.[3] Following puberty, the average young adult woman measures five feet, five inches tall, and the average man is five feet, nine inches tall.[4]

Building Blocks

Many social implications are associated with stature. For example, society has historically linked power, success, and athletic prowess to individuals of great build. However, today, all we have to do is look around us to see that this concept is flawed. Many notable leaders and Olympic champions, male and female, are simply not that tall!

Heredity has much to do with determining an individual's final height. The expected genetic contribution can be estimated by calculating the Mean Predicted Height (MPH) as follows: For girls: MPH = (*father's height – 5 inches + mother's height*) ÷ 2

For boys: MPH = (*father's height + 5 inches + mother's height*) ÷ 2

Normally, we would anticipate a person to be within three to four inches of the calculated MPH.[5] However, keep in mind that this is just a formula, and as interesting an idea as it is, many other factors determine your eventual height.

Why not test this formula out on your own immediate family? (It's probably easier to figure out if you perform the calculation with heights converted to inches.) Based on one author's parents' heights of five feet, nine inches (69 inches) and five feet, six inches (66 inches), this formula predicted that her adult height should be five feet, five inches, which is her exact height. Using this formula, her brother should be five feet, ten inches, five inches taller than she.

I started to diet and exercise shortly after I graduated from college because I felt that I was always walking around with a built in fat fanny pack. My boyfriend eats twice as much as I do and doesn't even have a hint of a spare tire. This does not seem fair.—Allison, age 29

While **androgenic** hormones enable pubescent males to build up their muscle mass, the **estrogenic** surge females experience results in increased body fat. Even for the same height, average body fat for men is 12 to 16 percent, compared to an average of approximately 26 percent for women.[6] Women also have their body fat distributed differently than men. You may have noticed that women seem to concentrate adipose tissue more in the hips and thighs and less in the abdomen and upper part of the body. Although it's not a rule, women do tend to be more pear-shaped, thanks to this extra padding on the hips. After menopause, a woman's body fat is redistributed and concentrated more like a man's—in the abdomen.[7]

DE-BULKING SOME MYTHS

I recently joined a gym and started lifting weights. I am not sure that I will continue because although I would like to tone up my muscles, I do not want to look like the Incredible Hulk. —Lynda, age 39

Hormonal differences account for the greater muscle mass found in males. The average female is 35 to 40 percent muscle mass, whereas the average male is 40 to 50 percent muscle mass.[8]

Many women who would like to pursue strength training have fears of "bulking up" and thus steer away from this activity. Weight training can benefit women by helping them to develop strength and improved muscle tone, but women are unlikely to "bulk up" like men because we have fewer androgenic hormones.[9] The larger muscles found in men reflect the increased size of the various muscle fibers. It has also been shown that women can increase their strength up to 44 percent without significantly increasing muscle mass.[10]

Carol Otis, M.D., an assistant team physician at UCLA, notes that the amount of muscle bulk a woman gains is based on heredity and body type. A tall, lean woman with tall, lean parents is less inclined to bulk up compared to a shorter, heavy-set woman whose parents are similarly built. More importantly, Dr. Otis assures us that most women will simply develop well-toned, well-defined muscles as a result of weight training.[11]

Muscle fibers are classified as **slow-twitch** or **fast-twitch**. The slow-twitch muscle fibers are better for endurance exercises, whereas the fast-twitch fibers provide short, rapid bursts of power.[12] (See Chapter 3 for more information.) Everyone, regardless of gender, has varying amounts of each muscle fiber type. Contrary to popular belief, it is not your sex, but your genetic makeup, that determines this difference. However, your ratio of fast- and slow-twitch fibers can be modified with athletic training and conditioning.[13]

You may have some athletic friends who excel in sprinting, whereas others are just natural long-distance runners. This difference may be related to the individual runner's percentage of fast- and slow-twitch fibers. Which category best describes you and your blood relatives?

How Strong Are You?

When I was in elementary school, I could easily pedal my bike as fast as, if not faster than, all the neighborhood boys my age. Now, as an adult, it is an effort just trying to keep up with my fiancé. It's even more embarrassing when we go kayaking.
—Marietta, age 23

Most women have observed that they are not as strong as men. Remember how, as girls, we performed modified push-ups and never could do as many chin-ups as the boys in gym class? This upper body strength difference probably became more apparent when you entered high school.

Before puberty, girls and boys of the same size have approximately equal muscle strength. When girls are 11 to 12 years old, they are about 90 percent as strong as boys. This decreases to 85 percent when they are 13 to 14 years old and drops to 75 percent at 15 to 16 years of age.[14] These percentages do not mean that girls are getting weaker and guys are becoming stronger. Let us explain.

Studies confirm that the average adult female is about one-half as strong as the average male in the upper body and about two-thirds as strong in the lower body. However, when strength is expressed relative to fat-free body weight (that is, comparing muscle to muscle), these differences in strength are minimized.[15]

Think back to your childhood. Do you recall much disparity in activities like running, which involved the lower body musculature? Most likely you will remember running as fast or kicking a ball as far as the boys in your elementary school class. Jog your memory for other athletic activities. You probably will recollect that young boys and girls of the same size were equally strong.

Gender differences in strength are related to the muscle groups measured and the training and conditioning level of the subjects studied.[16] These findings seem to imply that women are as strong as men—especially when strength is evaluated per unit size and type of muscle fiber.[17] *A sample of muscle fibers from the leg of an Olympic marathoner should be stronger than an equal-sized specimen from the leg of an unconditioned individual, regardless of gender.*

Tipping the Scales

Many of us probably know of women who began a diet and exercise program, only to discover to their dismay that they were gaining weight. Hopefully, these women did not get too discouraged and prematurely abandon their healthier lifestyles. Muscle is more dense than fat. In simpler terms, a cup of fat weighs less than a cup of muscle—and if given a choice, most of us would probably prefer the latter. Therefore, when you start to exercise and increase your muscle strength and mass (and simultaneously lose fat), your scale may not register a weight loss. So, rather than focusing on weight going up or remaining the same, exercising dieters should look at the inches being lost around the hip and waistline.

OTHER BENCHMARKS

Flexibility

Flexibility refers to your ability to bend a joint through a range of motion. As you get older, your flexibility tends to wane. Women tend to be more flexible than men of the same age because of differences in connective tissue and muscle mass. Women also participate more frequently in activities that foster flexibility, such as dance and gymnastics.

Heartbreak

It has been said over and over again that women have bigger hearts and are the more sensitive sex; however, structurally speaking, men have larger heart sizes compared to women. A larger heart implies greater stroke volumes and maximal cardiac output.[18] Not surprisingly, the size of the heart's left ventricle, which is the major pumping chamber, is also smaller in women. A slightly increased heart rate compensates for women's lower stroke volumes.

Take a Breather

Since men are larger, their chest cavities are also proportionately bigger. Consequently, men have greater lung volumes.[19] Men also surpass women in maximum oxygen consumption by approximately 20 percent. (Maximal oxygen consumption or VO_2 max is a measure of aerobic fitness. This term is explained in more detail in Chapters 3 and 4.) However, with conditioning, some women can actually exceed the endurance capacity of some men.[20]

Shaping Up

Up until recently, my 13-year-old daughter would borrow her twin brother's jeans and shirts. Right under my nose, she seems to have blossomed. Much to my son's delight, she can no longer wear his jeans as they no longer fit in the hips."

— Veronica, age 42, mother of teenage twins

Q Angle Illustration

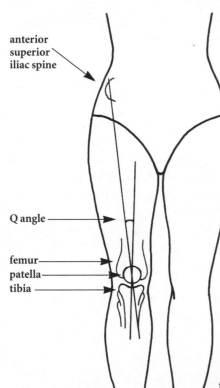

anterior
superior
iliac spine

Q angle

femur
patella
tibia

During puberty, boys experience broadening of the shoulders, while girls notice their pelvic bones getting wider. Hence, adult women have a wider hip-to-shoulder ratio compared to males, who have the reverse hip-to-shoulder ratio. You may think of the adult female skeletal structure as being shaped like a triangle with the apex pointing upwards, whereas her male counterpart would be an upside-down triangle.

Center of Gravity Changes. An individual's center of gravity is defined as the intersection of the three planes that can divide the body into equally weighted halves. Tracking this intersecting point is helpful in the analysis of individual sports performance. It was once believed that women had a lower center of gravity compared to men. However, center of gravity differences are now known to be determined by actual individual height and body type and not necessarily just by gender.[21] Because women are generally shorter (because of their shorter lower extremities) and have wider pelvises, they do tend to have lower centers of gravity and possibly greater stability—but this is based on each individual's body type, not simply their sex. Variations in center of gravity may help to explain why some folks excel in sports that require a sense of equilibrium, while others just don't seem to be able to handle a balancing act.

The Q Angle. Because women's hips are wider, our thighs slant more inward toward the knees. Physicians and athletic trainers frequently speak of the **Q angle**. The Q (quadriceps) angle is a measurement made by intersecting a line drawn from the anterior superior iliac spine (a prominence on the top part of the hip bone) through the middle of the patella or kneecap with that of a line drawn from the tibial tubercle (a prominent spot on the top of the lower leg bone) through the center of the patella.[22] Normally, the Q angle measurement is less than 15 degrees in women and less than 10 degrees in men.[23] The medical implications of this finding will be discussed in greater detail in Chapter 16: Understanding Aches and Pains.

What We Know

*Differences Between
Males and Females*

Females generally:
- are shorter,
- have shorter limbs, especially upper arms,
- have wider hips,
- have narrower shoulders,
- weigh less,
- have a higher percentage of body fat,
- have a different distribution of body fat,
- have less muscle mass, and
- have smaller hearts.

Limb Lengths.   Women also tend to have shorter limbs, especially arms, when compared to men—even when relative body length is taken into consideration. It seems that the humerus (upper arm), and not the forearm, accounts for this extremity size differential.[24]

Bosom Buddies.   One anatomical feature that clearly differentiates women from men is the presence of breasts. Breasts are not composed of muscular tissue—they are mostly fat.[25] A woman's breast size is essentially genetically determined, but can be altered by changes in body fat. While men can enlarge their chest sizes by developing their pectoral muscles, we would not expect to see major breast size differences in women who do the same, because they tend not to bulk up with exercise.

The search for a good sports bra has prompted biomechanical studies of breast motion. Women want good support and ideally want to limit breast movement during physical activity, in order to optimize performance and minimize discomfort. (For further details, see Chapter 8: Dressing for the Job.)

Plastic surgeon Norman S. Levine, M.D. presented a case report of a 46-year-old physical education teacher who underwent breast implantation and subsequently increased her bra size from 32A to 34B. The teacher was also a swimmer and noted that post-operatively her free-style time became slower and actually lengthened by nearly 25 percent. It was hypothesized that breast enlargement caused increased drag and resistance and resulted in slower swim times. It is also interesting that this woman's swim times for the backstroke did not change. Dr. Levine reassures us that his patient was happy with the surgery and felt that her breasts were a "ballast" and not a "drag."[26] More research is required to study whether large-breasted women are at any disadvantage in the sporting world.

Regulating Your Body's Thermostat

At one point in time, it was thought that women perspired less than men and therefore should not exercise in hot climates. Perhaps you still believe this. However, it is now known that our ability to cope in hot environments has a lot more to do with cardiovascular fitness level and body size and less to do with gender.[27]

Heat Syndromes.   Heat illness is recognized as a spectrum of disorders ranging from heat cramps to heat exhaustion to heatstroke, a life-threatening condition.[28] From basic science, we have learned that the incidence of heat syndromes increases when the temperature and humidity rise. Contrast taking a 5K run on a summer day in the sweltering south with one on a cool day in New England.

- **Who's at Risk.**   Certain individuals and body types are at a greater risk for suffering from heat syndromes. These include the very young and old, the obese, the unfit, and those unacclimated to the heat. For example, a short, husky, muscular person who generates more metabolic calories is at higher risk for heat illness than a tall, lean individual.[28]

It is difficult to interpret studies that report gender variations of heat tolerance and acclimation because of the different surface area-to-mass ratios between men and women. However, when adult men and women of similar size and fitness levels are matched, there are no real differences in response to heat stress.[29]

Body size makes a difference only when comparing one female to another. The larger athlete will generate more heat than a smaller athlete engaged in the same activity, and will dissipate heat less efficiently due to a smaller surface area-to-mass ratio. On the other hand, adult women tolerate exercise in hot climates more effectively than our smaller-sized young daughters.[30] Children, with their higher surface area-to-mass ratio, do fine in a temperate environment, but when the temperature is high or the sun is strong, they absorb relatively more heat from their surroundings than do adults. Young athletes also sweat less and require a higher core body temperature to trigger perspiration.

Fighting the Cold.   In cold climates, one would expect women, who have less heat-generating muscle mass, to be at a disadvantage. However, women, with their greater percentage of insulating body fat, tend not to lose body heat faster than men. When subjects of both genders were matched for percent body fat, no body temperature differences in a cold environment were observed.[31]

Putting on a Happy Face

Last winter, right before the holidays, I lost my job and broke up with my fiancé. I became very depressed and stayed indoors for days at a time. Spring arrived and I was still quite depressed. Fortunately, an older woman in my apartment complex was looking for a walking partner. She refused to take "no" for an answer and somehow convinced me to put on my athletic shoes and join her. Shortly thereafter, I got my life back in order. —Paula, age 30

The scientific evidence about the connection between exercise and depression is mixed. Contrary to popular belief, athletes are not immune to major depression. In fact, the rates of depression in athletes are roughly the same as those found in the general population. However, several studies have shown that women who play sports have lower levels of depression and improved self esteem.[32] While exercise has been shown to relieve depressive symptoms, stress, overtraining, and injury may actually trigger it in some athletes.[33]

Depression is one of the most common medical problems seen by primary care physicians today. The estimated lifetime prevalence of major depression is 21 percent for women and 12 percent for men.[34] Several explanations have been offered to help explain the nearly two-to-one female-to-male ratio of depression. Some of these possibilities include hormonal factors involving the menstrual cycle, menopause, and oral contraceptive use. Genetic factors, social stresses affecting women, and women's better recall about depressive symptoms could also contribute to this gender difference.

FOCUSING ON SOME IMPLICATIONS: THE ATHLETIC CONNECTION

Clearly, a woman is not a man, anatomically or physiologically. But what are the implications of these sex differences from a performance standpoint? (See Chapter 16, Understanding Aches and Pains, for a better understanding of the injury perspective.) We may also wonder if women can compensate for some of the skeletal and physiological differences. Can we, with better training, eventually surpass men in athletic accomplishments?

Stature

They've been called the "Magnificent Seven," the "Golden Girls," and the "Seven Sisters," but the 1996 Women's U.S. gymnastics team has more than team spirit in common—they are all short and petite relative to the general population.

A person of short stature has a lower center of gravity than a taller individual, which may help explain the good balance skills exhibited by gymnasts. A lower center of gravity may also be a distinct advantage for the skier who needs to maintain balance at high speeds. On the other hand, being shorter with a lower center of gravity may handicap the athlete involved in running and jumping sports.[35]

Arm Length

While on vacation at the beach last summer, my husband and kids were throwing stones back out to sea. My preschool-aged daughter asked me quite innocently: "Why does daddy always throw the stone farther than you?" As I paused to think of an answer, her older brother quickly chimed in, "that's because she's a girl and boys always throw better." —Debbie, age 34

There may be an ounce of truth to the above scenario. Perhaps it's not so much that men throw better, but more that they throw farther and more powerfully. There is an anatomical reason for this gender difference. An individual with a relatively short upper arm, combined with narrow shoulders, often produces less leverage and subsequently a less powerful throw.[35] This fits the skeletal profile of most women.

Body Fat

At the 1988 Summer Olympics in Seoul, Korea, swimmer Janet Evans finished the 400-meter freestyle swim two seconds faster than Mark Spitz swam it 20 years earlier. Being endowed with a high percentage of body fat often enables women to excel in swimming. It may be that the extra fat gives more buoyancy in the water, especially when it is distributed around the thighs, allowing the legs to stay higher in the water. A higher percentage of body fat is also helpful in cold-water activities because of the extra insulation it provides.

Muscle Mass

On the other hand, because women have less muscle mass compared to men, they usually do not have the power and strength required for lifting heavy weights. With proper training, women can improve their strength and power, but it remains to be seen whether women as a group will continue to make the rapid strength and speed gains they have achieved in the last several decades.

We Are Different

It's important for women to be aware of skeletal and physiological traits that make us different from men. Hopefully, this will enable us to continue to optimize our performances and enrich our lives while minimizing athletic injuries.

Developing a better understanding of some of the differences between the sexes is also the first step toward dispelling many of the myths surrounding women's athletic activities. It was also what prompted us to research and write this book. We hope that you can appreciate how certain anatomical features impact women's elite and competitive athletic performance. That's right: "a woman is not a man!"

1. Axthelm, P. The hustler outhustled. *Newsweek*, October 1, 1973, 63–64.

2. Sanborn, C. F., & Jankowski, C. M. Physiologic considerations for women in sport. *Clinics in Sports Medicine*, April 1994, 13 (2), 315–327.

3. Arendt, E. A. Orthopaedic issues for active and athletic women. *Clinics in Sports Medicine*, April 1994, 13 (2), 483–503.

4. Beim, G., & Stone, D. A. Issues in the female athlete. *Orthopedic Clinics of North America*, July 1995, 26 (3), 443–451.

5. Duck, S. C. Identification and assessment of the slowly growing child. *American Family Physician*, May 15, 1996, 53 (7), 2305–2312.

6. Beim, G., & Stone, D. A. Issues in the female athlete. *Orthopedic Clinics of North America*, July 1995, 26 (3), 443–451.

7. Stein, A. Pedaling to Freedom. *Women's Sports and Fitness*, November/December 1995, 27.

8. Fardy, H. J. Women in sport. *Australian Family Physician*, March 1988, 17 (3), 183, 185–186.

9. Cinque, C. Women's strength training: Lifting the limits of aging? *The Physician and Sportsmedicine*, August 1990, 18 (8), 123–124, 126–127.

10. Arendt, E. A. Orthopaedic issues for active and athletic women. *Clinics in Sports Medicine*, April 1994, 13 (2), 483–503.

11. Cinque, C. Women's strength training: Lifting the limits of aging? *The Physician and Sportsmedicine*, August 1990, 18 (8), 123–124, 126–127.

12. Lillegarde, W. A., and J. D. Terrio. Appropriate Strength Training. *Medical Clinics of North America*, March 1994, 78 (2), 457–475.

13. Lewis, D. A., Kamon, E., & Hodgson, J. L. Physiological differences between genders: Implications for sports conditioning. *Sports Medicine*, 1986, 3, 357–369.
    Cinque, C. Women's strength training: Lifting the limits of aging? *The Physician and Sportsmedicine*, August 1990, 18 (8), 123–124, 126–127.

14. Beim, G., & Stone, D. A. Issues in the female athlete. *Orthopedic Clinics of North America*, July 1995, 26 (3), 443–451.

15. Giel, D. Women's weight lifting: Elevating a sport to world-class status. *The Physician and Sportsmedicine*, April 1988, 16 (4), 163–167, 170.

16. Arendt, E. A. Orthopaedic issues for active and athletic women. *Clinics in Sports Medicine*, April 1994, 13 (2), 483–503.

17. Beim, G., & Stone, D. A. Issues in the female athlete. *Orthopedic Clinics of North America*, July 1995, 26 (3), 443–451.

18. Good, J. E., & Klein, K. M. Women in the military Academies: U.S. Navy (Part 1 of 3). *The Physician and Sportsmedicine*, February 1989, 17 (2), 99–102, 105–106.
    Fardy, H. J. Women in sport. *Australian Family Physician*, March 1988, 17 (3), 183, 185–186.

19. Beim, G., & Stone, D. A. Issues in the female athlete. *Orthopedic Clinics of North America*, July 1995, 26 (3), 443–451.

20. Fardy, H. J. Women in sport. *Australian Family Physician*, March 1988, 17 (3), 183, 185–186.

21. Sanborn, C. F., & Jankowski, C. M. Physiologic considerations for women in sport. *Clinics in Sports Medicine*, April 1994, 13 (2), 315–327.

22. Rubin, C. J. Sports injuries in the female athlete. *New Jersey Medicine*, September 1991, 88 (9), 643–645.

23. Ruffin, M. T., IV, & Kiningham, R. B. Anterior knee pain: The challenge of patellofemoral syndrome. *American Family Physician*, January 1993, 47 (1), 185–194.

24. Beim, G., & Stone, D. A. Issues in the female athlete. *Orthopedic Clinics of North America*, July 1995, 26 (3), 443–451.

25. Shangold, M. M. Gynecologic concerns in the women athlete. *Clinics in Sports Medicine*, October 1984, 3 (4), 869–879.

26. Levine, N. S., & Buchanan, R. T. Decreased swimming speed following augmentation mammaplasty. *Plastic and Reconstructive Surgery*, February 1983, 71 (2), 255–256.

27. Sanborn, C. F., & Jankowski, C. M. Physiologic considerations for women in sport. *Clinics in Sports Medicine*, April 1994, 13 (2), 315–327.

28. Knochel, J. P. Update on summer heat syndromes. *Patient Care*, June 15, 1989, 23 (11), 87–90, 95, 98, 103.

29. Lewis, D. A., Kamon, E., & Hodgson, J. L. Physiological differences between genders: Implications for sports conditioning. *Sports Medicine*, 1986, 3, 357–369.
    Cinque, C. Women's strength training: Lifting the limits of aging? *The Physician and Sportsmedicine*, August 1990, 18 (8), 123–124, 126–127.

30. Sanborn, C. F., & Jankowski, C. M. Physiologic considerations for women in sport. *Clinics in Sports Medicine*, April 1994, 13 (2), 315–327.

31. Beim, G., & Stone, D. A. Issues in the female athlete. *Orthopedic Clinics of North America*, July 1995, 26 (3), 443–451.

32. Lutter, J. M. History of women in sports: Societal issues. *Clinics in Sports Medicine*, April 1994, 13 (2), 263–279.

Lopiano, D. A. Equity in women's sports: A health and fairness perspective. *Clinics in Sports Medicine*, April 1994, 13 (2), 281–296.

33. Cunnien, A. J. Depression in athletes: Is the cure more troubling than the symptoms? *Family Practice Recertification*, January 1996, 18 (1), 39–54.

34. Endicott, J., Weissman, M. M., & Yonkers, K. A. What's unique about depression in women? *Patient Care*, August 15, 1996, 88–115.

35. Arendt, E. A. Orthopaedic issues for active and athletic women. *Clinics in Sports Medicine*, April 1994, 13 (2), 483–503.

3

Body Works: A Short Course in Anatomy and Kinesiology

SUSAN L. PURETZ, ED.D.

I recently started bodybuilding at home and am experiencing problems as I increase my weight-training program. I wish I worked out with someone who was experienced and had a trained eye. I'm sure that person could tell me exactly how to move my muscles to correct whatever it is I'm doing wrong. In the meantime, I have to rely on trial and error. —Wendy, age 25

A performer in any athletic activity should be able to take advantage of the greatest freedom of movement available. To do so, it is helpful to have an idea not only about the basic anatomy and physiology of bones, muscles, and joints, but also their mechanical actions (or **kinesiology**). This understanding gives you more of an awareness of the possibilities and limitations of your movements, and a greater recognition of the range of movements possible. For example, the elbow joint is constructed to permit movement in only one direction (up and down). However, by using two joints—the shoulder and the elbow—you can place the forearm in the best position for a more successful movement. By developing an understanding of anatomy and kinesiology, you may become more aware of the limitations of your joints, thereby possibly preventing joint strains and subsequent injuries. Knowledge is power!

ANATOMY: GETTING THE INSIDE PICTURE

Supported by bone and activated by muscle, the body enjoys an incredibly wide range of movements, as forceful as sledgehammering, as gentle as blinking. The same hand that pats a kitten can break a board in karate. The same foot that gingerly tests the bath water can kick a field goal.

Our skeletons are arrangements of **bones**. **Joints** are the places at which adjacent bones attach, and where the motion (for those bones) occurs; **muscles** span the joints and provide the force for moving the bones. Looking at bone-joint-muscle in mechanical terms, we see an intricate combination of levers which make possible the wide variety of coordinated movements we do.

Bones

Bones form the scaffolding that supports our body. We once thought of bone as being "hard as iron," but in recent years this conception has changed as we became aware of osteoporosis and realized that bone is a living structure with a state of hardness that varies over a lifetime.

Not only are bones not solid, they are dynamic little factories. For example, cells in the red bone marrow manufacture red blood corpuscles. In addition, bones support and protect the soft tissues of the body and give the body a definite shape. Bones anchor our muscles and serve as levers to allow those muscles to perform bodily movement.

Bone Composition. The 206 bones of the adult skeletal body begin their embryonic life as soft cartilage and harden with age. The essential difference between bone and any type of soft tissue can be found in the bone's inner composition—the **matrix**. The matrix is composed of about one-third various organic substances (chiefly collagen) and two-thirds inorganic salts, including calcium, magnesium, phosphorus, and sodium. These inorganic salts are constantly being deposited and withdrawn as the bone helps maintain the normal level of calcium in the bloodstream. We'll talk more about calcium interchange when we discuss osteoporosis in Chapter 14, Keeping It Going: The Older Athlete.

The presence of these inorganic compounds contributes to the bone's hardness, while the organic matter contributes to its flexibility. Bones of youngsters have a higher percentage of organic matter and are more flexible, less brittle, and more resistant to breaks. For example, a toddler may fall ten times a day without injuring a bone. As one ages, the amount of inorganic matter increases in proportion to the organic matter, causing the bones to be more brittle, break more easily, and heal more slowly. An old person may break a bone by simply stepping off a curb, stair, or stool.

Bone also reflects the influence of activity. For example, an athlete will develop more prominent bone surfaces than the sedentary individual. The athlete's bones will be stronger and maintain their flexibility longer than those of an individual who takes her sports as a spectator.

• **Bone Parts.**   Because bone is living tissue, it must constantly receive nourishment. The **osteocytes**—the living bone cells inside the hard matrix—receive nourishment through a fantastic system of tiny microscopic tunnels that permeate the solid bone tissue.

Bones come in two designer fashions: spongy and compact. The difference between them is that spongy bone contains spaces that are filled with marrow interspersed with the osteocytes and their surrounding matrix; compact bone has no marrow and appears as an apparently solid mass. All of our bones are a combination of spongy and compact; this works to our advantage because, fortunately, while compact bone is extremely strong, spongy bone is lighter in weight. Our bones would be unduly heavy if they were composed of only compact bone.

• **A Bone to Pick.**   Bones range in size from the powerful thigh bone, or femur—about twenty inches long—to the tiny bones of the middle ear. Although they may be distinguished by their size, bones are actually classified on the basis of their shape: long, short, flat, and irregular.

Long bones, like those found in the arms and legs, are quite strong given their relatively light weight. Those characteristics occur because compact bone alone is found in the bone's shaft, while a combination of compact and spongy tissue makes up the ends. Long bones are the only type of bone with this arrangement.

Short bones, found in the wrist and ankle, allow a great range of motion. They are small, chunky, and cubical in shape. In short bones, compact bone forms the protective outer coat surrounding the spongy bone.

Flat bones like the ribs, pelvic bones, and kneecaps are relatively thin but provide protection, while **irregular bones**, uniquely designed to suit specific assignments, include all the remaining bones such as the vertebrae and the bones of the jaw.

Joints

Joints are the unions between two or more bones, between two or more cartilages, or between cartilage and bone. This union is called an **articulation**. Joints provide the bones with a means of being moved while at the same time providing some stability.

Types of Joints.   Joints are categorized according to the amount of movement they permit. They range from immovable joints (like the sutures of the adult skull), to slightly movable (like the intervertebral disks of the spine or the point where the bones of the lower leg—the tibia and fibula—are united), to the freely movable. This last category covers most of the body's joints. As you can see in the following chart, our joints allow the variety of movements we have come to expect from our bodies.

CHART 3.1

··

Types of Joints

Type	Example	Movement
Hinge	Elbow	Flexion/extension
Gliding	Wrist bones	Gliding
Pivot	Forearm	Rotation
Condyloid	Wrist joint	Abduction/adduction Flexion/extension
Saddle	Thumb	Flexion/extension Abduction/adduction Circumduction
Ball and Saddle	Arm	Flexion/extension Abduction/adduction Rotation, Circumduction

Muscles

Three's a Team. Muscles are our bodies' engines, making up about 36 percent of the body weight in women. (In men it's about 42 percent.) The muscles that are involved in our bodily movements are known as **skeletal muscles** and are under our command as we move about at work or play. The two other types of muscle are **smooth** (found in blood vessels and the walls of visceral organs) and **cardiac** (heart) muscle.

Both smooth and cardiac muscle are involuntary—that is, they are not subject to our conscious control. Smooth muscle might be compared with a clock: geared for slow speed and constant use, it continues to function day after day in a slow and reliable manner.

Cardiac muscle is highly specialized and found only in the walls of the heart. Like smooth muscle, cardiac muscle works steadily day after day, but is also capable of vigorous responses for short periods, as when we exercise.

Skeletal muscles, which are voluntary (under our conscious control), are different in both structure and function from the other two types of muscle. Skeletal muscles can develop great power but, unlike cardiac and smooth muscle, they tire under constant use.

The more than 600 skeletal muscles have a combined weight about three times as great as that of all the body's bones.

Muscle Makeup.   If you took a muscle apart to its smallest component, you would find a threadlike cylinder (thinner than a human hair) about one to three inches in length, wrapped within a thin, delicate connective tissue sheath. Because these cylinders are longer than they are wide, they are called **fibers**. The biceps muscle in your upper arm is made up of some 600,000 muscle fibers.

Groups of muscle fibers are bound into bundles (much like strands of spaghetti) and each individual bundle of muscle fibers is enclosed in a fibrous tissue sheath—something like one pound of spaghetti strands wrapped in a cellophane bag. The groups of bundles are in turn encased within a tougher connective tissue sheath comparable to the grouping together of a dozen of the one-pound spaghetti bags into a large discount package. Thus a single muscle is made up of many fibers, ultimately all encased in one overall protective sheath. Skeletal muscles are also known as striated muscles, due to the striped appearance of the fibers when viewed under a microscope.

• **Twitchers.** There are two types of muscle fibers. One responds rapidly to stimulation and is called **fast-twitch**, whereas the other has a slower response, fatigues less quickly, and is known as a **slow-twitch** fiber. These fibers are further distinguished by their hemoglobin content as red or white—roughly comparable to the dark and white meat of chicken. Red muscle fibers contain a richer supply of hemoglobin and are associated with slow-twitch responses. They are more plentiful in the muscles responsible for the long-continued contractions necessary for aerobic activities. White, or fast-twitch, predominate in muscle responsible for relatively brief but forceful contractions. The oxygen consumption capacity of a muscle varies according to fiber type. For example, the ability to extract oxygen from blood is approximately three to five times greater in slow-twitch red than in fast-twitch white[1]; thus, each contributes a different response pattern, with slow-twitch fibers better adapted to endurance (aerobic) activities.

• **Arrangements.** Fiber arrangement varies considerably among different skeletal muscles. For example, the sartorius muscle, which slants across the front of the thigh and is the longest muscle in the body, is a **longitudinal muscle**. Longitudinal muscles are long strap-like muscles whose fibers lie parallel to their long axis and allow for the largest range of movement. In an average-size person, the sartorius can shorten about eight inches during a maximum kicking movement. This great range of movement is achieved at the sacrifice of strength.

In contrast to the longitudinal arrangement are the many diagonal variations of muscle fibers. For example, the muscle on the front of the chest, the pectoralis major, is an example of a **triangular** or **fan shaped muscle**, so called because it is relatively flat, with fibers radiating from a narrow attachment at one end to a broad attachment at the other. Other muscle fiber arrangements look featherlike (for example, the tibialis posterior muscle of the leg), or spindle-shaped, such as the brachialis muscle of the arm, whose sole function is to flex the elbow. The diagonal pulling position of these indirectly arranged muscles allows a greater number of fibers to act in unison, thus providing much strength; however, there is a loss of range of movement because the fibers, unlike the longitudinal ones, are shorter.

Naming Muscles.   Skeletal muscles all have names—some in English, others in Latin. The names have been assigned in a logical manner, for example: by location—the tibialis posterior muscle is behind the tibia (your shin bone); by shape—the neck, mid and upper back muscle, the trapezius, looks like a trapezoid. Other assigned names include those by size—maximus for largest, minimus for smallest; by length—longus and brevis; or by the number of points where the muscle originates, for example, biceps for two, triceps for three, and quadriceps for four points.

Muscle Properties.   **Extensibility, elasticity, excitability, tonus,** and **contractility** are the five properties of muscles. The first, *extensibility*, allows a muscle to be stretched, whereas *elasticity* is the ability of the muscle to return to its former size and shape. The average muscle fiber can be stretched or shortened by approximately one-half of its resting length.[2]

Tonus (generally referred to as muscle tone) is the capacity to maintain a state of steady, partial contraction. It is this property which produces the firm body and athletic look that comes from exercising. Muscle tone is often reduced as a result of ill health and especially when prolonged bed rest is necessary. Poor muscle tone leads to weakened muscles and that is why hospital patients are often encouraged to move and walk around as soon as possible.

Muscles are able to work because of *excitability*, their capacity to respond to a stimulus from the nervous system. The last property, *contractility*, is the ability to shorten, and this trait, unique to muscles, occurs whenever we use them.

Moving Muscles: A Two-Comb Strategy.   During muscle contraction, molecular changes occur involving proteins, which make up about 20 percent of muscle tissue (75 percent is water and the remaining 5 percent is a combination of fats, carbohydrates, and other substances). The main protein molecules contained within each muscle fiber are called **myosin** and **actin** filaments. They are precisely arranged in the fiber like two combs facing each other with their teeth partially interlocked. The thick myosin filaments are longitudinal in the middle but do not reach the ends, while the thin actin filaments extend from the ends but do not reach the middle of the muscle fiber. In that way, they overlap areas.

Powering Muscle. How do our muscles do the work we call on them to do? It boils down to energy. In order to power a muscular contraction, energy is necessary, and that energy is furnished by two biochemical events that occur within each muscle fiber. One provides the immediate "spark," while the other provides the "fuel" that is used to recharge the "spark."

The Spark. The immediate energy spark causing the interaction between the actin and myosin filaments is **adenosine triphosate (ATP)**. ATP is a molecule (composed of adenosine and three phosphate radicals), which, when it breaks down, releases energy and becomes **ADP (adenosine diphosphate)**. This reaction is reversible, which means that immediately after the contraction ends, the ADP can be and usually is converted back into ATP and the cell is, in a sense, recharged and ready to fire again.

The Fuel. The fuel for the muscular contraction comes from the breakdown of the food we eat. While proteins, fats, and carbohydrates can all be used for energy, carbohydrates are the more usual source. In a complex series of chemical reactions, all three nutrients are broken down. Ultimately, they are converted to one of two things: ATP (our spark—the good guy in this story) or **lactic acid** (in this case, the bad guy). The key to whether they become one or the other is oxygen. If oxygen is present, the muscle fibers get a resupply of ATP, but if not, lactic acid accumulates.

Unpowering Muscles: The Complications.

Lactic Acid. As lactic acid builds up in the muscle fiber due to inadequate oxygen, it causes muscle fatigue. Muscles fatigue because excessive amounts of lactic acid tend to depress muscle cell activity, leading to a decrease in the muscle's response to stimuli (lessened excitability), and interfering with its ability to contract. If the muscles can't contract, your activity will stop. Thus lactic acid buildup (caused by insufficient oxygen) is the limiting factor in strenuous activity. The less lactic acid there is, the more efficiently our bodies are working during exercise.

Oxygen Deficit. In any muscular work, there is normally a short transition during which the circulatory and respiratory adjustments lag behind and an **oxygen deficit** results. Sprinters can run short distances because they are capable of using their muscles for this scant period of lag time despite oxygen deficit. Physiologically, this happens because several of our sources of energy are not dependent on oxygen for their chemical conversion. For example: the spark (the breakdown of ATP into ADP) and the initial fuel breakdown of carbohydrates/fats/proteins do not require oxygen.

What We Know

The reason heart and breathing rates remain elevated after exercise stops is because you are paying back your oxygen deficit and debt. The more fit your cardiorespiratory system, the greater the ability to sustain an oxygen debt, and the faster will be the payback or the recovery.

Steady State. After the initial oxygen deficit, if our continued work demand does not call for greater amounts of oxygen, we enter into a condition known as **steady state**. In the steady state, the amounts of oxygen are adequate to allow for continued muscular activity. Distance running is an example of a steady state activity.

Oxygen Debt. When the exertion calls for larger quantities of oxygen, a different situation arises and you end up being forced to stop exercising. The reason: oxygen must then be present in sufficient quantities for the amount of work being done by your muscles. When you sprint or do a burst of some other strenuous activity for too long, sufficient oxygen is not available rapidly enough to handle the chemical conversions. Lactic acid accumulates, your muscles become physically unable to respond, and you must stop your activity.

In order to continue with the activity you must "pay back" the oxygen debt. You will continue to be "out of breath" and breathe hard until enough oxygen has been absorbed and provided to the muscle cells to change the lactic acid back—ultimately to ATP. Eventually, the initial oxygen deficit as well as any possible oxygen debt must be repaid.

In light exercise where there is sufficient oxygen and you are in a steady state, the debt at work's end may be entirely due to the oxygen deficit that occurred at the beginning of the exercise. But, when an exercise represents a true overload, the duration of the effort (or the level of performance) is limited by the athlete's ability to sustain an oxygen debt.

Connectors

Tendons and Ligaments. Move a muscle and chances are you will be using a tendon. Tendons connect some muscles to bones and function much like strings on a puppet. When the muscles to which they are attached contract, the ropelike tendons pull on bones and make them move.

Tendons and ligaments (which hold bones together at joints) are both constructed primarily of fibrous tissue. The fibers run, more or less, in the same direction, which provides for great strength and the ability to withstand tremendous pulling. But even tendons have breaking points, and ruptured Achilles tendons are the nemesis of athletes.

Nerves

Anyone who works with a computer knows that in order to get a hard copy (i.e., a paper document), you need a printer; but without the computer there would be no document in the first place. In order for the computer to talk to the printer, there must be cables or some connecting system. So it is with our bodies.

No matter how healthy your bone/joint/muscle connections may be, without ner-

What We Know

It is through constant feed-back from the proprioceptors during countless repetitions of various motor acts that we gain mastery of a particular movement or skill.

vous system involvement you would be unable to move. Sensory and motor nerves are our communication cables.

Sensory Nerves: Signal Carriers.   **Sensory neurons** transmit impulses from muscles, tendons, skin, and visceral and sense organs to the **Central Nervous System** (CNS—the brain and spinal cord), supplying it with information regarding our activity. Specific sensory nerve terminals, known as **proprioceptors**, respond to our movements and send signals to the CNS. For example, our proprioceptors enable us to know when we have gripped a paddle just right and when the swing of an arm or snap of the wrist are executed exactly the way we want. They also make us aware that we are doing a movement the wrong way, with insufficient strength, twist, speed, etc.

   • **Kinesthetic Sense.** Proprioceptors provide us with our **kinesthetic sense**—the muscular awareness of what is happening in our body parts. For example, even with your eyes closed, you can describe with substantial accuracy the position of your arms or legs. You are aware of both the position and movement of body parts. The recognition of position and feel of movements occurs both consciously and unconsciously, depending upon such things as whether it is a new or habitual movement, such as using a stair machine for the first time or simply climbing stairs. Your kinesthetic sensations may serve as stimuli for a different movement or they may help you correct or fine-tune an ongoing movement.

   Multiple muscular actions are often involved in producing a particular single movement. For example, in using a paddle ball racquet, muscles are required to hold the racquet, position the arm correctly, and provide the impetus for the movement. Feedback is constantly occurring throughout each swing during the entire time you are playing.

Motor Nerves: Signal Senders.   While our sensory nerves provide the feedback, the impetus for our movements is found in the **motor neuron**. Moving at a speed of nearly 350 feet per second, a signal travels from the brain to the muscle via the motor neuron. In the absence of motor nerves, there can be no initiation, modification, or coordination of muscular action. Motor neurons branch out when they reach their particular muscle, and each branch ends within a single muscle fiber.

   Nerve-Muscle Partnership. Together, neurons and muscle fibers form the neuromuscular system. The system's functional core is the **motor unit**, consisting of a single motor neuron together with all of the muscle fibers that its branches supply. Each motor neuron may service as few as 100 (or as many as 1000) muscle fibers. Muscles are capable of more precise movements when they have a large number of motor neurons, each serving a small number of muscle fibers. For example, a large muscle like the gluteus maximus (the buttock muscle) has a relatively small number of motor neurons and a large number of muscle fibers per neuron and so is capable of only large and strong muscular movements; in contrast, the thumb's muscles have many motor neurons controlling few muscle fibers, making fine and delicate movements possible.

KINESIOLOGY: MAKING THE MOVES

Action

Muscles are attached to bone, either directly or by ligaments or tendons. The muscles have an **origin** at one bone site and an **insertion** at a different bone location. When a muscle **contracts**, it moves its site of insertion closer to its site of origin and, in doing so, it moves the bones to which it is attached. A muscle does not favor origins over insertions (or visa versa), rather, it exerts equal force on the two attachments and attempts to pull them toward each other. Which bone moves and which remains stationary depends upon the purpose of the movement. For example, muscles that pull the trunk down toward the thigh, as in bending forward, also may pull the thigh up toward the trunk, as when you bring your knees upward.

   • **Muscle Movements.** When a muscle contracts, it causes **flexion, extension, abduction, adduction, rotation**, or **circumduction**. A muscle can do one or several of these actions, depending on the type of joint that it spans and the relation of the muscle's line of pull to the joint.

   Flexion brings bones closer together (decreases the angle at the joint), for example, when you do a biceps curl. *Extension* moves the bones farther apart and is usually the return movement from flexion. Straightening your fingers to open your hand (extension) after you've made a fist (through flexion) is an example. All parts of our body are in extension when we are standing: head facing forward, with our upper extremities at our sides and our palms turned forward (a stance known as the anatomic position). Flexion and extension are angular movements that occur in a forward and backward plane.

   Abduction and adduction are also angular movements but in a lateral (side-to-side) plane. *Abduction* is a movement away from the vertical midline of the body (for example, when you move your leg straight out to the side), while *adduction* is the return movement. In a jumping jack, you first abduct as you jump apart and move your arms and legs sideways, and adduct as you bring your arms to your sides and your legs back together.

   Circumduction occurs when all the angular movements are successively combined so that the movement segment as a whole describes a circle or a cone, for example, when you rotate your wrist or head in a circular motion.

What We Know

*A muscle, when it contracts, can result in movements which **flex**, **extend**, **abduct**, **adduct**, **rotate**, or **circumduct**.*

Movements in the horizontal plane about a vertical axis are known as rotations. Shaking one's head "no" is rotation, as is turning to look behind you while rotating your trunk. *Outward rotation* is a movement of the front side of a bone away from the midline of the body, for example, when a ballerina stands facing the audience with her legs "turned out." Standing in a pigeon-toed fashion (toes pointing inward) is an example of *inward rotation*, where the front side of the bone turns inward toward the midline of the body.

Coordination

Try the following experiment: Place your palm on the front of your thigh. First walk a few steps, then run a few steps, then bring your knee up toward your chest, then sit down and cross your legs. Repeat the sequence, but this time think about which of your thigh muscles are working, feeling the muscles that take part in some or all of those actions. For example, the sartorius acts as a hip flexor. (It draws your thigh towards your trunk and bends your knee.) When the knee is flexed, the sartorius rotates the lower leg (turns your thigh outward). Similarly, most other muscles can perform multiple movements as well.

While a muscle may have a particular role in one type of movement, its role changes in a movement which has a different requirement. Take the trapezius, the large muscle at the back of the neck and upper back, which is composed of four parts. When we raise our arms to reach an object on an overhead shelf, all parts of the trapezius are involved. But only certain parts are involved in the very different acts of turning our head and tilting our chin upward, extending our shoulders as when we pull oars back in rowing, bringing an arm back in preparation to release a bowling ball, or raising an arm in preparation for the "draw" in archery. One often overlooked role of the trapezius is its support of the clavicle (collar bone). If you've ever carried a heavy suitcase a long distance, you've no doubt felt the tension and subsequent soreness in parts of your "traps."

Most purposeful bodily movements involve not only the one set of muscles that is directly responsible for the movement itself but considerable activity from other muscles as well. The cooperative action of a relatively large number of muscles, each performing its own particular task, is necessary to produce a single well-coordinated movement. In order to permit us to "work" a single muscle, exercise machines often position us in such a way as to prevent muscle cooperation, thereby isolating the muscle being strengthened.

• **Muscle Roles.** Some of the roles muscles play include being **movers**, **agonists**, **fixators**, and **antagonists**.

Movers are the muscles directly responsible for affecting a movement. In the majority of movements there are several movers; the one or two of greatest importance are known as *prime movers*, while the helpers are known as *agonists*. The distinction is an arbitrary one, thus a designation can provoke arguments: "I'm the prime mover in flexing the hip," says the sartorius. "No, you're only the agonist," respond the hamstrings.

Fixators are the muscles that steady or stabilize a part of the body so that prime movers and agonists will contract more effectively in a desired movement. The trapezius acts as a fixator in the tennis forehand and backhand by stabilizing the scapula (shoulder blades), thus allowing the deltoids (located on your shoulders) to function more effectively as prime movers.

Antagonists are the muscles that cause the opposite movement from that of the movers and fixators. Thus, in a biceps curl, the flexors of the arm (including the biceps) are the movers, while the arm extensors (the triceps, located in the back of your arm) are the antagonists.

• **Reciprocal Innervation.** Reciprocal innervation describes how when a mover contracts, its antagonist automatically relaxes. In throwing a softball, if antagonistic muscles didn't check the movement at the end of the throw, we would dislocate our shoulder every time. However, in what might seem like a contradiction (exceptions always are part of the picture), when a movement is performed with great force and rapidity, the antagonistic muscles to the prime mover may contract to check the movement and thus prevent injury. Thus, in a vigorous movement, the antagonistic muscles have two functions. One is to relax so as to allow the prime movers to perform, and the second is to protect by acting as a brake at the completion of the movement.

Communicating Movement

While I was thru-hiking on the Appalachian Trail, two wheels of an 18-wheel tractor trailer ran over my foot. Needless to say, I couldn't walk for awhile! In the process of rehabilitation, the simple act of getting my toes to stretch up or curl down took such intense concentration that it would leave me breathless and sweating—as if I had run a mile. Fortunately for me, I recovered, and now, several years later, am hiking again. —Gloria, age 54

How We Move. The intricate task of coordinating our body's movements in response to stimuli from inside and outside falls to our nervous system. Some signals we react to consciously, as when we put our hands up to catch a ball. Others, like those involved with our heart, are usually outside of our conscious control.

• **Nerve Meets Muscle and Begins to Talk.** Briefly, skeletal muscles respond (excitability) to nerve impulses coming from the brain and spinal cord. When these impulses reach the junction of the nerve and muscle, a chemical substance, **acetylcholine**, is

What We Know

When muscles contract, they accomplish work either isotonically or isometrically. In an isotonic contraction we can see the muscle working, which is not so for the isometric contraction.

released. Acetylcholine acts as a messenger, exciting the muscle fiber and thereby initiating the process of contraction.

Once stimulated, the muscle fiber transmits an electrochemical impulse along its membrane. These transmissions, called muscle impulses, produce an "action current" that releases calcium ions, which allow the start of the process of the breakdown of ATP (see page 40). The energy from that breakdown of ATP powers the interaction between the "two combs," actin and myosin, causing the fibers to contract. *Note:* The body maintains a constant calcium level in the blood. If the calcium present in the diet is insufficient, the body removes calcium from its main storage area, the bones.

Contractions: The Power of Pull.   Muscles contract to accomplish work. By "work" we include **isotonic** as well as **isometric** exertions. The terms come from the Greek language and mean, respectively, "equal tension" and "equal length." In an isotonic contraction, motion is permitted in the direction of the contraction and the muscle shortens. If you isotonically contract your biceps, the forearm will move toward the upper arm.

In contrast, an isometric contraction is one in which motion does not occur, yet the muscle contracts. An example is if you press your palms together and contract the biceps but do not allow the movement of your forearm upward toward the upper arm. While you do not see a movement externally, the muscles are contracting internally. Bodybuilders are expert at bulging—that is, contracting their muscles isometrically without moving the body parts.

In most physical activities, a **concentric**, or shortening, contraction occurs whereby the muscle actually shortens—as the back muscles do when you lift a weight from the floor. There are instances, however, when there is a gradual release of the contraction whereby the rate and range of movement is checked, moderated, or controlled. This type is known as an **eccentric contraction** and occurs, for example, in your back when you slowly lower the previously lifted weight to the floor.

• **Grading a Pull.** We have the ability to use our elbow flexors to pick up a piece of paper or to lift a 50-pound bundle. How do we make such gradation changes? The ability to adapt to either circumstance is based first on how many motor units within a muscle are stimulated.

Numbers Make a Difference. Remember that one skeletal muscle may consist of several hundred motor units. For each motor task we attempt, from a simple act like scratching our face to any of the more complicated motor actions we engage in, an evaluation is made through our senses (sight or touch, for example) and an appropriate number of motor units within a particular muscle are stimulated. All of us can remember making an error in evaluating a task's need, for example, serving a volleyball with so much force that it lands way out of bounds. In this case, too many motor units were brought into play. Conversely, our kinesthetic sense may have been caught off guard when attempting to lift an object that looked light but was far heavier than expected.

Frequency Counts. A second factor at work is how frequently the muscle is stimulated. If nerve impulses are discharged at a low frequency, the muscle fibers will partially relax between impulses; but if the nerve impulses come at a high frequency, the fibers will have insufficient time to relax and the result is a maximal contraction of those fibers. Frequent stimulation may increase the tension by as much as four times.

Adding Them Together. If these two factors are combined, that is, if our senses tell our muscles that the maximum number of fibers must be stimulated and the impulses are discharged at a high frequency, then the resulting contraction will be of maximal strength and you may lift a 50-pound weight bar. On the other hand, if a minimal number of fibers are stimulated and the impulses are discharged less frequently, you may gently dab at a piece of dust in your eye. The simultaneous and cooperative action brings about the very fine gradations in response of which we are all capable. Fortunately for us: Think what would happen if we put our finger to an eye with the same force we use to lift those fifty pounds!

• **Speedy Responses.** Our voluntary movements may be rapid or slow. Slow is when the tension is maintained throughout, like lifting weights or pulling back the bow string in archery as you carefully take aim. Rapid movements are usually **ballistic**, which means they are initiated by a vigorous muscular contraction and completed by momentum (generated by that vigorous contraction). In the beginning stages of practicing or learning a new movement—before it becomes automatic—we are usually uneconomical and unskillful. That's because the action is performed in its entirety with a constant muscular contraction (rather than being ballistic and letting momentum take over). This substitution of non-ballistic movement often occurs in those early stages of learning because we are concentrating on accuracy rather than form.

Although momentum from a ballistic movement usually runs its course, there are three ways a ballistic movement can be ended. We can contract the antagonistic muscles, thus applying a braking action, as when in the tennis forehand we shorten our stroke (pull back with deltoids and traps) in order to place the ball to a specific area of the court. The moving part also can be stopped by the body's passive resistance, i.e., the physical (anatomic) impossibility of going any farther as in a *grand battement*, the high kick in ballet. Finally, the momentum can be stopped by the interference of an obstacle, for instance, a boxer's punching bag.

Range of Movement (Flexibility)

Flexibility is the range of movement possible around a joint. If you're a dancer you need the best possible hip flexion so you can get your leg to almost reach your head; if you're a tennis player, you need good shoulder and ankle flexibility for full extension and power on the racquet and to stop and turn sharply; if you're a diver, you need spinal flexibility to execute a deep pike position. Although the need for range of movement may vary, whether you're an armchair athlete or a competitor, basic flexibility is necessary.

Girls are more flexible than boys, but this difference seems to disappear after puberty. Older people in their sixth decade (male and female) are ten times stiffer (less flexible) than those in their first decade. As a result of exercise, joint mobility is maintained or increased and the potential for injury is reduced.[3]

When we say someone is flexible, she may just be flexible in a movement that we admire, for example, a gymnast doing a back bend. Because flexibility is specific to a given joint and since our bodies are composites of many different joints, it is technically incorrect to say that an individual is flexible. Thus the gymnast may be unusually flexible in some joints, but in other joints may be of average or even less-than-average flexibility.

Improving Flexibility. Flexibility is determined by a variety of factors, including the anatomy of the joints, the extensibility of the muscles, and the elasticity of the surrounding muscles, tendons, and ligaments. It can best be improved through the use of a stretching program. Stretching techniques for improving flexibility have evolved over the years. See Chapter 4, Focus on Fitness, for more information about flexibility and stretching.

Muscle Considerations

Muscular Strength and Muscular Endurance. A marathoner who can run at top speed for long distances without tiring, now lifts weights as part of a training program. Conversely, a boxer who relies on arm strength includes road running as part of the workout. The reason: there is a difference between muscle strength and muscle endurance, and in many sports, both are necessary for maximum performance outcomes.

Muscle strength is the amount of force or tension that a muscle or muscle group can exert during one maximal effort. **Muscle endurance** is the ability to perform many repetitions of a movement. While a weight lifter has the muscular strength to lift huge amounts of weight overhead once, it takes muscular endurance to repeat that feat several times. The test for muscular strength involves measurement of a single maximum contraction, while a test for muscular endurance requires the measure of the number of times you can repeat an act. Although you might overall have a great deal of one but little of the other, it is also possible that you may have extraordinary strength in one muscle group but not in other muscles. Muscle strength and endurance are specific to a particular muscle or muscle group, for example, while ballerinas have very strong leg muscles, their ability to do push-ups or pull-ups may be minimal. Chapter 4, Focus on Fitness, has more information about muscular strength and endurance.

Muscular Hypertrophy.   As a result of a strength training program, you can expect an increase in the size of the muscles exercised (muscular hypertrophy). This occurs as a result of the enlargement of the muscle fibers.

Generally, women have lower absolute strength levels than men, as a result of a smaller muscle fiber area (as we saw in Chapter 2, A Woman Is Not a Man); however, the trainability of women's muscles for strength and endurance performance is similar to that of men.[3]

With proper training, women can increase their muscular strength, but will not enlarge their muscles as much as men will.[4] This finding is quite important for women who want to increase their strength but are worried about "bulking up."

The "Muscle Bound" Myth.   Until the early 1950s, there was a belief that heavy weight training resulted in a condition known as "muscle-bound." Being muscle-bound was rumored to limit both range and speed of movement and, therefore, weight training was anathema to most athletes. The newest research has resulted in the debunking of this old fallacy and has allowed us to achieve a higher level of conditioning through the use of muscle strength training. Chapter 5, Routines: The Stars Are the Limit, provides more information.

Muscle Fatigue.   Researchers have long noted that samples of excised muscle, when tested in the laboratory, will show a decreased response if they are caused to contract repeatedly and with very short rest intervals. This finding also applies to the intact muscle. Exercise physiologists have found that fatigue does not occur at the nerve-muscle junction, or because of faulty nervous transmission, but instead occurs within the muscle itself. As we discussed earlier in this chapter, the culprit appears to be the lactic acid buildup within the muscle. We discuss general body fatigue in Chapter 5, Routines: The Stars Are the Limit, and relate it to workload, physical fitness, and depletion of energy sources.

Exercise is a vital part of my life. It keeps the energy moving in my body. It releases stress and energizes me. I love to get my heart rate up and feel my blood pumping through my body. —Rhonda, age 37

Until now, this chapter's focus has been on bones, joints, muscles, and nerves, but another component of motor activity—our cardiovascular respiratory capacity—also needs to be considered. Presented here is a brief introduction to terms and concepts which are explored in greater depth in Chapters 4 and 5.

The cardiovascular respiratory aspect of human movement involves the ability of the heart to deliver oxygen to the muscle cells. This defines the limits of our physical work capacity. In exercise, endurance boils down ultimately to oxygen. The more oxygen you get while you exercise, the greater is your ability to sustain high exercise intensity levels. Since oxygen cannot be stored, it is crucial that adequate amounts of it be supplied to the tissues. That is the heart's main function: it is a pump and its performance is measured by its output.

Cardiac Output

Cardiac output is how much blood the heart is capable of pumping. During exercise, cardiac output increases to approximately four times that of the resting level (it increases up to six times in the elite endurance athlete). Maximum cardiac output (the volume of blood ejected by the heart per unit of time) for the average individual at rest is approximately five liters per minute—but during activity, it can be increased to 34 to 42 liters per minute in an elite athlete.[5] Cardiac output is determined by two factors: the heart rate and the amount ejected with each beat (known as the **stroke volume**).

Heart Rate.   The **heart rate** is what you measure when you put your fingers on one of your arteries in either your wrist or neck and count the pulses. (Your thumb echoes your heart, so when you count someone else's pulse, avoid using your thumb or you will pick up your pulse and not the other person's.) Heart rate reflects how effective the heart muscle is in performing its work. The lower your resting and exercise heart rates, the more efficient your heart, because it's accomplishing tasks with less effort. While the average normal heart rate at rest is about 65 to 80 beats per minute, it has been observed to be as low as 40—in highly trained endurance athletes—and as high as 100. Resting heart rate varies not only from individual to individual but also within an individual from one observation to another. It can be affected by exercise, emotion, food, environmental factors, smoking, posture, etc. Women have higher heart rates than men, averaging five to ten beats faster. See Chapter 4 to learn how to measure your resting heart rate.

Your resting heart rate is different from your **maximum heart rate**, which is the biologically fixed fastest rate that your heart can beat. The maximum heart rate is largely determined by heredity and age, and it becomes lower as you age. (See Chapter 14, Keeping It Going, for more information.)

Typical Heart Rate Response to Exercise. As you begin to exercise, your muscles need more oxygen and your heart must pump more oxygenated blood to meet this increased demand. Your body's response is an elevated heart rate and an increase in your stroke volume. Your heart rate is increased by the intensity and duration of the exercise as well as the type of exercise. For example, exercises like running and swimming, which involve rapid and vigorous muscular contraction, result in large increases in heart rate. In contrast, isometric exercises like weight lifting, which involve a held position or straining against a heavy load, result in only a slight increase in heart rate.

As you begin to exercise, the heart rate elevates very rapidly. If the exercise is light or moderate, a leveling off (steady state) is seen in two to three minutes, and this rate continues until you stop exercising. If the work load is heavy, the rate increases until exhaustion (caused by oxygen debt and lactic acid buildup) intervenes.

When exercise ends, the next two to three minutes produce a decline in heart rate that is almost as rapid as the initial increase. After this initial decline, further decline occurs more slowly. Because of this rapid decline, you should take your pulse immediately after stopping your exercise, if you wish to measure your highest rate.

Stroke Volume.   The average man has a larger heart size and heart volume than the average woman. This results in a greater output (**stroke volume**) during maximal exercise and contributes to the sex differences observed in oxygen consumption (for more information on gender differences, see Chapter 2, A Woman Is Not a Man).

Stroke volume is controlled by a physiological interplay of blood and heart muscle. It is a product of the cardiac muscle's ability to contract with great force (the stronger the muscle, the more complete the emptying of the heart chambers), venous return of blood to the heart, and blood volume. Endurance training increases all of these things.

Measuring Cardiac Output.   Cardiac output can be evaluated by several methods that monitor oxygen consumption. The most accurate involves catheterization; however, several non-invasive techniques which estimate oxygen consumption are also available.

The best measure of cardiovascular capacity is considered to be **maximal oxygen** consumption (VO_2max). VO_2max is the point at which oxygen consumption does not rise despite increased exercise intensity or, put another way, the greatest rate at which oxygen can be taken in and utilized during exercise. Chapter 4, Focus on Fitness, provides more information on VO_2max including techniques for its evaluation.

The higher your VO_2max, the greater your ability to sustain high exercise intensity levels. A high VO_2max is a prerequisite to performing at winning levels in endurance events. As you increase your training, your VO_2max increases. Changes in your VO_2max are due largely to changes in your stroke volume, which is increased through exercise. If you are running in your first marathon, the higher your VO_2max compared to other novice marathoners, the faster you will tend to run.[6] However, if you ever become a world class marathoner (in the league of Grete Waitz, for example), then all your competitors will, more than likely, have high VO_2max. At that competitive level, other physiological factors such as lactic acid clearance capacity, maximal muscle blood flow, and performance economy become increasingly important to gain a winning edge.[7]

GOING FORWARD

In closing this chapter, we are reminded of an engineering professor who said that the human machine has an advantage over the manufactured one because while the latter wears out with use, the former improves with use (within limits), provided it is used in accordance with the principles of efficient human motion. In succeeding chapters you will discover how the principles we discussed here get translated into the goal of efficient human motion.

ENDNOTES

1. Tesch, P. A. Short-and long-term histochemical and biochemical adaptations in muscle. In P. V. Komi, (ed.). *Strength and Power in Sport*. London: Blackwell Scientific Publications, 1992, 250–265.
2. Arkin, A. M. Absolute muscle power: Internal kinesiology of muscle. *Archives of Surgery*. 1947, 42, 395–410.
3. O'Toole, M. L., & Douglas, P. S. Fitness: Definition and development. In M. M. Shangold & G. Mirkin, (eds.). *Women and Exercise: Physiology and Sports Medicine*, 2nd ed. Philadelphia: F. A. Davis Co., 1994, 3–26.
4. Clark, D. H. Training for Strength. In M. M. Shangold & G. Mirkin, (eds.). *Women and Exercise: Physiology and Sports Medicine*, 2nd ed. Philadelphia: F. A. Davis Co., 1994, 60–72.
5. de Vries, H. A. Physiology of Exercise for Physical Education and Athletics, 2nd ed. Dubuque, IA: William C. Brown Co., 1974.
6. Christensen, C. L., & Ruhling, R. O. Physical characteristics of novice and experienced women marathon runners. *British Journal of Sports Medicine*, 1983, 17, 66–72.
7. Fahey, T. D. Endurance Training. In M. M. Shangold & G. Mirkin, (eds.). *Women and Exercise: Physiology and Sports Medicine*, 2nd ed. Philadelphia: F. A. Davis Co., 1994, 73–88.

4

Focus on Fitness

SUSAN L. PURETZ, ED.D.

I started exercising four years ago only because my doctor suggested it. I had low back pain and was 40 pounds overweight. I started slowly with low impact aerobics and didn't like it for awhile—however, something happened. I started having more energy, eating less, losing weight (very slowly), feeling more positive, and came to look forward to my exercise class. —Judy, age 43

Many of us have the idea that we should be healthy and fit; as in Judy's case, the two are often intertwined. While we think we understand the words healthy and fit, their meanings have changed over the years. In the past, if you weren't born with a congenital disease, had no symptoms of disease, and were free of pain and disability, you were considered healthy. That was the best you could hope for. To be fit wasn't even an issue. Nowadays, as a result of medical science, many communicable diseases that plagued us have been conquered, degenerative diseases can be helped by new treatments, and our life expectancy has risen.

As a result, our view of health has changed so that now, one of the more popular definitions of health comes from the World Health Organization and is "a state of complete physical, mental, and social well-being and not merely the absence of disease or infirmity."[1]

Fitness contributes to that state. Keeping fit is a necessity, not an option. This chapter should provide you with the essentials to help in your pursuit of healthy fitness.

FITNESS FOR FEMALES

What is Fitness?

There are five components of fitness: **cardiorespiratory endurance**, **muscular endurance**, **muscular strength**, **flexibility**, and **body composition**. Performance in any activity will

TABLE 4.1

....

Activities for Physical Fitness Development

Cardiorespiratory Endurance

Aerobic Dancing	Hiking
Backpacking	Jogging
Basketball	Racquetball
Bicycling	Rowing
Calisthenics	Running
Cross-country Skiing	Skating
Downhill Skiing	Squash
Field Hockey	Stair Climbing
Fitness Walking	Swimming
Handball	Tennis (singles)

Muscular Strength

Aerobic Dancing	Gymnastics
Backpacking	Rowing
Calisthenics	Swimming
Cycling	Weight Training

Muscular Endurance

Calisthenics	Rowing
Fencing	Running
Handball	Swimming
Jogging	Weight training

Body Composition (Body Mass)

Aerobic Dancing	Running
Cross-country Skiing	Swimming
Jogging	

Flexibility

Aerobic Dancing	Karate
Calisthenics	Modern Dance
Gymnastics	Stretching

both influence and be influenced by one's health and physical fitness. See Table 4.1 for a list of some physical activities broken down by fitness components.

Cardiorespiratory Endurance.   Our lungs, heart, and blood vessels must function efficiently if they are to deliver adequate amounts of oxygen to meet the demands of prolonged physical activity. For a given amount of exercise, a woman with a low level of cardiorespiratory endurance must work much harder than one who is fit. That is because her heart pumps more often to supply the same amount of oxygen as the heart of the fit woman, who has a high level of cardiorespiratory endurance. Consequently, the less fit woman will fatigue faster. Remember, the heart is a muscle, and the fit heart, like other muscles, is strengthened by exercise.

Exercise that improves cardiorespiratory endurance helps your body perform the same amount of work with lower heart and respiratory rates and with a lower systolic blood pressure.[2] Exercise makes you more efficient by causing the heart to pump more blood per beat (known as stroke volume) so that you get maximum amounts of blood with minimum effort. At the same time, your resting heart rate decreases, which means that, when you are not exercising, your heart does not beat as frequently because it pauses longer between beats.[3] A reduction of 20 beats per minute can save your heart about 10,432,200 beats per year. All of these changes contribute to a healthier heart, and some studies show that effects occur after as little as four weeks of training.[4] While you can live without big muscles or a nice figure, you can't live long and well without a healthy heart.

Muscular Endurance.   Muscular endurance is the muscle's ability to perform without fatiguing over a set period of time. The more repetitions of a weight training exercise you can perform successfully (for example, lifting 80 pounds 20 times instead of 10 times), the greater your muscular endurance. Having muscular endurance is critical in carrying out everyday activities. We do not typically perform a motion only once. For example, it's not enough to be able to lift one shovelful of dirt. You have to be able to keep shoveling until you've dug the required hole. A test for muscular endurance usually involves measuring the number of repetitions of a specific exercise or movement.

Muscular Strength.   Whether you're hitting a tennis ball, lifting a heavy suitcase or dumbbell, unscrewing a jar's tight lid, or pulling a 110-pound archery string, you need muscular strength. While muscle strength and muscular endurance are interrelated, they are different. Muscular strength refers to the amount of force that a muscle (or muscle group) is capable of exerting. Weak muscles can't repeat an action several times, nor can they sustain it for a long time, because they lack strength and endurance. When you enhance strength you usually also influence muscular endurance.

Power. The difference between strength and power is important, but it's a distinction seldom made. For example, if two women can each lift 50 pounds, but one does it twice as fast as the other, they are both equally strong, but the one who does it twice as fast is twice as powerful. Strength is the ability to move heavy objects without regard to the time it takes, whereas power refers to the ability to move those objects in the shortest time possible. Power combines strength and speed.

Muscle Specificity. When you develop muscular strength or endurance it is usually muscle-specific. Thus, when you do bicep curls, you are working on increasing the strength and endurance of the biceps and not the triceps, the hamstrings, or the abdominals.

Flexibility. Touching your nose to your knees while standing may be considered by some to be the ultimate test of flexibility, but it is not the gold standard. Flexibility is a measure of the range of motion—or the amount of movement possible—at a particular joint. It is joint-specific and is important in order to perform tasks that require reaching, twisting, turning your body, or lifting and moving objects. We are most flexible until our late twenties, when a gradual loss of mobility begins.[5] As we get older, muscles, ligaments, and tendons shorten and become tighter if not used through their full range of motion.[6]

Body Composition. An overweight person might not only find it difficult to tie her shoelaces because of a bulging stomach, she might also be less flexible, weaker, and tire more easily with exertion. Being overweight, besides placing us at risk of developing health problems, puts extra stress on our joints and heart. Determining whether we are overweight is somewhat subjective and depends on our self-image, cultural factors, body structure, and how our weight is distributed, as well as the method we use to make the decision. Traditionally, we have compared our weight with data from a standard height-and-weight chart. However, height-weight tables do not provide an indication of body composition.

Body composition refers to the amount of fat versus the amount of lean tissue in the body. Lean tissue includes everything except fat: muscles, bones, organs, fluid, and so on. It is the ratio of body fat to lean muscle tissue that is the true indicator of how fat we really are.

Assessment of body composition is based on comparing our recommended body fat with our actual body fat percentage (or percent body fat mass). While there is agreement on a general range of body mass that is consistent with good health, there is no consensus on exactly where the cutoffs between normal and overweight should be drawn. Because there is no agreement, you will see some variation in body mass recommendations. In general, however, a woman with more than 25 percent body fat is considered overweight, and over 30 percent is considered obese. One researcher has proposed that the numbers should get slightly higher as you age. Accordingly, a score in the range of 19 to 25 percent for women through age 34 (and 21 to 27 percent for those over 35) is considered acceptable.[7] However, many researchers disregard age and simply use 27 percent as the overweight cutoff point. *Note:* Although weight and body composition are interrelated, they are different. Female body builders who are 15 to 20 pounds overweight according to the charts (and thus considered obese) probably have very little body fat; rather, the scale is reflecting the heaviness and relative density of muscle tissue. Similarly, a 45-year-old woman who weighs the same 135 pounds that she did in high school may be surprised to learn that almost one-quarter of her total body weight is now fat (compared to 18 percent when she was sweet sixteen).

Assessing Fitness

Whether we are first starting to improve our physical fitness or are already fit, an assessment that provides baseline values is always a good idea. Since physical fitness is based on the five distinct components just discussed, an assessment of each will provide us with an overall fitness profile. *Note:* For those who have been sedentary or are older, it's strongly recommended that you consult a physician before doing a fitness evaluation or starting a training program.

Cardiorespiratory Endurance Assessment.   As you remember from Chapter 3, the level of cardiorespiratory endurance (aerobic capacity) is determined by the maximum amount of oxygen we are able to utilize per minute of physical activity, usually expressed as milliliters per kilogram of total body weight per minute (ml/kg/min). This aerobic capacity is known as **VO_2max** (V for volume, O_2 for oxygen, and max for maximum). The higher our VO_2 max, the more efficient is our cardiorespiratory system.

The most precise way to determine VO_2max is in a laboratory, through direct gas analysis while exercising on a treadmill or bicycle. As an alternative to this maximal aerobic capacity treadmill test, several submaximal exercise tests have been developed, such as the Rockport Fitness One-Mile Walk Test, the 1.5-mile run test, the Harvard step test, and the 12-minute swim test. Although less reliable, they have the advantage of allowing you to do them outside of the laboratory and on your own. Your choice of a test should be based on which one fits both your present physical condition and the activity you do. For example, the Rockport One-Mile Walk Test is good if you are just beginning an exercise

TABLE 4.2

....

Rockport Fitness One-Mile Walking Test

Purpose: To evaluate aerobic capacity (VO_2max) without expensive equipment.

Equipment: Watch with a second hand, digital watch, or stopwatch, and a measured, level one-mile surface.

Procedure:
1. Before starting the test, you should warm up—a slow walk is an appropriate warm-up.
2. To begin the test, note the time (or start the stopwatch) and begin walking.
3. Stop walking after one mile and note your time to the nearest minute.
4. Immediately locate your pulse, and take it for 15 seconds. Multiply that nuber by 4 to get your heart rate in beats per minute.

Evaluation:
1. Select the fitness chart on page 59 that matches your age.
2. Draw a vertical line through your time and a horizontal line through your heart rate. The point where the lines intersect will determine your cardiorepiratory fitness level.

Reprinted with permission of The Rockport Company.

regimen, because all that is required is a brisk walk, fast enough to produce a heart rate of at least 120 beats per minute at the end of the test. The run and the swim tests are more demanding and not appropriate if you are an unconditioned beginner, smoke, or can't swim. If you have heart problems or risk factors such as obesity or hypertension, consult a physician before taking any of the tests. A description and scoring scale for the Rockport One-Mile Walk Test appear in Table 4.2 and on page 59. *Note:* Level 1 places you in a low fitness category, Level 3 is average, while Level 5 is high.

Muscular Endurance and Strength Assessment. While a number of tests can be used to assess muscular strength and endurance, several of them require specific equipment, such as a chinning bar or a 16-inch bench. To avoid these requirements, we've selected two tests that don't require special equipment. A key concept in muscle testing is to use several different body sites, because our specific muscular development will probably vary. A

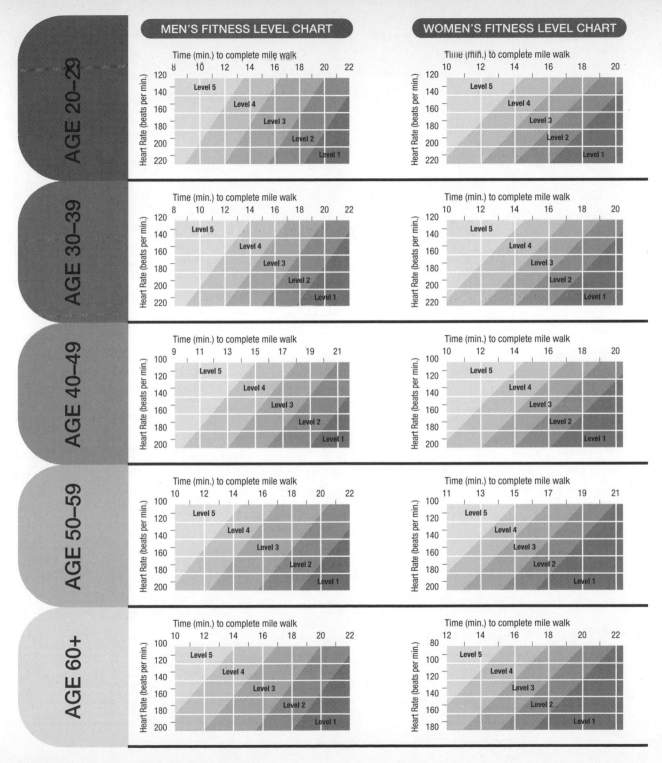

TABLE 4.3A

One-Minute Modified Push-up Test

Purpose: To test muscular endurance and strength in the arms, shoulders, and chest.

Equipment: Watch with second hand, digital watch, or stopwatch. A partner would be helpful.

Procedure:

1. Begin in the modified push-up position with your weight on your hands and knees. Hands should be flat on the floor and directly under your shoulders.
2. Lower yourself (by bending your elbows) until your chest touches the floor. Then push yourself back up to the starting position.
3. Do as many correct push-ups as possible in one minute. Evaluate your score against the standards listed below.

Pointers:

Don't hold your breath: exhale each time you push yourself up. Keep your body straight—don't just lower your chest and keep your hips in the air.

Evaluation:

Age	Poor	Average	Excellent
18–29	<16	16–35	>35
30–39	<11	11–30	>30
40–49	<7	7–25	>25
50–59	<5	5–20	>20
60 plus	<3	3–10	>10

< means less than
> means more than

Adapted from: National Fitness Foundation Test, cited in W. E. Prentice, *Fitness for College and Life*, 3rd edition. St. Louis: Mosby Yearbook, 1991.

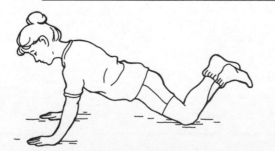
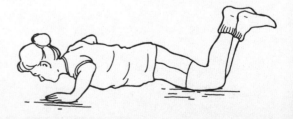

TABLE 4.3B

··

One-Minute Curl-up Test

Purpose: To measure the strength and endurance of the abdominal muscles.
Equipment: Watch with second hand, digital watch, or stopwatch.

Procedure:
1. You should come up less than halfway (about 30 degrees).
2. Lie down with your knees bent and your shoulders touching the floor. Your arms should be completely extended by your sides with palms facing down. It is helpful to have someone hold your feet down and time you.
3. With your arms fully extended, lift your head, shoulders, and upper trunk off the floor and slide your hands forward. Then return to the lying position—it is not necessary to return your head to the floor with each curl-up. Do as many as you can in one minute.

Hints:
Exhale as you curl up—don't hold your breath. Rest at any time, but don't stop the clock. If you don't have a partner to hold your feet, try not to slide back during the test.

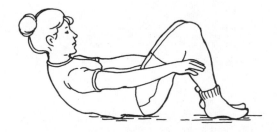

Evaluation:

Age	Poor	Average	Excellent
18–29	<25	25–45	>45
30–39	<20	20-40	>40
40–49	<16	16-35	>35
50–59	<12	12–30	>30
60 plus	<11	11–25	>25

< means less than
> means more than

··

Adapted from: National Fitness Foundation Test, cited in W. E. Prentice, *Fitness for College and Life*, 3rd edition. St. Louis: Mosby Yearbook, 1991.

TABLE 4.4

....

Sit-and-Reach Test

Purpose: To evaluate the flexibility of muscles in your lower back and the back of your legs.

Equipment: Yardstick and a piece of tape. A partner would be helpful.

Procedure:

1. Place a piece of tape on the floor. Place the yardstick alongside the tape with the 15-inch mark at the tape.

2. Sit down with your legs extended, knees flat on the floor, and your heels about 5 inches apart. Make sure that you have the yardstick between your legs—with the zero mark closest to you. Place your heels on the near edge of the tape alongside the 15-inch mark.

3. Keeping your knees straight, slowly reach forward with both hands as far as you can. Have your partner read the yardstick to see how far you reach.

Evaluation:

Age	Poor	Average	Excellent
18–29	<16	16–22	>22
30–39	<15	15–21	>21
40–49	<14	14–20	>20
50–59	<13	13–19	>19
60 plus	<12	12–18	>18

< means less than
> means more than

....

Adapted from: National Fitness Foundation Test, cited in W. E. Prentice, *Fitness for College and Life*, 3rd edition. St. Louis: Mosby Yearbook, 1991, and from *ACSM Fitness Book*, 1992.

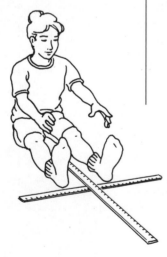

TABLE 4.5A

Body Mass Index

Purpose: To evaluate your body composition.
Equipment: Scale and a ruler.

Procedure:
1. Measure your body weight. Weigh yourself several days in a row, at the same time of day, and then average the results. Wear minimal clothes and no shoes.
2. Measure your height. Remove your shoes and stand tall with your heels together.
3. Compute your Body Mass Index by doing the following mathematical calculations:
   a. Convert your weight in pounds to kilograms (kg) by dividing it by 2.2. For example, if you weigh 125 pounds, your weight in kilograms is:
      125 lbs/2.2 = 56.8 kg
   b. Convert your height in inches to meters (m) by multiplying it by 0.0254. For example, if you were five feet tall, you would be 60 inches, and:
      60 in x 0.0254 = 1.52m
   c. Multiply your height in meters by itself. Using the same number as in b, you would have:
      1.52 x 1.52 = 2.31
   d. Now plug these numbers into the formula for BMI which is
      $BMI = weight\ (kg)/height\ (m)^2$ and you would have:
      BMI = 56.8/2.31 = 24.58
4. If you are mathematically challenged, you can use Table 4.5B to determine your BMI.

Evaluating your BMI:
Acceptable: 19 to 25 (under age 34)
                   21 to 27 (34 and over)

Adapted from National Institutes of Health (NIH), Methods for voluntary weight loss and control. *Nutrition Today*, 1992, 27(4), 27–33.

high degree of strength or endurance in one group of muscles does not necessarily indicate a high degree in another group. The arms of runners are usually not so strong as those of swimmers; however, swimmers' legs are not so well-developed as those of runners. The two tests we recommend are: modified push-ups (for the arms) and curl-ups (for the abdominals). See Tables 4.3A and 4.3B for descriptions of these tests.

Flexibility Assessment. We have included only one test in this assessment; however, remember that flexibility, like muscle strength and endurance, is specific. Good flexibility in one joint area is not indicative of flexibility in another. The modified sit-and-reach test is designed to measure the flexibility of the muscles in the lower back and the back of the legs. A description is found in Table 4.4.

Body Composition Assessment. The percentage of body fat can be determined by skin fold thickness, underwater weighing, bioelectrical impedance, and girth measurements. To avoid the elaborate hydrostatic test or the equipment necessary for the bioelectrical impedance or skin fold thickness assessment, we have included an easy way of determining body composition by calculating your Body Mass Index (BMI). See the directions in Tables 4.5A and 4.5B to determine your BMI.

The Body Mass Index is a measure based on your height and weight. Even though this value can't determine how much body weight comes from fat tissue and how much from muscle, bone, and water, the Body Mass Index correlates highly with direct measures of body fat.[8]

BMI is often used as an estimate of critical fat values at which the risk for disease increases. Since risk is approximately proportional to degree of overweight, the degree of risk has been classified on a scale (see Table 4.5C, Body Mass Index and Weight/Health Risks) from very low risk to very high risk.[9] It is important to note that it is possible to have a health risk associated with too little body fat—a BMI of less than 20 (see the discussion on eating disorders in Chapter 18, Beware of the Danger Zones).

Your Fitness Profile. Recording all your scores in Table 4.6 will give you a quick overview of your current status. Now that you have your report card, it should give you a clearer picture of your fitness profile. Fitness for health and the greater fitness necessary for participating in moderate to vigorous physical activity are not equivalent. Building a fitness or training program will be easier because you now know which areas need work. The scorecard also provides you with a baseline that can be used for future comparisons to see how effective your training regimen has been.

TABLE 4.5B

Determining BMI from Height and Weight

Body Mass Index

Height (in)	19	20	21	22	23	24	25	26	27	28	29	30	35
					Body Weight (lbs)								
58	91	96	100	105	110	115	119	124	129	134	138	143	167
59	94	99	104	109	114	119	124	128	133	138	143	148	173
60	97	102	107	112	118	123	128	133	138	143	148	153	179
61	100	106	111	116	122	127	132	137	143	148	153	158	185
62	104	109	115	120	126	131	136	142	147	153	158	164	191
63	107	113	118	124	130	135	144	146	152	158	163	169	197
64	110	116	122	128	134	140	145	151	157	163	169	174	204
65	114	120	126	132	138	144	150	156	162	168	174	180	210
66	118	124	130	136	142	148	155	161	167	173	179	186	216
67	121	127	134	140	146	153	159	166	172	178	184	191	223
68	125	131	138	144	151	158	164	171	177	184	190	197	230
69	128	135	142	149	155	162	169	176	182	189	196	203	236
70	132	139	146	153	160	167	174	181	188	195	202	207	243
71	136	143	150	157	165	172	179	186	193	200	208	215	250

Each entry gives the body weight in pounds (rounded off) for a person of a given height and body mass index.

Find your height in the left-hand column. Move across the row to your weight.

The number at the top of the column is the Body Mass Index for the height and weight. Adapted from National Institutes of Health (NIH), Methods for voluntary weight loss and control. *Nutrition Today*, 1992, 27(4), 27–33.

TABLE 4.5C

....

Body Mass Index and Weight/Health Risks

Body Mass Index	Weight/Health Risk
Below 20	Underweight / moderate to very high health risk
20 to 25	Acceptable weight / low to very low health risk
25 to 30	Overweight / low to moderate health risk
30 to 35	Obese / moderate health risk
35 to 40	Obese / high health risk
Over 40	Obese / very high health risk

....

Adapted from Wilfley, Grilo, & Brownell. In *Women and Exercise: Physiology and Sports Medicine*, Shangold, M. M., & Mirkin, G. (eds.), 1994 and from G. Bray, M.D.

THE GOLDEN RULE FOR FITNESS

The Overload Principle

The overload principle, the golden rule for developing overall physical fitness, states that our bodies must be stressed beyond their normal levels of activity if they are to improve. To increase the overload, and consequently our level of physical conditioning, we must gradually increase either **intensity**, **duration**, or **frequency** of activity.

Intensity. By intensity we mean the rate, degree of vigor, or how hard an exercise is performed. The amount of weight lifted is the intensity measurement used in weight training activities, while heart rate is usually used as a measure of intensity in aerobic activities such as walking, running, and swimming. For aerobic activities, exercise intensity can be calculated easily by checking the pulse. According to the American College of Sports Medicine, cardiorespiratory improvement occurs when working between 60 to 90 percent of your maximum heart rate during aerobic exercise.[10] This area is known as your **training intensity** (or target training zone). The higher the percentage, the more optimal the training results—although gains are made at the lower levels as well.

    • **Upping the Ante.** To increase the intensity, you must raise your target training number, for example, from 60 percent to anywhere from 65 to 90 percent. This means that you will need to exercise more vigorously to get to your new targeted heart rate. If

TABLE 4.6

....

Personal Fitness Profile

	First test	Follow-up test
DATE:	_____	_____
BODY WEIGHT:	_____	_____
Cardiorespiratory Fitness		
Rockport One-Mile Walking Test	_____	_____
Muscular Strength and Endurance		
One-Minute Modified Push-up Test	_____	_____
One-Minute Curl-up Test	_____	_____
Flexibility		
Sit-and-Reach Test	_____	_____
Body Composition		
Body Mass Index	_____	_____

What We Know

The more intense the training, the greater the training effect.

you have been physically active, you might consider raising your intensity to increase your training effect. If, on the other hand, you have been sedentary, you may consider training at around 60 percent intensity during the first two months before gradually increasing the intensity.

The same principle of increasing the intensity applies to weight lifting, but in this case it means increasing either the amount of weight lifted or the number of repetitions at each of the weights chosen (see Chapter 5, Routines: The Stars Are the Limit, for more information).

• **Figuring It Out.** To use heart rate as the measure of intensity for achieving a strong cardiorespiratory training effect, you must know your **Target Heart Rate** (**THR**). There are several methods for determining THR.

1. In the percent of heart rate maximum (%HRmax) method, you would use the formula THR = MaxHR x TI (where THR = Target Heart Rate, MaxHR = Maximum Heart Rate, and TI = Training Intensity). To get that final figure, you must first calculate your Maximal Heart Rate (MHR). An easy approximation of that rate is achieved

by subtracting your age from 220. Second, you must choose a Training Intensity (TI) between 60 and 90 percent. That number represents how hard you should be exercising. Both of these figures then are entered into the formula.

Let's substitute some numbers: If a woman of 40 were to choose a 60 percent training intensity level, then her Target Heart Rate would be 220 – 40 x .6 = 108. In order to achieve a minimum conditioning level from the aerobic activity she has chosen, our 40-year-old woman's heart rate would have to be at least 108 beats per minute during the exercise period.

2. Some exercise physiologists prefer to use the heart rate reserve method (HR-reserve), which takes into account cardiac reserve and is another way of determining exercise heart rate.[11] Also known as the Karvonen Method (after its developer), it requires a few simple calculations before using the formula THR = HRR x TI + RHR (where HRR = Heart Rate Reserve, and RHR = Resting Heart Rate).

First, to use this formula, your RHR must be determined. Because your RHR is affected by many factors (caffeine, nicotine, anxiety, food), the best way to determine yours is to standardize the procedure. Take your pulse in a sitting position after waking up in the morning—before you get out of bed. Repeat this procedure for four to five consecutive days and average the readings.

Second, to get your HRR, subtract your RHR from your MHR (220 minus your age). Third, decide which TI you want to use and then plug the numbers into the equation. Using the previous example, our hypothetical woman would subtract her RHR (let's assume it is 70) from her MHR of 180 (220 - 40) to get her cardiac reserve rate (HRR) of 110. Her Target Heart Rate would look like: THR = 110 x .6 + 70 or 136.

You'll notice that the numbers aren't the same for the two methods. The advantage of using the Karvonen formula is that the use of RHR gives a better estimate of your fitness level. Generally, the lower the RHR, the more fit the individual. The advantage of the %HRmax method is that it's a little easier to compute. One drawback of both methods is that they use an estimated maximum heart rate. The estimated MHR has the distinct disadvantage of being based on population averages and as a result has a range of plus or minus 10 to 12 beats per minute.[12]

• **Double Checking**. A simple way of checking whether you have achieved your target is to **immediately** monitor your pulse (heart) rate when you have stopped the activity. After 15 seconds, heart rates drop rapidly as the body recovers. The pulse can be taken either at the neck or wrist. At the neck, place your index and middle fingers at the base of your neck, on either side of your windpipe (but don't exert too much pressure) until you feel the strong pulse of the carotid artery, the brain's main feeder. At the wrist, place your index and middle fingers on the artery on the underside of your wrist and find your pulse. Count for 15 seconds and multiply that number by four.

• **Perceived Exertion.** If you've spent time in health clubs, you may have noticed posters that depict the target heart rates we have just described. Some cardiologists believe that target heart rates have little meaning and that when we slavishly take our exercise pulse, we are wasting our time. Instead they believe (and some studies support them) that the body knows what its target heart rate is and that we intuitively begin to sense the level of activity we can safely withstand.[13]

This self-selected pace of exercise is known as perceived rate of exertion, and exercise researchers have reported that it equates well with VO_2 max targets.[14] So, if you are one of those exercisers who chafe at being regimented, trust your body to tell you what pace is suitable for you. See Chapter 14, Keeping It Going: The Older Athlete, for further discussion of perceived rate of exertion.

• **Try Using METs.** METs are another intensity concept whereby physical exertion can be measured. One MET (for metabolic equivalent) is the energy expended in a minute by somebody resting quietly. Using METs, the cost of a particular exercise can be calculated. The American College of Sports Medicine has constructed tables listing the energy cost in METs for walking, jogging, and running.[15] For example: light exertion, such as strolling at 2 miles per hour, is approximately 2 to 3 METs; moderate exertion, like walking at 4 miles per hour, is approximately 3 to 6 METs; while hard/vigorous exertion, for example, a fast walk/jog at a 5-miles-per-hour pace, is considered to be above 6 METs.

Duration. Duration refers to the length of time of the workout. By increasing the amount of time we exercise, we can contribute to the overload principle. In general, the intensity of an exercise is inversely related to its duration, that is, as one increases, the other usually decreases. *Note:* As we age (or when we first begin an exercise program), it is advisable to increase duration rather than intensity.

It is generally recommended that we exercise from 20 to 60 minutes per session, depending on the intensity of the session.[16] If training is at 90 percent of the maximum heart rate, 20 minutes may be sufficient; at 60 percent, a minimum of 30 minutes is recommended. This period of time does not include warm-up and cool-down, which are discussed later in this chapter.

Frequency. Frequency refers to the number of days per week of exercise. Exercising three to five times per week, for 20 to 30 minutes each session, is normally sufficient to maintain a training effect.[16] Training more than five days per week may only contribute minimally to further improvement. The other two days might be better used as rest days.

What We Know

The greater the duration of training (up to a point), the greater the training effect. Duration can compensate for lower intensity in aerobic conditioning.

The intensity and/or duration of activity should be gradually and continually increased to reach optimum levels of fitness.

Recuperation between exercise days is important, to allow our bodies to adapt to and recover from the stress placed on them during exercise.

Where to Go from Here?   Yesterday's newspaper said: Longevity is fostered by vigorous exercise. Today's paper says that moderate exercise is best. So what's the story, what's enough?

The seeming conflict comes from two recommendations by the American College of Sports Medicine. The first, made in 1990, gave recommended guidelines for developing and maintaining physical fitness.[17] The second, issued in 1995, seemingly urged a more moderate level of exercise.[18]

To understand the difference between these recommendations requires that we realize that the less formidable recommendation was designed, in part, to present less of an obstacle to exercise in the predominately sedentary U.S. population. Less than 27 percent of women in this country meet the Centers for Disease Control minimum guidelines for physical activity.[19]

Be that as it may, everyone agrees that exercise is good for you (see Chapter 1, Why We Exercise, for the specific reasons). **Don't "sit it out."** The best attitude toward exercise is that for those who can exercise, more is better than less, but less is better than none at all. To move out of the least-fit category does not require intensive exercise. The 1995 recommendations from the American College of Sports Medicine and the Centers for Disease Control and Prevention (ACSM-CDC) are to do at least 30 minutes or more of moderate activity on most days of the week, preferably every day of the week.[20]

Moderate vs. Vigorous Exercise. It is important to keep in mind that good health resulting from an active way of life is different from physical fitness. Moderate activity will not produce the capacity for hard physical work or play, but it will promote general health.[20]

Moderate exercise is clearly healthful, but it may take longer to achieve physical fitness benefits than if you exercised intensely. For example, in one study of women who did moderate levels of exercise, it took 24 weeks to see an improvement in HDL cholesterol levels; the same benefit occurred in 8 to 10 weeks with vigorous exercise.[21] However, a 14-week difference doesn't amount to much, since exercise should be a lifetime goal.

THE WORKOUT

No matter what activity you pursue, and whether you do it moderately or vigorously, you should try to think of each workout as a unit consisting of a **warm-up, stretches, your particular activity/exercise/sport**, and a **cooldown**. A warm-up prepares your body for a workout, while a cooldown following an activity helps your body begin its recovery. Stretching allows your muscles to gradually become more flexible.

Warm-up

When children want to get somewhere fast, they just break into a run. Try that as an adult, and you could pull a muscle. Tight muscles may invite disaster when they are suddenly called upon for vigorous activity. The remedy: Ease into exercise through a warm-up.

Physiology of Warm-up. As the term "warm-up" suggests, these preparations for exercise are helpful in several ways. A warm-up increases body and muscle temperature, may increase oxygen delivery to the muscle cells, and decreases resistance to blood flow. Finally, a warm-up may increase the speed of nerve impulses and may increase blood flow traveling to muscles and tendons. All these factors might help explain the importance of a warm-up.

    Controversy. But are warm-ups effective? Despite universal agreement that warming up is beneficial, little scientific evidence proves that it enhances performance or reduces injuries.[22] The major reason for thinking muscles would be protected by a warm-up was the belief that muscles were injured because they received inadequate amounts of blood flow and therefore, less oxygen. But an injury is now seen as a mechanical trauma to the muscle fibers, and in one recent study, there was no evidence indicating that warming up helps prevent those injuries.[23]

    However, if your activity requires flexibility and a wide range of motion, warm-ups may improve your performance. And if they don't improve performance, the warming up and stretching of connective tissue surrounding muscles might help prevent soreness that can occur even if your muscles are not injured.[24]

    Further, warm-ups may help prevent excessive strain on the heart.[25] Warming up lowers blood pressure and increases blood flow to the heart, thereby reducing the risk of heart problems when you start vigorous activity. Unfortunately, many times it is the poorly conditioned individual (someone possibly more prone to heart problems) who decides to engage in activity without warming up first.

Types of Warm-up. Warm-ups may be task-specific or general. The **task-specific warm-up** uses less intense levels of the actual exercise or skill you will be doing. If you are going to be engaging in a particular sport, then your task-specific warm-up is tailored to that sport: a tennis player hits some gentle shots, a basketball player does some easy runs while dribbling the ball, a softball player throws balls, a runner jogs. If you are not engaged in a

What to Do

- *Individualize your warm-ups. Experiment and determine the right amount for you. If you are not very flexible or are in poor physical condition, you may need more warm-up time. If you are competing, you might want to time your warm-up so that it is close to the time of the competition, or do a general warm-up earlier and then a short, task-specific warm-up prior to the event.*

- *You will need to warm up more in cold weather.*

- *When it's cold, you might warm up inside to avoid bundling up in clothing that you'll want to remove later.*

specific sport, then a general warm-up is all you should need. The **general warm-up** uses a total body exercise like brisk walking or jogging in place. All warm-ups should be followed by some stretching, and these too can be task-specific or general. For example, a swimmer stretches arm muscles, and a soccer player stretches leg muscles.

Intensity and Duration of Warm-up.   As a rule, your warm-up should start slowly and then escalate. The entire warm-up should last from 5 to 15 minutes. Keep in mind that this movement is preliminary to what you are about to do, so you don't want to exhaust yourself during your warm-up. As you warm up, there is an increase in both core body temperature and the temperature of your skeletal muscles. Use your sweat as a thermometer. When you begin to sweat lightly, your body is probably ready. A combination of intensity and duration produces the desired warm-up effect. Too little of either does not achieve optimum levels of temperature and too much can result in impaired performance due to fatigue.

Stretches

> *To stretch my hamstrings, I lie flat on my back and pull one leg straight up and over until my knee is even with my ear. I am a dancer and I do these stretches before and after classes, rehearsals, and performances.* —Melissa, age 22

To Stretch or Not to Stretch?   Mark Allen, who has won the Ironman Triathlon six times, supposedly never does stretching exercises. Who is correct, Melissa or Mark?

For years, exercisers of all ages have tried to follow Melissa's example and stretch before and after their activity. But now there is a growing debate about the merits of all this stretching, as well as about the most effective stretching methods.

Most trainers still believe that some stretching helps to lower the incidence of musculoskeletal injuries, and improves the body's flexibility. And flexibility is one of the components of fitness. Remember, flexibility means you can move your joints through a full range of movement—something necessary when you participate in exercise or sport. Although stretching may help flexibility, not everyone can expect the same results. Women seem to be more supple than men, but whether or not that's true, the older you are (past about age 30) the more difficult it is to increase flexibility.[26] Regardless of age or sex, your flexibility also is determined by the type and amount of physical activity in which you are involved (See Chapter 7, The Competitive Edge, for more information).

Proponents of stretching are convinced that it is crucial in preventing injuries; they reason that a short muscle that lacks flexibility is more vulnerable to damage than a long, supple one. Others feel that susceptibility to muscle pulls and injuries caused by sudden forceful movements has more to do with muscular strength than flexibility. Some even go so far as to say that increasing one's flexibility can be more harmful than helpful.

Many exercisers in the '70s and '80s became caught up in a "cult of flexibility." It was not uncommon to see runners trying to be contortionists before beginning their runs. On the other hand, the idea that everyone had to stretch in this manner before and after a run was termed "just nonsense" by Dr. Richard H. Dominguez, an early outspoken critic of static stretching for everyone. He is convinced that more injuries are caused by over-stretching than by lack of flexibility.[27]

We are not all born equally supple, and stretching to the limit may be risky and often unnecessary. For example, jogging/running does not place great demands on range of motion; it doesn't require the amount and degree of stretching that had become commonplace. A high degree of flexibility is not necessarily a sign of fitness and, in reverse, we can be very fit and not be able to contort like a human pretzel. Stretching to make ourselves flexible beyond our limit makes our joints vulnerable to injury.

After reviewing the discussion for and against flexibility, it is clear that everyone doesn't need the same kind of stretching routine. Stretching does increase range of motion, and that is particularly important as we become stiffer with age. Find the stretching routine that best suits your fitness level, goals, and lifestyle, but do not take it to an extreme.

A Warm-up Is Not a Stretch.   Many people confuse stretching with warming up, but they are not the same. You should warm up **BEFORE** you stretch. Stretching will not warm you up, it will stretch you. It should be done either after a rhythmic cardiorespiratory warm-up, or following the cooldown after a workout. Some studies show that the warmer muscle tissue is, the more it can be stretched without risk of tears.[28]

What Kind of Stretch?   Prior to about 1970, ballistic stretching was routinely used to warm up the body before exercise. Ballistic stretching consisted of movements such as bending over, touching your toes, and "bobbing"—using small, bouncing, repetitive motions—while trying to reach further with each bounce. Unfortunately, we didn't know then that a muscle stretched in this fashion responded with a reflex contraction (rather than a stretch), whose amount and rate varied directly with the amount and rate of the bounce. Thus the jerking motion was more irritating to the muscle than helpful.

Static stretching was introduced in the '70s. In this type of stretch, you assumed a position and held it for approximately 15 to 30 seconds, until you felt a mild tension (not pain) in the muscle, at which point you relaxed. At one time the goal was to gradually increase the time that the stretch was held; however, experts who still recommend static stretches have now reduced the time that you hold the stretch to 15 seconds.[29]

Static stretches have now been augmented by a technique collectively known as **PNF** (known to physical therapists and exercise physiologists as **proprioceptive neuromuscular facilitation** techniques). PNF is a variation on passive stretching (someone holds you in a stretched position) and involves alternating contractions and stretches. The disadvantage of this technique is that it usually requires a partner. PNF techniques include slow-reversal-hold, contract-relax, and active isolated (a term that has been copyrighted) stretches. All involve some combination of alternating the contraction and relaxation of two opposing sets of muscles. For example, to stretch hamstring muscles at the back of the thigh, you would also contract the quadriceps muscle at the front of the thigh. The stretch is held for under ten seconds and the procedure is repeated 8 to 10 times.

Putting PNF Technique Into Practice. To stretch your hamstrings using, for example, the slow-reversal-hold technique, you lie on your back. While your leg is relaxed, a partner passively pushes your leg toward your upper body (in effect flexing your leg at the hip joint) to the point at which you feel slight discomfort in your hamstring muscle. Now you begin pushing against your partner's resistance by contracting the hamstring muscle. After pushing for 10 seconds, the hamstring muscles relax. You then contract your quadriceps muscle while your partner applies passive pressure to further stretch the quadriceps. This should result in increased hip flexion. This relaxing phase lasts for approximately 10 seconds, at which time you again push against your partner's resistance—repeating the sequence—but at an angle closer to your face. You might find this difficult to achieve without guidance from someone trained in this method, as distinct from "just a partner."

Two mechanical principles underlie the support for using PNF stretching techniques. First, by decreasing the length of time that you hold the stretch, it's less likely the stretch reflex—where the muscles tighten rather than relax—will kick in. Second, since muscles work in opposition (as one contracts, the other relaxes), it makes sense to utilize this phenomenon to achieve a better stretch. Some researchers have found PNF techniques to be more effective than static stretching for increasing the range of motion.[30]

How to Stretch?   Avoid bouncing. If you choose static stretches, hold for about 15 seconds; if you are using a PNF technique, hold each about 10 seconds, and repeat 8 times. Discomfort that doesn't dissipate is a sign that you're probably overdoing it. Reject the "no pain, no gain" philosophy. Pain is the body's way of communicating and means something is wrong. STOP. *Note:* There is a difference between discomfort you may feel when you exercise and pain. Only common sense permits you to recognize a potentially hurtful pain. However, if your pain (or discomfort) lasts for an hour or longer after you stop exercising, you may be overdoing your exercise and you should cut back on intensity or duration. If the pain persists despite cutting back, it is prudent to have the pain checked out.

Suggested stretches include:

For the Neck

Side-to-Side Look: Stand comfortably. Slowly turn your head to look over your shoulder, and hold. Return and repeat to other side.

Shoulder Shrug: Stand comfortably. Keeping your shoulders relaxed, lift them toward your ears. Hold, and slowly return.

Forward and Downward Look: Stand comfortably. Gaze down toward your toes, but don't put your head on your chest. Hold and then slowly return.

For the Shoulders, Chest, and Upper Back

Arm Extension: Stand comfortably. With arms overhead and palms crossed and together, stretch your arms upward and slightly backward. Breathe in as you stretch upward, hold, and return.

Shoulder Stretch: Stand comfortably. Place one hand on or behind your opposite shoulder. Gently pull your elbow across your chest and towards your opposite shoulder. Hold and then return.

Tricep Stretch: Stand comfortably. With your arms overhead, hold the elbow of one arm with the hand of the other arm. Slowly and gently pull the elbow behind your head. Hold and return.

Side Stretch: Stand with your knees slightly bent. Gently pull your elbow behind your head as you bend to the side. Hold and then switch sides. Stretch gently.

For the Lower Back

Back Stretcher: Lie on your back with hands clasped at the back of the thigh of your bent right leg. Pull your leg to your chest and hold. Return and switch legs.

Back Stretcher II: From the same position, clasp your hands behind both thighs and pull both bent legs to your chest, hold, and then return.

Trunk Stretch: Stand erect with feet shoulder-width apart and arms extended over head. Reach as high as possible while keeping heels on floor and hold for 10 to 15 seconds. Bend knees slightly and bend slowly at waist, touching floor between feet with fingers. Hold (if you can't touch the floor, try to touch the tops of your shoes). Repeat entire sequence two to five times. This will place a stretch on your hamstrings as well.

For Front of Thighs (Quads)

Thigh Stretcher: While standing, bend your right leg up in back of you, and grasp it with your left hand. Slowly pull your foot toward your buttocks. Use your right hand to keep your balance. Stretch gently and steadily, and do not bounce. Hold, and then switch legs.

For Back of Thighs (Hamstrings)

Modified Hurdler's Stretch: Sit with your right leg fully extended, with the sole of the left foot against the inner right thigh. Keeping your right leg straight, lean forward as far as you can and attempt to reach your foot with the extended arm. Hold, and then switch legs. Version II—Same position, but reach forward with the opposite hand. This will place some stretch on the lower back. Hold, and then switch.

For Inner Thigh and Hips:

Butterfly Stretch: Sit with your knees bent and the soles of your feet together. Place your forearms on your legs. Lean forward. A variation is to push the knees gently to the floor as you lean forward.

Spinal Twist: Sit with your right leg straight. Bend your left leg, cross your left foot over, and rest it to the outside of your right knee. Then bend your right elbow and rest it on the outside of your upper left thigh, just above the knee. With your left hand resting behind you, slowly turn your head to look over your left shoulder, and at the same time rotate your upper body toward your left hand and arm. Hold, and reverse sides. Don't hold your breath. **Hints:** As you turn your upper body, think of turning your hips in the same direction—they won't move because your right elbow is keeping the left leg stationary; during the stretch, use your elbow to keep your leg stationary with controlled pressure to the inside.

For the Calf and Achilles Tendon

Lower Leg Stretch: Stand facing the wall, arm's length away. Lean forward and place palms of hands flat against wall, slightly below shoulder height. Keep back

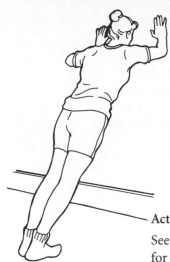

straight, heels firmly on floor, and slowly bend elbows until forehead touches wall. Tuck hips toward wall so that your body remains straight, and hold. *Note:* In order to best stretch your calf muscle you need to stretch three structures: the two calf muscles (gastrocnemius and the soleus) and the Achilles tendon. Stretching with the knee straight or locked stretches only the gastrocnemius muscle. To get the most complete and beneficial stretch, you must bend the back knee, hence the following variation.

Variation: Rest your forearms on the wall with your forehead on the back of your hands. Bend one knee and move it toward the wall. The back leg should be straight with the foot flat and pointed straight ahead. Move your hips forward until you feel the stretch. Stretch gently and steadily. Do not bounce. Hold and then switch legs.

Activity/Exercise/Sport

See Chapter 5, Routines: The Stars Are the Limit, and Chapter 6, A Sampler of Activities, for a full discussion of this part of the workout.

Cooldowns

Cooling down (or warming down) is often ignored, but is just as important as warming up. Phidippides—the first endurance athlete, famous for his run to Athens from the site of the battle of Marathon to announce the Greek victory over the Persians—supposedly gasped "rejoice, we conquer," and died. He died *after* he had stopped running. Who knows if he would have survived if he had "cooled down?"

The worst possible strategy for exercise cessation is to abruptly stop and stand still. We work hard to get our pulse to high levels during exercise, and it takes a while for this natural "hyping-up" to return to our pre-exercise rate. The best strategy is to diminish the workload slowly, thereby allowing for a gradual decrease in pulse rate.

Although the type of cooldown often depends upon the specific sport or exercise just completed, it is usually a gradual tapering of exercise intensity and perhaps some gentle stretching as well.

Physiology of Cooldowns.   If you continue to move after your main activity, the circulatory system has the time to remove some of the by-products—such as lactic acid—that were created during exercise. More importantly, a cooldown, according to some researchers, helps reduce levels of adrenaline and norepinephrine produced during vigorous exercise, which could stress the heart during rest.[31]

What to Do

Don't stand still or sit imme-diately after exercise. A car-diorespiratory cooldown should be a minimum of three or more minutes of continual, rhythmical, low-level activity. If you've run several miles, an effective cooldown would be a light jog followed by a walk, continued until breath-ing and pulse return to pre-exercise levels.

Sudden rest also might cause blood to pool, especially in the legs. This pooling may cause muscle cramps or even shock. Additionally, it may lower blood pressure precipi-tously, which could lead to light-headedness and possible inadequate flow of blood to the heart while the heart rate remains high.[32]

Tip: During cold weather, do your cooldown stretches indoors. It's more comfortable and will slow the loss of body heat and prevent a chill.

Last But Not Least

If you are involved in an activity program or if you are about to start one, a supplemen-tary exercise program to strengthen your abdominals and improve the flexibility of your lumbar, or lower back, region is advisable.

Lower Back (Lumbar) Muscles. You might have been lucky so far and have avoided an affliction common to many Americans—lower back problems. (See Chapter 16, Under-standing Aches and Pains, for more information.) Low back pain occurs more frequently as we get older. Back pain can often be prevented, and an existing problem helped, by fol-lowing two guidelines. First, develop abdominal muscular strength and flexibility, and second, avoid behaviors that may increase the risk of back injury or reinjury.

The usual behavioral causes of low back injury are mechanical harm due to incorrect lifting techniques, lifting too heavy a load, or improper posture. Avoiding or correcting problems involves using proper lifting techniques, improving posture, and gaining greater flexibility.

Lifting Techniques. To lift properly, keep your back relatively straight rather than stooped over. You should use your leg muscles rather than back muscles as the main source of power; that is, bend at the knees when lifting. Avoid lifting objects that are too heavy for you, and keep objects being lifted as close to your body as possible. Further, when you pick up objects (or touch your toes), slowly bend over and remember to bend your knees at the same time.

Posture. The major cause of poor posture is inadequate muscle tone with accompa-nying shortening and tightening of certain muscles and concurrent lengthening and weakening of the opposite set of muscles. Posture in which your lower back (butt) pro-trudes contributes to lengthening and weakening of the abdominal muscles and a con-comitant tightening of the lower back muscles. This exaggeration of the natural curve of the lower back is called lumbar lordosis or hollow back. In addition to avoiding move-ments that increase this curvature of the lumbar spine (like slouching while standing or sleeping on your stomach), you should consciously work to increase both the strength of your abdominals and the flexibility of your lower spine.

Flexibility. For flexibility of the lower spine, include exercises that flatten out the curve of the lumbar spine. For example, while sitting with your legs extended straight in front, reach as far towards your toes as possible; hold that position for 15 seconds, then relax and repeat three times.

Abdominals. Weak abdominal muscles often contribute to back injuries. The abdominals are comprised of three major muscle groups: the internal and external obliques, and the rectus abdominis. The rectus abdominis serves the upper and lower abdominal areas, helping to hold the internal organs in place and drawing the pelvis and rib cage to each other. The internal and external obliques are the muscles that form the waist and act as the rotational muscles of the abdomen when twisting the trunk and bending to the side.

An exercise program to achieve abdominal strength includes curl-ups or sit-ups with knees bent and feet flat on the floor. For a description of abdominal exercises, see sidebar on next page. Other abdominal exercises include variations that aim at the specific abdominal muscle group you want to strengthen. Two precautions to keep in mind when doing abdominal exercises: Don't hook your feet under an object, and don't perform straight-leg exercises where both legs are lifted or lowered simultaneously. In both movements, the hip flexors, not the abdominals, are the main muscles used. Any straining can cause excessive and possibly painful arching of the lower back—the condition these exercises are designed to help prevent or cure!

ACHIEVING RESULTS

Body Sculptors

Exercise today has been made easy with mechanical equipment that does almost everything. These machines can be motivational, and they can also boost the quality of the workouts. However, an individual trainer can give your workout a personal touch. For a fee, you can hire a trainer who will provide hands-on attention during your entire workout. Exercising one-on-one can be a gratifying experience, maximizing your workout. At worst, it can be a humiliating hour spent half-dressed.

Most trainers are affiliated with fitness centers or will meet you at your own gym or in your home. Their major focus will be on weight training, and they will expect you to do your cardiorespiratory workout on your own. That makes sense—why should you pay someone $40 to watch you walk on a treadmill?

Finding a Trainer. Personal training is a self-regulated business. Legally, all it takes to become an $80-an-hour personal trainer is a client willing to pay $80. Trainers do not need

Exercises for Abdominals

Here we've listed several versions of the sit-up in reverse order of difficulty (easiest one listed first, most difficult one last). Start with the sit-up that you can do 3 times without undue strain. When you are able to do 10 repetitions of the exercise without great difficulty, move on to a more difficult version.

1. *Lie flat on back with arms at sides, palms down, and knees slightly bent. Curl head forward until you can see past feet, hold for three counts, then lower to start position. Repeat exercise 3 to 10 times. This is sometimes called a bent-leg curl-up.*

2. *Lie flat on back with arms at sides, palms down, and knees slightly bent. Roll forward until upper body is at 45-degree angle to floor, then return to starting position. Repeat exercise 3 to 10 times.*

3. *Repeat either exercise 1 or 2, but with arms crossed on chest and knees slightly bent.*

4. *Repeat either exercise 1 or 2, but with hands laced behind head and knees slightly bent.*

to fulfill specific education requirements, nor do they need to know cardiopulmonary resuscitation (CPR). What all this means is that the potential exists for your trainer to do you more harm than good.

Although many people simply choose their favorite aerobic instructor as their trainer, another common way of finding a trainer is from a friend's recommendation. If you live in New York City, check out *The Jones Guide to Fitness and Health in New York*, a book by Kathy Myers Jones.[33] The book offers a comprehensive listing of dozens of training centers and gyms in New York City. (Other cities may have similar guidebooks.) Bear in mind that the information requires regular updating and is just one person's opinion.

Certification. When choosing from the myriad trainers out there, one way of winnowing the selection is to choose one who is certified. By 1995, approximately 15,000 trainers worldwide had been certified by the American Council on Exercise after passing a written examination, whereas in 1990 there were just 2,000 ACE-certified trainers.[34] Thousands more trainers are not certified. You can call the American Council on Exercise at (800) 529-8227 for the names of three trainers located within or near your zip code.

You should be aware that certification does not guarantee competence. Of the organizations that use certification tests, many are tests of minimum competency, and even then there is marked variability in test difficulty. For example, while all examinations have a written portion, only a few organizations require that trainers physically demonstrate that they can help exercisers in strength training.

Sometimes certification may be a minor consideration compared to where and how the trainer was educated. The younger the trainer, the more likely he/she has undergone some relevant formal education. However, that education can vary dramatically in quality and depth: There are college programs of two to four years; non-college courses offered by the Cooper Institute for Aerobic Research or the Equinox Fitness Training Institute; and home study courses which may or may not be supplemented by a weekend cram course. On the other hand, an older trainer may have had years of hands-on experience.

While certification is not enough to prove competence, it is a start. Certification by most organizations means that those trainers at least have passed a CPR course.

Choosing a Trainer. First, find out the trainer's education and certification. Second, check out the trainer's experience and references. Third, assuming the trainer passes the first two hurdles, will the two of you work well together? The best way to answer this question is to hire the trainer on a trial basis for, say, a month or less.

Divorcing a Trainer. Because the relationship with a personal trainer can be intense, many trainers become not just coach but confidant as well, so that ending the association may be psychologically difficult. Some people have changed clubs rather than risk running into a trainer they've fired. Others have spent months agonizing over the decision. If you and your trainer's styles, schedules, or goals don't mesh, you'd be advised to cut your losses and end the relationship!

New Trends

I wish my women friends would give physical activity at least six weeks. They will spend years and hundreds of dollars worrying or trying to lose weight, yet they won't give exercise a mere six weeks. —Justina, age 33

Trends and tastes in exercising change with bewildering speed. Many contemporary exercisers engage in basic cardiorespiratory activities on machines such as the treadmill or bike (check out Chapter 9, Gearing Up, for information on machines). "**Spinning**" is an example. Under the teacher's shouts of "sprint," or "uphill," or "jump," a group of men and women, in unison, pedal specially designed stationary bikes to music for a high-intensity cardiorespiratory workout. The special bikes allow for movements like "running" (cycling while standing on the pedals), "jumping" (alternately quickly standing up then sitting down), "sprinting" (pedaling with all-out intensity while seated or standing), "going up hills" (using increasingly harder resistance), and "rhythm presses" (pressing the upper body toward the handlebars).

High-impact aerobic dance classes appear to be making a comeback. High-impact, where both feet can be off the ground, was replaced for a while by low-impact classes, where one foot is always on the floor at any given time. Both of these classes may use show tunes, disco music, live drumming, or reggae, and often feature new and innovative choreography. However, one of the reasons for the original switch away from high-impact classes has not changed—injuries. For example, inner-ear damage has been linked to jarring high-impact aerobics but not to regular aerobics.[35] Thus it's hard to explain why it has become popular again.

Jumping Rope. In 1996, the *New York Times* reported on a new fitness phenomenon, jumping rope.[36] However, rope jumping actually is an old activity, long confined to kids and boxers, that is now back "in."

Devotees of rope jumping point out that it can be done just about anywhere, is inexpensive, and is considered to be a very good cardiorespiratory exercise. Dr. Ken Solis, an emergency room physician who has held two Guinness world records in jumping, claims that jumping rope is relatively injury-free. According to him, the stress to the knee is less than in running because the calves and shins absorb the impact of the rope jump.[36] Rope jumpers expect the activity to gain in popularity as people realize its benefits.

Fitting Fitness In

On the Job.   Below are some suggestions for the working woman who has time constraints but would like to fit fitness in. *Note:* If you are pregnant, Chapter 12 (Fitness for Two) has suggestions for incorporating fitness while pregnant; Chapter 13 (Starting Early) is geared to giving you options for exercising with children.

Walk to Work: Park your car a mile or two from your office or the train station and walk briskly to your destination.

Take the Stairs: Don't use elevators or escalators. Walking up and down stairs is better than a stair machine.

Change Menu and Venue: Instead of eating a large lunchtime meal, eat modestly and spend the "saved" time walking, before or after lunch. Barbara, an acquaintance of the authors, changed her lifestyle several years ago. During her lunch-hour break, she substitutes fruit for her regular meal and eats as she walks around campus. She attributes this simple change with helping her lose (and keep off) approximately 20 pounds.

Traveling Light.   You don't have to come home from a vacation several pounds heavier and flabbier. Following the next few suggestions may help you keep in shape while traveling.

Getting There. Utilize the time spent en route to exercise by trying to walk every two hours. If driving, plan to stop to stretch, and if in a plane, walk up and down the aisle. Between flights, walk around the airport—as if you were mall-walking. Even while seated you can get some exercise: stretch arms and legs, roll your shoulders, rotate your head and your hands and feet.

Checked In. Before you make hotel reservations, consider finding out what pool and fitness facilities are available on site or nearby. Even if your hotel has no designated exercise area in which to do your usual workout, you can still walk, jog, or run. That's a good way to stay fit and at the same time get a feel for the new location.

A Word About Food. The solution to not being overly self-indulgent is easy to prescribe—but, as many overweight Americans know, is hard to follow. Some suggestions for eating on vacation include: Sample or share dishes with your companion, thereby spreading the calories; drink plenty of water with your meals—it might make you less likely to overeat; order food that seems least likely to be loaded with fat. Sometimes eating like a native instead of a tourist works because there are few countries in the world which match our overabundant style of eating.

With some planning and effort, you can be one of those people who return from your vacation in as good (or better) shape than when you left.

Where Do You Go from Here?

You're convinced. You want to be fit and healthy. Once you've made the decision to get fit, you need to choose an activity and a method. The next two chapters on routines and activities will help you do just that.

1. Constitution of the World Health Organization. Chronicle of the World Health Organization, Geneva, Switzerland: WHO, 1947.

2. Drinkwater, B. L. Women and exercise: Physiological aspects. *Exercise and Sport Sciences Reviews*, 1984, 12, 21–29.

3. Haskell, W. L. Cardiovascular benefits and risks of exercise: The scientific evidence. In R. H. Strauss (ed.). *Sports Medicine*. Philadelphia: W. B. Saunders, 1984, 57–76.

4. O'Toole, M. L., & Douglas, P. S. Fitness: Definition and development. In M. M. Shangold, & G. Mirkin (eds.). *Women and Exercise: Physiology and Sports Medicine*, 2nd ed. Philadelphia: F. A. Davis Co., 1994, 3–26.

5. Garnett, L. R. Stretching it to the limit. *Harvard Health Letter*, July, 1996, 4–5.

6. DeVries, H. A. *Physiology of Exercise*, 2nd ed. Dubuque, IA: Wm. C. Brown, 1974.

7. Bray, G. A. Pathophysiology of obesity. *American Journal of Clinical Nutrition*, 1992, 555, 488S-494S.

8. Wilfley, D. E., Grilo, C. M., & Brownell, K. D. Exercise and regulation of body weight. In M. M. Shangold, & G. Mirkin (eds.). *Women and Exercise: Physiology and Sports Medicine*, 2nd ed. Philadelphia: F. A. Davis Co., 1994, 27–59.

9. Bray, G. A., & Gray, D. S. Obesity, part I: Pathogenesis. *Western Journal of Medicine*, 1988, 149, 429–441.

10. American College of Sports Medicine. Position stand on recommended quantity and quality of exercise for developing and maintaining cardiorespiratory and muscular fitness in healthy adults. *Medicine and Science in Sports and Exercise,* 1990, 22(2), 265–274.

11. Davis, J. A. A comparison of heart rate methods for predicting endurance training intensity. *Medicine in Science and Sport*, 1975, 7, 295.

12. Thompson, G. D., & Franks, B. D. Developing a personalized exercise program: Prescription guidelines. In J. A. Peterson, & C. X. Bryant (eds.). *The Stair Master Fitness Book*. Indianapolis: Masters Press, 1992, 109–120.

13. Dishman, R. K. Prescribing exercise intensity for healthy adults using perceived exertion. *Medicine and Science in Sports and Exercise*, 1994, 26(9), 1087–1094.

14. Thomas, T. R., Ziogas, G., Smith, T., et al. Physiological and perceived exertion responses to six modes of submaximal exercise. *Research Quarterly for Exercise and Sport,* 1995, 66(3), 239–246.

15. American College of Sports Medicine. *Guidelines for Graded Exercise Test and Exercise Prescription*, 4th ed. Philadelphia: Lea & Febiger, 1991.

16. O'Toole, M. L., & Douglas, P. S. Fitness: Definition and development. In M. M. Shangold, & G. Mirkin (eds.). *Women and Exercise: Physiology and Sports Medicine*, 2nd ed. Philadelphia: F. A. Davis Co., 1994, 3–26.

17. American College of Sports Medicine. Position Stand on the recommended quantity and quality of exercise for developing and maintaining cardiorespiratory and muscular fitness in healthy adults. *Medicine and Science in Sports and Exercise*, 1990, 22(2), 265–274.

18. Pate, R. R., Pratt, M., Blair, S. N., et al. Physical activity and public health: A recommendation from the Centers for Disease Control and Prevention and the American College of Sports Medicine. *Journal of the American Medical Association*, 1995, 273(5), 402–407.

19. Prevalence of recommended levels of physical activity among women—Behavioral Risk Factor Surveillance System, 1992. *MMWR Morbidity Mortality Weekly Report*, 1995, 44, 105–7,113.

20. Pate, R. R., Pratt, M., Blair, S. N., et al. Physical activity and public health: A recommendation from the Centers for Disease Control and Prevention and the American College of Sports Medicine. *Journal of the American Medical Association*, 1995, 273(5), 402–407.

21. Blair, S. N., Kohl, H. W., & Barlow, C. E. Physical activity, physical fitness, and all-cause mortality in women: Do women need to be active? *Journal of the American College of Nutrition*, 1993, 12(4), 368–371.

22. Blakeslee, S. Warm-up may not protect muscles. *New York Times*, September 27, 1990, c8.

23. van Mechelen, W., Hlobil, H., Kemper, H. C. G., et al. Prevention of running injuries by warm-up, cool-down, and stretching exercises. *The American Journal of Sports Medicine*, 1993, 21(6), 711–719.

24. Blakeslee, S. Warm-up may not protect muscles. *New York Times*, September 27, 1990, c8.

25. Barnard, R. J., Gardner, G. W., Diaco, N. V., et al. Cardiovascular responses to sudden strenuous exercise—heart rate, blood pressure, and ECG. *Journal of Applied Physiology*, 1973, 34, 833–837.

26. Rosato, F. D. *Fitness for Wellness*, 3rd ed. Minneapolis: West Publishing Co., 1994.

27. Shyne, K. Richard H. Dominguez, M. D. To stretch or not to stretch? *The Physician and Sportsmedicine*, 1982, 10(9), 137–140.

28. Safran, M. R., Seaber, A. V., & Garrett, W. E. Jr. Warm-up and muscular injury prevention: An update. *Sports Medicine*, 1989, 8(4), 239–249.

29. Madding, S. W., Wong, J. G., Hallum, A., et al. Effects of duration of passive stretch on hip abduction range of motion. *Journal of Orthopaedic and Sports Physical Therapy*, 1987, 8, 409–416.

   Wilkinson, A. Stretching the truth: A review on the literature of muscle stretching. *Australian Physiotherapy*, 1992, 38, 283–287.

30. Etnyre, B. R., & Lee, E. J. Chronic and acute flexibility of men and women using three different stretching techniques. *Research Quarterly for Exercise and Sport*, 1988, 59(3), 222–228.

31. Cooper, K. H. *Running Without Fear*. New York: M. Evans & Co., 1985.

32. DeVries, H. A. *Physiology of Exercise*, 2nd ed. Dubuque, IA: Wm. C. Brown, 1974.

33. Jones, K. M. *The Jones Guide to Fitness and Health in New York*. New York: City and Company, 1995.

34. Steinhauer, J. Test-driven by trainers. *New York Times*, August 9, 1995, c8.

35. Weintraub, M. I. High-impact aerobic exercises and vertigo—a possible cause of bilateral vestibulopathy. *New England Journal of Medicine*, 1990, 323(23), 1633-e (letter).

36. Zimmer, J. New in aerobics: Pumping rope. *New York Times*. October 9, 1996, c1, 6.

5

Routines:
The Stars Are the Limit

SUSAN L. PURETZ, ED.D.

As a child and teenager I was always very physically active but did not view my activity as exercise, per se. In my twenties and in the "real working world" I found I have to make an effort to exercise and do the same activities I did as a teen. Now I consider them a form of exercise whereas in my teens it was just something I did for fun. —Connie, age 28

Women's exercise routines are as individualized as the reasons for pursuing physical activity. Routines are born out of necessity, motivation, and goals. Factors such as time, competitive level, finances, pressures and stresses, and physical condition all enter into decisions about routines. The routines that we create are as varied as we are; what might be right for us when we're twenty, might be inappropriate at 40, and possibly harmful when we're 60. Similarly, what was considered an adequate workout in the 1950s is inadequate by 1990s training standards. One of our respondents said, "I'm working harder (and with weights) now at age 59 than I did at 20."

LOOKING AT THE STARS

Running Greats.   It would seem evident that recreational fitness runners are going to put in less effort than world-class athletes, but that's not necessarily so. Nor is it true that all world-class athletes train the same; they often devise individualized routines. For example, when Lynn Jennings (the holder of the American record in the 10,000 meter run since 1992) was training in the 1980s, she ran up to 80 miles a week, although 60 to 70 miles per week was a more usual amount. Such distances were typical among world-class runners. She didn't do any weight training at that time, just lots of sit-ups and push-ups twice a day.[1]

On the other hand, during that same time period, Joan Benoit, the winner of the first Olympic women's marathon in 1984, was doing as many as 120 miles per week (with no days off). Benoit generally would not run more than 22 miles at a time because she had found that to do more would begin to damage her bones and Achilles tendons. She, like Lynn Jennings, also didn't lift weights at the beginning of her career. However, in recent years, Ms. Benoit has supplemented her running with other sports—swimming, cycling, and cross-country skiing—to improve her cardiovascular fitness system.[2]

Back in 1982, Tim Wendel wrote in *Women's Sports* about Mary Decker-Slaney that "when the 24-year-old runner stays healthy, nobody can catch her."[3] However, besides stellar track performances, she had also suffered three shin operations, a torn back muscle, and surgery on her Achilles tendon in the years since she started running competitively at the age of 11. Decker-Slaney, who holds the American record for the 800 and 1,500 meter runs, had known but one way to run—as hard as she could—even in practice. That attitude had caused her to race well and then get hurt.

Decker-Slaney was 37 when she competed in the 1996 Olympics. To prepare for the Olympics, Alberto Salazar, the great marathoner and now Decker-Slaney's coach, pulled the reins in and put her on a program of controlled and gradually progressive workouts, which included weight lifting. Salazar observed that "the greatest athletes want it so much, they run themselves to death. You've got to have an obsession, but if unchecked it's destructive."[4]

Uta Pippig, the first woman to win the Boston Marathon three years in succession, trains up to 180 miles a week at high altitude in Boulder, Colorado.[5] She came in first in 1996 despite suffering from menstrual cramps and diarrhea.

Just as demanding, but with a different emphasis, was the routine the great sprinter Valerie Brisco-Hooks followed to prepare for the 1984 Los Angeles Olympics. Brisco-Hooks won gold medals in the 200 and 400 meter runs, and was the first person, man or woman, to capture that double gold. She went on to win another gold medal in the 1,600 meter relay, thereby joining Wilma Rudolph as the only American female track and field athlete ever to capture three gold medals at a single Olympics.

Brisco-Hooks' weekly schedule included running five days a week and three to four days of weight training, and looked like this:

Monday
Weight training 1.5 hours; Track 1.5 hours—hill and stair work; weight training if needed for another hour

Tuesday
Running day emphasizing mechanics, road runs, and Fartlek workouts (speed interspersed with slow jogging)

Wednesday
  Day off
Thursday
  Same as Tuesday
Friday
  Same as Monday
Saturday
  Pick up day, jump rope, weights, run
Sunday
  Day off
**As the season progressed, Saturdays were replaced with track meets and there was more emphasis on track work during training. For example: sprinting sixteen 150s in a 19- to 20-second range.[6]

Weight Lifting Greats.   On the opposite end of the spectrum from the aerobic activity of running, is the muscular strength and power required for weight lifting. Looking at the stars in weight lifting, we find women like Dawn Reshel, who did a squat with 633.9 pounds in an official powerlifting competition. That record has survived for ten years—the next closest lift is 628.3 pounds. Mary Ellen Warman has lifted a "measly" 518 pounds, but since she weighs a mere 132 pounds, her lift is, pound for pound, one of the more notable ones.[7] In 1994, Tamara Grimwood made weight lifting history with the first 400-pound bench press, although that record is already being challenged. In 1996, several women set new American deadlift records with lifts of 291 pounds.[8]

To prepare for competition, women powerlifters work out with very heavy weights and a minimum number of repetitions while following a workout cycle of anywhere from 8 to 20 weeks. In a 15- to 20-week cycle, for example, the first several weeks are spent doing high-volume, medium-intensity workouts. That means performing perhaps up to 500 lifting repetitions per week at 80 to 90 percent of the maximum amount they are able to lift. During the next four to five weeks, the powerlifters do fewer repetitions (200 to 300 per week) but at a higher intensity (using heavier weights that are 90 to 100 percent of their capacity). In these five weeks, the athletes are building power and strength on top of the base from the first several weeks of training.

As the event approaches, they work at maximum intensity to consolidate the gains of the previous 15 weeks. Then, with little more than a week before competition, they focus on tapering. During tapering, the athletes reduce the volume and intensity of the workout, thereby allowing recovery from the stress of training while retaining the benefits.[9]

And Back on Earth

I compete in running not for the sake of competition alone, but rather as motivation to stay in shape. It's easier to not slack off when you know you have a race coming up and you don't want to be last! —Cheryl, age 27

Any training regimen we adopt will probably be a step down from "the stars." However, whether you are a recreational exerciser or a competitor, you need to create a training routine that is safe, effective, and fun.

The important thing to remember about routines is that they are not cast in stone. They are simply guidelines. When they don't work, they should be abandoned or redesigned.

DEFINING YOUR TRAINING

Quantity and Quality

We need to focus on sustained activity that will, over time, result in overall fitness and, for those of us in competition, help develop muscles adapted to ever-increasing levels of stress and ready for peak performance. In creating a training regimen, our efforts should lie somewhere between the recommended minimum amount necessary for maintaining physical fitness and the maximum as exemplified by the training programs of the world-class athletes previously described.

The Minimum Amount.   The American College of Sports Medicine guidelines for developing and maintaining cardiorespiratory fitness, body composition, muscular strength, and endurance in the healthy adult are:

1. **Frequency:** 3 to 5 days per week.
2. **Intensity:** 55 to 90 percent of maximum heart rate or 40 to 85 percent of maximum oxygen uptake (VO_2max).
3. **Duration:** 15 to 60 minutes of continuous aerobic activity. Duration is dependent on the intensity of the activity; thus, lower intensity activities should be conducted over a longer period of time.
4. **Activity:** any activity that uses large muscle groups, can be maintained for a prolonged period, and is rhythmical and aerobic in nature.
5. **Resistance training:** strength training of a moderate intensity should be an integral part of an adult fitness program. Strengthening exercises should be done two to three times per week.[10]

TABLE 5.1

Frequency of Activity in Women Surveyed

	1–2 Days Per Week	3–4 Days Per Week	5–7 Days Per Week	Total
HOBBYIST				
Number	42	178	147	367
Percent of total	9.09	38.53	31.82	79.44
COMPETITOR				
Number	4	28	63	5
Percent of total	0.87	6.06	13.64	20.56
TOTAL				
Number	46	206	210	462
Percent	9.96	44.59	45.45	100

The numbers in this table are based on the authors' survey, Puretz, S., Haas, A., and Meltzer, D. Profile of exercising women. *Perceptual and Motor Skills*, 1996, 82, 890. The totals in each table differ because not every participant answered all questions.

Conflicting Guidelines.   In Chapter 4, we described how in 1995, four years after the recommendations outlined on page 89, the American College of Sports Medicine and the Centers for Disease Control published a different type of recommendation—one that urged moderation in exercise. That different recommendation created needless confusion.

Unfortunately, many people believe that the new moderate recommendation supersedes the old vigorous one and that high-intensity exercise offers no additional benefit over moderate-intensity physical activity. Not so! In fact, the recent guidelines for moderate activity state that "the recommendation is intended to complement, not supersede, previous exercise recommendations."[11] The report then goes further and states "people who already meet the recommendation are also likely to derive some additional health and fitness benefits from becoming more physically active."[11] A study of male Harvard alumni added additional support to the theory that vigorous exercise was necessary for health and longevity,[12] while the Nurse's Health Study found the same thing for women.[13] Those who exercised vigorously lived longer!

TABLE 5.2

Intensity of Exercise in Women Surveyed

	Mild	Moderate	Intense	Total
HOBBYIST Number	60	252	66	378
COMPETITOR Number	3	59	31	94
TOTAL Number	63	311	97	472
Percent	13.35	65.89	20.55	100

The numbers in this table are based on the authors' survey, Puretz, S., Haas, A., and Meltzer, D. Profile of exercising women. *Perceptual and Motor Skills*, 1996, 82, 890. The totals in each table differ because not every participant answered all questions.

Which guidelines are for you? Your goals will determine whether you should do 30 minutes of moderately intense physical activity every day or vigorous endurance exercises three to five days and weight training on two days. However, the basic message is the same: Americans—especially women—are too sedentary; either routine is better than nothing. You be the judge of how much you need.

Interpreting the Recommendation (Our Sample)

Frequency. In our study, almost 91 percent of the women exercised three or more days per week. Women who defined themselves as hobbyists are about equally divided between those who exercise three or four days per week and those who exercise five to seven days per week; the majority of competitors exercise five to seven days per week. Table 5.1 shows exercise frequency comparisons for hobbyists and competitors.

Intensity. Approximately two-thirds of the hobbyists exercised at the moderate level recommended by the American College of Sports Medicine. However, there was a major difference at the next level of intensity. Whereas 33 percent of the competitors (31 of the 94) indicated that they exercised intensely, only 17 percent of the hobbyists (66 of the 378) judged their workouts to be intense. See Table 5.2.

TABLE 5.3

Duration of Activity

	About 15 minutes	About a half hour	About an hour	More than an hour	Total
HOBBYIST					
Number	13	90	199	81	383
Percent of total	2.73	18.91	41.81	17.02	80.46
COMPETITOR					
Number	0	13	46	34	93
Percent of total	0.00	2.73	9.66	7.14	19.54
TOTAL					
Number	13	103	245	115	476
Percent of total	2.73	21.64	51.47	24.16	100

The numbers in this table are based on the authors' survey, Puretz, S., Haas, A., and Meltzer, D. Profile of exercising women. *Perceptual and Motor Skills*, 1996, 82, 890. The totals in each table differ because not every participant answered all questions.

Duration. Fifty-one percent of all the women in our study exercised for about one hour per workout. Table 5.3 summarizes the differences in the duration of workouts for competitors and hobbyists. Proportionately more competitors than hobbyists indicated they work out for one hour or more, whereas more hobbyists than competitors exercised for about a half-hour per session.

DANGER IN EXERCISING TOO MUCH

Is there a point where strenuous exercise or too much activity becomes a problem? Newer findings seem to indicate a possible "yes" for certain individuals and sports; for running, the one activity that has been studied frequently, the risk appears fairly substantial.[14]

No Pain, No Gain? Injuries to the muscles, ligaments, joints, and bones caused by overuse become more problematic as exercise intensity, frequency, and duration increase.[15] Each year approximately 35 to 65 percent of runners are injured.[16] For example, some 50 to 70 percent of runners are alleged to suffer from knee or foot injuries. There also appears to be a direct relation between the risk of musculoskeletal injury and the distance run per week. One survey of a large group of runners found that only 20 percent of those who ran less than nine miles a week developed musculoskeletal problems, as compared to 50 percent of those who ran 30 miles a week.[17] In cycling, overuse injuries were reported in 85 percent of the recreational cyclists studied by researchers at California State University, Northridge.[18] The odds of female cyclists developing overuse injury/complaints at the neck and shoulder were 1.5 and 2.0 times more, respectively, than their male counterparts. See Chapter 16, Understanding Aches and Pains, for more about the physical problems of cyclists.

The Athletic Triad. Another set of problems afflicting some individuals is the female athletic triad—menstrual irregularities, anorexia or bulimia, and osteoporosis. Whether or not these are exercise-related or individual problems is still unclear. Chapter 18, Beware of the Danger Zones, provides more details.

Exercise Junkies. Then there are the exercise addicts—the "fitaholics" or exercise junkies (we talk about this in Chapter 1, Why We Exercise, and Chapter 18, Beware of the Danger Zones). Since society applauds physical activity, this dependency may go undiagnosed or unrecognized. *Note:* Time spent working out is not in itself the sign of an addiction.

Tips for Finding a Balance

- Push yourself, but know where the line is between good hard training and over-training.
- Listen to your body. One good indicator is your pulse—if you find that your resting pulse rate has changed by just a few beats one way or the other, you could possibly be training too hard.[19]
- Sudden weight loss, restlessness in bed at night, and frequent colds (reflecting diminished immune system functioning) are signs that you might be training too hard.
- Know the difference between mere soreness and bona fide injury—sometimes a bit tricky. If by the next day, your soreness hasn't improved, back off on your training. If it's better, go back to training. Unless, that is, you have chosen that day to rest.

IMPROVING PERFORMANCE

Most of us want to improve in whatever we do. This may be common to human nature. When we no longer ask "can we compete and finish?" but are determined to finish better or faster, we are looking to improve our performance.

Prerequisites. Better performance must be built upon a solid base of endurance and strength. We cannot really expect to improve if we have been inconsistent in our training. Plan to train all year round, because fitness is lost when you are not training. Your chosen sport/exercise/activity will dictate what training program to follow. Some will require either a more efficient cardiovascular system, stronger muscles, or better technique; others will require all of them.

Goals. Before beginning, set realistic goals in order to measure progress. Remember that when you started exercising, you started gradually. Do the same thing with your new training program: step by step, inch by inch. It's better to be able to pat yourself on the back and move on to the next set of goals than to set yourself up for failure because your goals are not sensible.

Going the Distance

In order to go the distance you have to improve your endurance, and that's best accomplished with LSDs—long, slow distance workouts.

Long, Slow Distances (LSD). Although the acronym LSD may conjure up drugs, long, slow distances are relaxed, comfortably paced workouts done at about 75 percent of your maximum heart rate. These long, slow distances, whether in biking, running, swimming, or other aerobic sports, are the nuts and bolts for building fitness and endurance in your activity. (For more information on running, see Chapter 6.)

The Bottom Line. To build endurance, you must **gradually** increase your long, slow distance per workout or per week. For example, after about two months of training, beginning runners should aim for a minimum of two to three miles per workout (or approximately ten miles per week). Once you've built your endurance base, any mileage above that minimum will increase your endurance.

Speeding Up

While some women dreamt of being "Jeannie in a Maidenform bra," I had dreams of running faster than a speeding bullet. —Ann, age 26

When you race, you want to go fast. Once you have trained for endurance, you can then go for speed.[20] Two methods to increase your speed are **interval** and **fartlek training**.

Interval Training. Interval training, also known as speed training, is appropriate if you are: looking for a way to lower your performance times, seeking more aerobic fitness with less expenditure of time, or searching for a little variety and challenge in your daily training routine. Anyone can speed train. The purpose is to help your body adapt to moving comfortably for longer distances at faster speeds.

Interval training has played a time-honored role in athletic conditioning since the 1960s. At that time, it was found that if runners included rest intervals, they could run for an hour at a pace (intensity) that would ordinarily have caused exhaustion in nine minutes.[21] Interval training often intimidates the recreational athlete; it is physically and psychologically hard to exercise more intensely than we are accustomed. Thus many people end up exercising longer and slower rather than pushing themselves with speed training.

Interval training can be applied to almost any exercise or sport. For example, it can be done indoors on the exercise bicycle, stair, rowing, or cross-country machines, as well as while walking, jogging, running, swimming, or biking. The ideal speed training workout doesn't exist. The variations are endless and they are all beneficial when performed properly.

• **The Basics**. The basis of interval training is a series of short, measured distances done at a race pace or faster (approximately 90 percent of your maximum heart rate), alternated with rest periods—about as long timewise as the speed interval you just did. Using running as an example, let's say your speed workout consists of running a total of two to four miles. If you ordinarily run a ten-minute mile (two and a half minutes per quarter), you would plan to run quarter-mile intervals at an eight-minute-mile pace (two minutes for each interval). You would rest for two minutes in between each quarter-mile interval. This process would be repeated several times and would be your total workout. You should try to run each of the intervals at the same fast speed and slowly walk during the rest period to maintain body warmth and keep the blood circulating. *Note:* An interval workout is best done on a track or a flat stretch of road or grass.

Fartlek Training. Fartlek is a Swedish word for speed play. The idea is to add bursts of speed to your slower, steadier, continuous aerobic workout (running, swimming, biking, etc.). Between these fast segments, you continue your workout at a relaxed pace until your regular breathing returns. Whether you measure the bursts of speed by timing them, or by setting distance goals, such as a certain house, tree, or telephone pole down the road (or, when swimming, by laps in a pool), they provide your workout with periodic anaerobic bursts of speed.

What We Know

Fartlek training has you speed up while you continue traveling; interval training is a run with a series of starts and rests.

Tips for Speed Training:

• Remember that less is often more! To gain speed, you should occasionally sacrifice distance.
• Never let speed training become more than 10 to 15 percent of your total weekly program. Your regular training workouts are the most important.

- Include only one session of speed workout every week to ten days—especially if you are new at it.
- If you are experienced and prefer to speed train more often, you will want to schedule two easy days between speed sessions.
- To see results, you must be consistent over the long run. One speed session will not improve your pace.

IMPROVING STRENGTH

Not so long ago, women who worked out with weights were thought of as body-builders, who in turn were considered weird. Now if you don't do weight training you're not "with it." —Samantha, age 35

Weight Training

Popular opinion, in just over 25 years, has gone from an avoidance and disdain of weight training to its complete acceptance. While some may disagree as to which one—free weights or machines—produces better muscle strength and endurance, there is no question about the benefit of including weight training in one's workout regimen.[22]

Weight training is now considered integral to obtaining better performance results in aerobic activities despite the fact that it does little specifically for aerobic (cardiovascular) fitness. What weight training does is provide muscular fitness, which helps protect against injury while we pursue aerobic fitness through running, racquet sports, aerobic dance, swimming, or cycling. Also, weight training is currently viewed as a worthwhile strategy for pre-and postmenopausal women to increase bone mass[23] and reduce the long-term risk of osteoporotic fractures.[24] However, researchers have yet to fully identify the optimum exercise prescription (moderate versus high intensity) necessary for bone loading. Initial research points to high-intensity weight training, something that may not appeal to many women.[25]

One further use for weight training has been found by space scientists grappling with the daunting problem of keeping astronauts healthy for extended periods in space. New research on how people react to long spans of weightlessness points to the problem of continuous loss of bone mineral in space—especially from the hip and lower spine. However, NASA scientists are seeing a possible solution with something as simple as pumping iron. Although the astronauts currently do endurance exercise while on board, there is a growing consensus that those exercise regimens need to be supplemented by resistance workouts that increase the mechanical stress on astronauts' muscles.[26]

Don't Worry About Bulking Up. Despite the fact that women have approximately two-thirds of the absolute overall strength of men (see Chapter 2, A Woman Is Not a

Man), both respond to strength training in very similar ways, although women tend not to develop the muscle mass characteristic of males.[27] Current research presents no evidence that women should train differently than men; rather, training programs should be tailored for each individual.[28]

Who Weight Trains?

Competitive Lifters. Weight lifting can be a competitive sport for women. In one type of competition, Olympic-style weight lifting, the object is to see who can lift the most total weight overhead using two different lifts (the snatch and the clean-and-jerk). In powerlifting competition—more popular for women—there are three lifts: the bench press, the squat, and the dead lift. While some women are competitive lifters, they are in the minority of women who strength train.[29]

Bodybuilders. Bodybuilders participate in competition that is more art than sport. Through weight training, bodybuilders mold their bodies into living sculptures. Their goal is to develop maximum muscular size while maintaining symmetry (a balanced appearance) and a high degree of definition (individual muscular visibility). Increasing numbers of women are entering this arena, often as a natural progression from their interest in weight training.

Athletes. Most coaches now require their athletes to lift weights to improve performance and prevent sports injuries. Weight lifting is also a tool used by physical therapists to help athletes recover from sports injuries.

Patients. Doctors and physical therapists often prescribe weight training (progressive resistance exercise) as part of a rehabilitation program.

Physical Fitness Enthusiasts. Those of us who exercise for health and physical fitness have discovered the benefits of weight training either as cross training to supplement an aerobic sport, or as part of a workout routine that focuses on muscle strength and endurance.

Principles of Weight Training

Weight lifting is a resistance exercise: Put a muscle under a heavy load, slowly contract and then relax it. Typically, this is repeated a given number of times or **repetitions**— known as one **set**—and each set is repeated, usually three times in one session. In future sessions, the weight can be increased. The amount of weight you lift is dependent upon whether you are trying to develop muscular strength or muscular endurance. For muscular strength, a resistance of approximately 80 percent of your maximum capacity is recommended, while less than 80 percent (but not under 50 percent) will help increase muscular endurance. *Note:* Your maximum capacity, also known as 1-RM (one-repetition

TABLE 5.4

....

Suggested Exercises for Specific Body Parts

	Free Weights	Machine[1]
CHEST	Bench Press	Bench Press Machine
	Incline Bench Press	
	Bent Arm Flys	Chest Machine
CHEST / BACK	Bent Arm Pullover	Pullover Machine
BACK		
Lats	Pull-ups	Lat Pulldown
	Chin-ups	Pull-up Machine
Upper Back / Triceps	Shoulder Shrug	Shoulder Shrug Machine
Lats and Triceps	Barbell Rowing	Seated Rowing Machine
	One-Dumbbell Rowing	Low Pulley-Cable Rowing Machine
LEGS	Hip and Knee Extension	
	Squat	Squat / Leg Press Machine
Hip Extension	*machine exercise only*	Hip Extension Machine
Hip Flexion	*machine exercise only*	Hip Flexion Machine
Knee Extension	*machine exercise only*	Leg Extension Machine
Knee Flexion	*machine exercise only*	Knee Curl Machine
Ankle Plantar Flexors	Calf Raises	Heel / Calf Machine
SHOULDERS	Military Press	Overhead or Shoulder Press Machine
	Upright Rowing	Upright Rowing Machine
	Lateral Raise	Lateral Raise Machine
	Front Raise Dumbbells	*free weights only*
	Bent-Over Lateral Raise (Dumbbells)	*free weights only*

....

1. There are many brands of machines available, so we have used only generic rather than trade names.

Suggested Exercises for Specific Body Parts

	Free Weights	Machine[1]
ARM		
Upper Arm	Barbell Curl	Arm Curl Machine
(Elbow Flexion)	Dumbbell Curl	Low Pulley Curl Machine
Upper Arm	Triceps Extension	Triceps Extension Machine
(Elbow Extension)	Parallel Bars or	Dip Machine
	Bench Dips	
Forearm	Wrist Curl	*free weights only*
	Reverse Wrist Curl	*free weights only*
ABDOMINALS AND BACK		
Trunk Flexion	Bent-leg curl-ups	Abdominal (crunch) Machine
(Abdominals)		
Trunk and Hip Flexion	Bent-leg sit-ups	
(Abdominals and Hip Flexors)		
Trunk Extension	Back Extension	Back Extension Machine

1. There are many brands of machines available, so we have used only generic rather than trade names.

maximum), is the heaviest weight you can lift one time while maintaining correct exercise techniques. This amount will fluctuate depending upon which muscle group you are testing, and it will also change as your level of conditioning improves. Because finding 1-RM requires a trial-and-error method of manipulating weight loads until a maximal effort is achieved, it can be time consuming, inaccurate, and may cause injuries. Because of the likelihood of injuries, we recommend estimating your 80 percent level rather than doing 1-RM trials.

Practicality. What makes a set? Experts disagree about the number of repetitions that comprise a set. Numbers range from 6 to 20, although most exercise researchers suggest 8 to 12 repetitions. Highly trained athletes seeking maximum muscular strength development often use 3 to 6 repetitions with very high resistance (a weight which takes effort, but

TABLE 5.5

Summary of Types of Weight Training Programs

Weight Training Program	Repetitions	Sets per Exercise	Rest Between Sets	Workouts per Week	Number of Exercises
Health & Fitness	8–12	1–3	2 min.	2–3	8–10
Muscular Strength	1–6	3–6	3 min.	2–3	8–12 or more
Muscular Endurance	10–20	3–6	2 min.	3–6	8–12
Body Building	8–20	3–8	1 min.	5–12	8–12 or more

not strain, to lift 6 times); training with lower weights, but more than 12 repetitions, primarily develops muscular endurance. Since the number is not sacred, and since it depends upon what you want to achieve, our recommendation is that you choose a number from 8 to 12 and then use it consistently. We usually do sets of 10 repetitions in our workouts.

While the number of repetitions comprising a set is in dispute, the traditional prescription is that each exercise be repeated for 3 sets.[30] Regarding weight, a quick rule of thumb is to use a weight with which you can only do 12 repetitions. When you can lift that weight more than 12 times comfortably, then the weights should be increased slightly, and the process of building up begun again. If you are a beginner and using free weights, you might consider starting with 2.5 pounds for the arms and 10 pounds for the legs, so that you learn proper form. Gradually increase it in increments of 2.5 and 10 pounds for the arms and legs, respectively.

Frequency and Routine. The recommendation for frequency and type of routine varies depending upon your reason for weight training. For health and fitness purposes, the American College of Sports Medicine recommends a minimum of 8 to 10 exercises involving the body's major muscle groups at least 2 times per week (see Table 5.4 for suggested exercises for specific body parts). Use enough resistance to perform 8 to 12 repetitions per set, with effort but not strain.[31] Each workout, then, will consist of approximately 30 sets and 300 repetitions. If the purpose of your weight training is to go beyond minimal health and physical fitness benefits, you might consider working out 3 times a week with approximately 48 hours of rest between training sessions.

If you are weight training for reasons other than health and fitness, then different approaches are recommended. For example, if you are using weight training to improve your sports performance, the exercise combinations will more likely concentrate on the muscles used in your sport.

If you are trying to sculpt your body, you will want to do more than one exercise per body part. Serious bodybuilders usually alternate between legs and chest on one day, and shoulders and back at the next day's session. Abdominals and calves are usually exercised at each session. Table 5.5 presents a summary of guidelines for various weight training programs.

Guidelines for Weight Training

1. **Smooth Movements**: Don't jerk the weights. All exercises should be done with smooth, continuous movements.

2. **Speed of Movements**: Don't throw the free weight upward or lift the machine stack of weights too quickly, nor allow the weights, in either case, to drop back. Raise and lower the weights in a smooth, controlled manner. Lifting should take about 2 seconds and lowering should take about 2 to 4 seconds. With the machines, the weights should return gently and quietly. If you can't control the speed of the weight, it is too heavy for you. You will be better off decreasing the weight and gradually building back up.

3. **Full Range of Motion**: For maximum benefit, whenever possible, exercise the muscle from full extension to full contraction, and then back to full extension. Using a full range of motion results in strength gains throughout the muscle.

4. **Breathing**: A good general rule is to exhale during the greatest exertion (the lifting phase) and inhale when lowering the weights. Don't hold your breath. Physiologically, this is not healthy and may be dangerous since it can cause dizziness, blackout, or hernias.

5. **Concentration**: Focusing full attention on the working muscles helps performance. Dream of your love life or worry about paying your bills some other time. You need to be continually aware of position, breathing, and range of motion.

6. **Correct Exercise Form and Body Position**: These are important so that the muscles you want to work on are in the right position to receive maximum benefit from the exercise. If form and body position are incorrect, you increase the risk of injury by placing muscles in positions which stress them unnecessarily or improperly.

    If you are using a machine, body position is also important because each machine is designed with a pivot point to work specific muscles. For example, on the seated leg curl machine you need to line up your knees with the machine's pivot point. Some machines have a seat belt to hold you on the machine and in the correct body position. Using the seat belt makes the exercise more effective and safe.

7. **Training Partners**: When lifting free weights, there are some exercises in which a partner who "spots" for you is essential for safety. While spotters will generally simply encourage you, they are in a position to help if you get into trouble.

Building a Program. It's best to begin cautiously. As a beginner, start with very light weights and learn to do each exercise correctly before you add resistance. Don't overdo it at the beginning—the resulting soreness will decrease your next performance attempts and may discourage you from continuing. If any muscles, joints, or tendons have been prone to injury in the past, avoid putting added stress on them when you start your program. While a weight as low as 10 pounds on the bar may seem ridiculously light for an overhead lift, resist the temptation to pile on more weights in the beginning.

Recommendations

Weeks 1 and 2: During your first six sessions, perform 1 set of 10 (or a number from 8 to 12) repetitions of each exercise. That's 1 set of 10 repetitions for each of the major muscle areas (see Table 5.4).

If the weight you started with at the first session feels very light and the repetitions are easy, a significant increase in the weight for the next session may be appropriate. However, if it was slightly difficult, a smaller increase in weight is recommended. Experiment, but by the end of two weeks, you should be using a weight that makes it possible to do your chosen number of repetitions with effort but not strain.

Weeks 3 and 4: During the next two weeks, add a second set of repetitions. We recommend starting the second set of 10 repetitions 2 to 3 minutes after the first set. A couple of minutes' rest allows energy stores in the exercised muscle to be replenished.

Weeks 5 and 6: Add a third set of repetitions. During this time you might start to increase your resistance. A six-week introduction is conservative; you may condense to three weeks if you are finding no problems during or after your workouts.

Tips for Weight Training

- To make your routine more time effective, try alternating two or three exercises that work different muscle groups. For example, by alternating bench press, leg extensions, and abdominals, you can go directly from one set to the next with little or no rest in between.

- Choose between what is known as a **fixed load**—where the resistance, repetitions, sets, and rest remain the same—or a **variable load**, where they change for each set. For example, if you were intermediate to advanced in the bench press, you might do a fixed-load workout by lifting 120 pounds for 10 repetitions of 3 sets, with 2 minutes' rest between sets. If you used a variable load, you might lift 120 pounds, 10 reps, 1 minute rest; then 130 pounds, 8 reps, 2 minutes' rest; then 140 pounds, 6 reps, 3 minutes' rest. *Note:* In the fixed-load workout you would have lifted a total of 3,600 pounds, and in the variable-load workout, a total of 3,080 pounds. Though 520 pounds less, the variable load in this example would increase your strength more than the fixed-load workout.
- After a maximum strength workout, rest your muscles for 48 hours to allow adequate recovery. If you have not completely recovered in two or three days, it is possible that you are overtraining. Cut back, either on sets or total number of exercises performed.
- It takes approximately a minimum of eight weeks of consecutive training to start to achieve results.[32]
- Abdominal exercises call for more repetitions and sets and can be done daily.
- About 3 minutes of rest between sets that work the same muscles are necessary for people who are trying to maximize their strength gains, while 2 minutes is sufficient for anyone training for health and fitness. Bodybuilders should rest no more than 1 minute to maximize the "pumping" effect.

Free Weights or Machines

Should you use barbells and dumbbells, known as free weights, or machines? Either is okay and will accomplish the same gains in strength. There is also nothing wrong in using either or both methods.[33] Each has its own advantages and disadvantages (see Chapter 9, Gearing Up, for more information).

Machines permit easier adjustment in weight totals and may be considered safer—because you can't be trapped under the weight. They are faster to change from one weight to another, an advantage if you have a limited time for your exercise. Learning the movement is easier and faster because the direction of the movement is controlled by the machine.

Free weights develop balance because you use a variety of other muscles to stabilize your body during the exercise. The variety of exercises is greater because you are not limited by the specific mechanics of the machine. Free weights are less expensive than most exercise machines, and enable you to exercise at home rather than at a health club.

Spicing Up Your Routine

Cross Training. Joan Benoit, winner of the 1984 Olympic marathon, inadvertently discovered the benefits of cross training after having Achilles tendon surgery on both feet. Exactly one week after surgery, she began riding a stationary bicycle as seriously as she ran. Then she increased her weight training schedule, which had accounted for no more than 2 percent of her training time prior to surgery. When her casts were removed, she started swimming. "My overall fitness increased considerably," she says. "My whole body felt in sync. Yet it was the longest time off (from running) I've ever had."[34]

In her first race after surgery, the Old Kent River Bank 25K, Ms. Benoit missed her American record by just nine seconds. She had regained her former performance with relatively low training mileage, 70 miles a week versus her usual 120. Joan Benoit had also discovered the beauty of cross training—achieving more aerobic work without the stress and abuse.

The pioneers of cross training were triathletes who ran, swam, and cycled. Prior to the popularity of triathlons, each sport disparaged any serious participation in another activity as being detrimental to training and performance in the first sport. Times have changed. Or have they?

Despite rave reviews from some athletes about the benefits of cross training, no definitive study has yet demonstrated that cross training improves performance in a specific sport.[35]

Because of the principle of muscle specificity (where only the muscle worked will increase in strength and endurance), which we discussed in Chapter 3, Body Works, some exercise physiologists feel that training must be tailored specifically for your sport.[36] If you are going to run, then the muscles involved in running need to be made stronger and more adept at performing the task you have chosen. If you use them repeatedly to perform that specific task (repetitions for muscular endurance) and place increased demands on them over time (duration for muscular strength), then your performance should improve because your muscle physiology has changed due to those workouts.

Some exercise scientists go so far as to say that cross training takes away from total training time for specific muscles and doesn't allow them to achieve maximum changes at the cellular level.[37] Peak performance is thereby not achieved.

Why the Raves? Then why do top competitive athletes praise cross training? The answer may be that they had been overtraining. For them, pushing too much and reducing overall performance as a result of overtraining is a constant problem. There's a fine line between training too much and not training enough. A recent study of competitive triathletes, who may log up to five hours of training every day, reinforces the notion of overuse. Three out of four of the triathletes studied experienced a musculoskeletal overuse injury while training.[38] These results suggest that perhaps the benefits from cross training are more psychological than anything else; at that level of training perhaps it doesn't make any difference whether an athlete runs 100 miles a week or runs 60 miles a week combined with miles of cycling and swimming.

When top athletes reduce an intense training schedule and engage in cross training, they often improve their performance. Cross training seems to allow muscles time to recover between training sessions. *Note:* We need almost 48 hours for complete recovery of muscle glycogen stores between workouts, and it helps to eat a diet containing at least 60 percent carbohydrates (see Chapter 10, Food for Fitness, for more nutritional information).

Cross training could also be effective because it may reduce overuse injuries caused by continuous stress on the same muscles and joints. Cross training also introduces variety, which keeps workouts from being boring. One last explanation for the effectiveness of cross training is that it can strengthen other muscles which, although not directly involved in a specific movement, may aid in the biomechanical efficiency of the total movement. The result: better performance with less effort.

Why Cross Train? Cross training also makes sense for those among us who are not super competitors. Ideally, we should do a mix of activities over a week's period in order to exercise all our muscles and joints, and possibly avoid injury. Running, swimming, or bicycling in themselves are incomplete exercise programs, but when used as cross training, they enhance overall fitness by providing complementary workouts. For instance, running builds your lower body, and swimming primarily works your upper body. Alternating them can help give the benefits of both while also building aerobic endurance. The variety of activities that cross training embraces can provide a tonic for the boredom and staleness often engendered by a one-activity pursuit. Variety is the spice of life! Swim today, run tomorrow, and cycle the day after that.

And for those of us who are single-minded in our competitive pursuits (the Jenny-One-Notes of exercise), cross training may be the brake on a possibly deleterious exercise program. While hard workouts where we push our bodies to the limit are a must if we are to develop our potential to the fullest, we don't want to injure ourselves.

How to Cross Train. The best method is to pair sports that train different parts of your body. Table 5.6 has some suggested complementary activities. Depending on the activities, you can do them on alternate days or, perhaps work them in on the same day. For example, instead of three or more 50-minute runs per week, run for 25 minutes and spend the remaining time cycling.

Hint: Regardless of what exercise you choose, new research suggests that you should swing your arms for more exercise benefit. Whether you are on a treadmill or a stationary

TABLE 5.6

....

Complementary Cross-Training Activities

Major Activity	Cross Train with	Helps
Walking/Running	Swimming/low impact aerobic classes	Upper body strength
	Weight training	Leg and upper-body strength
	Abdominals	Good for hills / prevents back problems
Cycling	Running / swimming	Endurance
	Weight training	Leg and upper-body strength
	Abdominals	Prevents back problems
Swimming	Walking, running, cycling	Leg strength
	Weight training	Stronger arms and legs
Aerobics	Walking, running, cycling, swimming	Endurance
	Weight training	Muscle strength and tone

....

Source: Adapted from UC Berkeley Wellness Letter, May 1995.

bicycle, walking or running, it has been shown that using both arms and legs is not only more beneficial to overall fitness, but burns more calories than using the legs alone.[39]

Finding a Workout

The best exercise is the one that you enjoy and will pursue with some regularity.

Know Yourself. Figuring out why you choose to work up a sweat (in addition to looking and feeling good) can help you find your ideal exercise. Some things to consider are:

1. **Level of competitiveness:** If you like to excel and tend to drive yourself to win, pursue activities where there are competitions, such as racquetball, tennis,

softball, volleyball, running, swimming, etc. If you run, consider different types of racing events, often sponsored by running clubs, which may add an incentive to your workouts.

2. **Need for tension release:** If you turn to exercise to relieve mental and physical tension, an activity that is fast paced or totally absorbing may be for you. Try aerobic sports or activities that require steady concentration.

3. **Amount of self-discipline:** Are you lax at regulating yourself? If so, solo sports or repetitive endurance sports such as running, race walking, swimming, or cycling are not for you. It takes motivation to work out and it's very easy to talk oneself out of exercising. Choosing a team activity where the training and competition schedules are externally imposed will help to get you to toe the line and stick it out. Another suggestion is to pay for a membership in a "Y" or health club. You might work out just to get your money's worth.

4. **Sociability:** If you like to be social while you work out, swimming is probably not for you, but tennis, bowling, or golf might be. You might also consider joining a health club or "Y" where you can take advantage of workouts in a group setting.

5. **Going solo:** If your desire for personal space is paramount, consider activities you can do alone, such as walking, running, cycling, or swimming, which allow you time to reflect, meditate, or simply be alone with your sport.

6. **Need for aesthetic or creative expression:** Choosing dance, gymnastics, or fencing, for example, may be the outlet for this important part of you.

7. **Quality of life:** If you exercise because it provides variety and excitement to your life—besides making you look and feel good—then any activity that appeals to you will most likely be a good choice and will satisfy that need.

Other Considerations

• **Affordability.** Can you afford the activity you choose? You might love swimming, but joining a health club may be prohibitively expensive. Low-cost activities include walking or running (shoe replacement is the major expense), bicycling and cross-country skiing (the initial outlay is the major expense), and some team sports such as volleyball or softball.

• **Accessibility.** Is what you want to do available in your neck of the woods? If you live in Florida, you can pursue cross-country skiing by flying north occasionally, but you would be better served finding an activity which you can easily do year round—beach volleyball, maybe?

• **Time Framework.** You do not find the time for exercise, you MAKE the time. Rearrange or make your schedule more flexible so that you can fit in your activity. Most of us have extra time, which we fritter away. Turn that time into exercise time—30 minutes is often all you need.

Where there's a will, there's a way. The time is now for you and your exercise routine.

AVOIDING INJURY

How people gauge their training routine remains one of the mysteries of exercise. What constitutes overuse in one person and ideal training in another is not fully understood, thus it is difficult to make individual training recommendations. But there are some givens. Increasing the duration too quickly, for example, increasing total weekly running miles from 20 to 40 from one week to the next, may cause an injury. Your body will probably communicate that sudden overuse with early warning signs such as strained or inflamed muscles and tendons. Don't "work through" the injury. Adjust your workout. See Chapter 17, Fixing Things: An Approach to Rehabilitation, for more information.

No Rest, No Gain.   All work and no play makes Jenny a dull girl. That should be the theme song for athletes and fitness enthusiasts who push themselves too hard or work out seven days a week. Resting is necessary. As a matter of fact, it's such an important part of improving fitness and ability that it's now being called the other half of a workout.

Resting provides an opportunity for the body to get used to the stress put upon it during the workout. To increase your prowess in whatever activity you do, you must challenge your body by increasing the frequency, intensity, or length of your workout. Rest allows a consolidation of the gain you made during that challenge.

How Much Rest? At a minimum, one day a week. But depending on the activity you do, it may be more. For example, people who do weight training are usually advised to train several times a week and rest 48 or 72 hours between workouts; if you've run a marathon, you shouldn't run for several days and then only lightly for the next two weeks.

Active Rest. While it may sound like an oxymoron, the term "active rest" is used by exercise researchers to describe the less rigorous participation in activities other than the exerciser's usual sport or workout. It's the theory behind cross training!

PUTTING IT TOGETHER

In this chapter and Chapter 4 we have provided the basic information necessary to begin or enhance an already existing exercise program. In the next chapter, we provide a sampler of activities for your consideration.

1. Louise Mead Tricard, personal communication

2. Morton, C. Through alternative training, recovered runners are better, stronger and faster than before. *Running*, March/April, 1983, 24–25.

3. Wendel, T. Fragile: Handle with care. *Women's Sports*, October, 1982, 45–47.

4. Longman, J. Slaney slows down to speed things up. *New York Times*, May 1, 1996, B9,14.

5. Longman, J. Pippig comeback keeps Kenyans from a sweep. *New York Times*, April 16, 1996, B9,12.

6. Teper, L. Born to Run. *Sports Fitness*, April, 1985, 29–32, 94.

7. Glossbrenner, H. Commentary: USA men and women top 25. *Powerlifting USA*, February, 1996, 20.

8. Powerlifting USA. Meet results. *Powerlifting USA*, July, 1996, 75.

9. Rhonda O'Conner, personal communication (1991 World Record Holder in Bench Press for age 35 and over—weight 122 pounds and under).

10. American College of Sports Medicine. *Guidelines for Graded Exercise Test and Exercise Prescription*, 4th ed. Philadelphia: Lea & Febiger, 1991.

11. Pate, R. R., Pratt, M., Blair, S. N., et al. Physical activity and public health: A recommendation from the Centers for Disease Control and Prevention and the American College of Sports Medicine, 1995. *Journal of the American Medical Association*, 1995, 273(5), 404.

12. Lee, I-M., Hsieh, C. C., & Paffenbarger, R .S. Exercise intensity and longevity in men: The Harvard alumni health study. *Journal of the American Medical Association*, 1995, 273(15), 1179–1184.

13. Rich-Edwards, J. W., Manson, J. E., Hennekens, C. H., et al. The primary prevention of coronary heart disease in women. *New England Journal of Medicine*, 1995, 332(26), 1758–1766.

14. Manson, J. E., & Lee, I-M. Exercise for women—how much pain for optimal gain? *New England Journal of Medicine*, 1996, 334(20), 1325–1326.

15. van Mechelen, W. Running injuries: A review of the epidemiological literature. *Sports Medicine*, 1992, 14(5), 320–335.

16. Bouchard, C., Shephard, R. J., & Stephens, T., (eds.). *Physical Activity, Fitness, and Health*. Champaign, Ill: Human Kinetics, 1994.

17. Hunt, M. Too much of a good thing. *New York Times*, February 7, 1988, 42–44.

18. Wilber, C. A., Hollard, G. J., Madison, R. E., et al. An epidemiological analysis of overuse injuries among recreational cyclists. *International Journal of Sports Medicine*, 1995, 16(3), 201–206.

19. Levin, S. Overtraining causes Olympic-sized problems. *The Physician and Sportsmedicine*, 1991, 19(5) 112–116.

Rosato, F. D. *Fitness for Wellness*, 3rd ed. Minneapolis: West Publishing Company, 1994.

20. Fahey, T. D. Endurance Training. In M. M. Shangold, & G. Mirkin, (eds.). *Women and Exercise: Physiology and Sports Medicine*, 2nd ed. Philadelphia: F. A. Davis Co., 1994, 73–88.

21. Astrand, P. O., & Rodahl, K. *Textbook of Work Physiology*, 3rd ed. New York: McGraw-Hill, 1986.

22. Holloway, J. B., & Baechle, T. R. Strength training for female athletes: A review of selected aspects. *Sports Medicine*, 1990, 9(4), 216–228.

23. Dalsky, G. P., Stocke, K. S., Ehans, A. A. Weight-bearing exercise training and lumbar bone mineral content in postmenopausal women. *Annals of Internal Medicine*, 1988, 108, 824–828.

Heinrich, C. H., Going, S. B., Pamenter, R. W., et al. Bone mineral content of cyclically menstruating female resistance and endurance trained athletes. *Medicine and Science in Sport and Exercise*, 1990, 22(5), 558–563.

Notelovitz, M., Martin, D., & Tesar, R. Estrogen therapy and variable-resistance weight training increase bone mineral in surgically menopausal women. *Journal of Bone Mineral Research*, 1991, 6(6), 583–590.

24. Sinaki, M. Loading exercises affect muscle strength earlier and more than bone density in healthy, active, young women. *Journal of Bone and Mineral Research*, 1994, 9(S1), abstract #B145.

25. Nelson, M. E., Fiatarone, M. A., Morganti, C. M., et al. Effects of high-intensity strength training on multiple factors for osteoporotic fractures. *Journal of the American Medical Association*, 1994, 272(24), 1909–1914.

26. Broad, W. J. Space doctors decide pumping iron is key to astronauts' health. *New York Times*, December 10, 1996, c 1, 3.

27. Staron, R. S., Malicky, E. S., Leonardi, M. J., et al. Muscle hypertrophy and fast fiber type conversions in heavy

resistance-trained women. *European Journal of Applied Physiology*, 1990, 60(1), 71–79.

28. Holloway, J. B., & Baechle, T. R. Strength training for female athletes: A review of selected aspects. *Sports Medicine*, 1990, 9(4), 216–228.

29. Garhammer, J. A comparison of maximal power outputs between male and female weight lifters in competition. *Journal of Applied Sport Science Research*, 1989, 3(3), 73–78.

30. Berger, R. A. *Introduction to Weight Training*. Englewood Cliffs, NJ: Prentice-Hall, 1984.

31. American College of Sports Medicine. Position Stand on the recommended quantity and quality of exercise for developing and maintaining cardiorespiratory and muscular fitness in healthy adults. *Medicine and Science in Sports and Exercise*, 1990, 22(2), 265–274.

32. Stone, W. J., & Kroll, W. A. *Sports Conditioning and Weight Training*. Boston: Allyn and Bacon, Inc., 1978.

33. Clark, D. H. Training for strength. In M. M. Shangold, & G. Mirkin, (eds.). *Women and Exercise: Physiology and Sports Medicine*, 2nd ed. Philadelphia: F. A. Davis Co., 1994, 60–72.

34. Morton, C. Through alternative training, recovered runners are better, stronger and faster than before. *Running*, March/April, 1983, 24–25.

35. O'Toole, M. L., & Douglas, P. S. Fitness: Definition and development. In M. M. Shangold, & G. Mirkin, (eds.). *Women and Exercise: Physiology and Sports Medicine*, 2nd ed. Philadelphia: F. A. Davis Co., 1994, 3–26.

36. Cross-training may be good for the psyche, but will it prevent overuse injuries? *Sports Medicine Digest*, December 1995, 7.

37. Stockton, W. Can cross-training improve your fitness? *New York Times*, April 18, 1988, c10.

38. Wilk, B .R., Fisher, K. L., & Rangelli, D. The incidence of musculoskeletal injuries in an amateur triathlete racing club. *Journal of Orthopaedic and Sports Physical Therapy*, 1995, 22(3), 108–112.

39. Butts, N. K., Knox, K. M., & Foley, T. S. Energy costs of walking on a dual-action treadmill in men and women. *Medicine and Science in Sports and Exercise*, 1995, 27(1), 121–125.

6 A Sampler of Activities

SUSAN L. PURETZ, ED.D.

Exercise should be a way of life for everyone. It should be like brushing your teeth, something you must do to survive. You should not think about it, just go do it.
—Yvonne, age 65

Women exercise in many ways and, like the women in our survey, have different reasons for participation in physical activity (see Chapter 1, Why We Exercise, for the variety of reasons). However, it doesn't really matter how you get your daily dose of movement—whether you work out just to stay in shape, or participate in sports as your exercise. The bottom line is that you are physically active. Likewise, it doesn't matter what activity you choose, as long as the choice gets you moving.

The activities covered in this chapter are just the tip of the iceberg. They were chosen to illustrate a range of weight-bearing, relatively simple and inexpensive, popular physical activities. While we have concentrated on mainly two-legged pursuits, we have also gone off-track and introduced a section on horseback riding. It was included initially as an extension of running activities (when you read about ride and tie you'll understand), but then became enlarged as we focused on making riding as much of an exercise for the rider as for the horse.

THE WALK-JOG-RUN CONTINUUM

Walking, jogging, and running are a continuum of activities where the legs—the primary mode of locomotion—are in direct contact with the ground (unlike cycling). The physical differences between ordinary walking and running seem obvious, and yet, a fast race walk may cover more ground in a given period of time, be more vigorous, and result in better fitness than a slow run. The difference between jogging and running is also not so simple. While jogging can be classified simply as a slow run, at what point does a slow run become a fast run? One way to think about the difference is that jogging involves endurance training at a noncompetitive level.

Walking, jogging, and running all develop cardiorespiratory endurance; the extent is dependent upon intensity, frequency, and duration. We will describe all three activities in this chapter.

Walking

I have often started off on my walk mad—soreheaded, bored, or confused. I begin walking, dull, lifeless, and discouraged. But I never come back in the same frame of mind. It is my sovereign remedy. —Melissa, age 39

Fitness Walking: Slower but Surer. We used to think of walking as merely a way to get from the front door to the car or to get from one golf hole to the next. But now that America has gone through its jogging craze, fitness walking has emerged as a great alternative.

The attractions of walking are as seductive as ever. Testimonials abound; it is perhaps the easiest, healthiest, and safest physical activity, and it requires no special equipment except for a pair of well-fitted athletic shoes. Moreover, walkers are not subjected to the musculoskeletal dangers of running, the traffic hazards of cycling, or the problem of finding a swimming pool. Walking can be done nearly anywhere and at any time. It is also one of the most effective and cheapest emotional therapies available—a psychophysical alchemy that transforms the body and the mind.

If you are worried that fitness walking is not as beneficial as running, worry no more. Walking at a brisk rate of 4 to 5 miles per hour for 30 to 45 minutes exercises the heart at the same rate as 20 to 30 minutes of medium-paced jogging. Your heart prospers without the possible painful shin splints, stress fractures, Achilles tendinitis, plantar fasciitis, chondromalacia, and other ailments suffered by many who run seriously.[1]

Energy Costs. The amount of energy we use while we walk depends largely on our speed and weight. For example, at a speed of 3 miles per hour (that's one mile in 20 minutes), a 140-pound woman will use 114 calories while walking for 30 continuous minutes. If that same woman increased her pace to 3.5 miles per hour, she would expend 27 more calories in the same time. Of two women walking at that same 3.5 miles-per-hour speed, the heavier of the two would expend more calories.

Note: Since the minimum energy expenditure necessary for a training effect has been estimated to be around 300 calories, a hypothetical 140-pound woman would have to walk approximately an hour on level ground at 3.5 miles per hour to improve her fitness.

Fitness Walking Technique

While the thought of instruction in walking may seem absurd (after all, we've been doing it since we were about a year old), fitness walking 2 or 3 miles a day requires some attention to technique so as to derive the most from the activity.

Four things separate strollers from those who get aerobic benefit from their fitness walking. They are (1) good posture, (2) heel-toe roll, (3) stride, and (4) arm pump. Remember: Although a physical fitness benefit is important, it is better to stroll for your health than to do nothing.

Posture. Good walking posture means that your ears, shoulders, hips, knees, and ankles are in a vertical line. Leaning forward won't help you go faster and may cause back strain. To help get into that correct postural alignment, you should keep:

- your head erect and centered with your eyes looking forward (focused about 15 to 20 feet ahead) and your chin tucked in.
- your shoulders square (relaxed and not slumped forward or raised upwards towards your ears) and your back straight.
- your arms bent at the elbows at 90 degrees and close to your torso. Your wrists should be straight with your fingers curled gently to form a loose fist.
- your buttocks and your stomach tucked in to avoid arching your back. This position is known as the pelvic tilt, and people with weak backs use it to strengthen muscles in the lower back while also preventing undue stress in that region.

Heel-Toe Roll. When you walk, land on your heel and roll forward to the ball of your foot, which then pushes off (called the toe-off) for the next step. You should not land flat-footed because you won't get the necessary momentum for the next step; nor should you lift your foot from the knee (it should be lifted from the hip). The heel-toe roll will exercise the front of your legs and your calves.

Stride. In a normal strolling walk, your feet land in two parallel tracks on either side of an imaginary line. In fitness walking, your footsteps should fall almost in one straight line, that is, they land closer to the imaginary line. (See diagram, next page.)

You should pick up your leg at the hip for maximum extension (the hip of your back leg will push forward to accommodate this movement). To increase your pace, you will want to step more frequently rather than trying to stretch your stride, although some authorities recommend both more steps and a lengthening of the stride.

Arm Pump. The arm pump is what transforms walking from a lower-body to a total-body aerobic exercise. You should swing your bent arms in a straight forward-and-back plane with an ever so slight brushing of the sides of your body. The hand opposite the forward leg travels to chest height in front, while the other hand moves to the top of the

What to Do

If you do lengthen your stride, be aware that it may lead to injury by placing an additional stress on the knees. If you want to lengthen your stride, practice stride stretching and remember to keep your back straight and your pelvis tucked under— this should let you take a longer step and reduce stress on your joints.

Changes in foot placement for various walking speeds

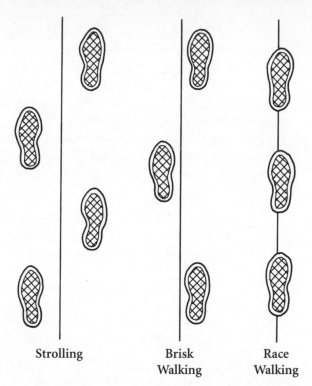

Strolling   Brisk Walking   Race Walking

buttocks in the backswing. *Note:* When you walk normally, your arms are straight and swing freely at your side, which requires almost no muscular strength. If you pump your arms, you increase the aerobic benefits of your walk, and strengthen the arms and upper torso. At the beginning this new technique may tire you; if your arms, shoulders, or back begin to ache, let your muscles rest by going back to your normal arm swing for a few minutes until your muscles recover. After several weeks of training, you should not notice fatigue in those muscles.

Common Fitness Walking Errors (How and Why They Occur)
- Droopy head—from watching the road directly in front of you.
- Overreached arms—from using a straight arm reaching-to-the-sky swing in order to gain speed.
- Chicken wings—from thrusting the elbows out to the side and letting the arms fly across the chest.

- Shoulders slumping or by the ears—the former from poor posture, the latter from tension as you pick up speed.
- Overstriding—from thinking that it's the way to move faster. It can cause your hips to swivel sideways and place stress on your lower back. You shouldn't reach further than the distance reached when you lean forward and your foot automatically goes out to catch you.
- Wide stride—from walking with your feet too far apart.
- Faulty footing—from landing on flat feet (this will also send shock waves to your knees and back). Practice landing on your heel and rolling in a straight line through the ball of your foot to the toe.
- Forward tilt—from assuming it will get you to your goal faster. To counteract the tilt tendency, keep your pelvis under your shoulders.

Special Equipment

Shoes. Ordinary shoes are not recommended for fitness walking. You should select a shoe that has:
- a low back tab to reduce pressure on the Achilles tendon;
- flexible, non-sticky soles (running shoes are not suitable because they usually have stiffer soles and more rigid sides);
- well-cushioned heels (about half to three quarters of an inch) and good arch support (*note*: neither heels nor arch support needs to be as thick as for running shoes);
- a toe box that is roomy enough to allow for expansions of the foot during your heel-toe roll. For more shoe information, see Chapter 8.

What to Do

Select shoes specifically designed for walking. Many running shoe companies now manufacture them. When you choose a shoe, it should be comfortable the first time you put it on. Try shoes on at the end of the day and wear the same kind of socks you wear when walking. Once you're using them, check for evenness of wear. If discomfort develops, see a podiatrist or sports medicine specialist.

Weights. The consensus is not yet clear, but most experts do not recommend wearing or carrying extra weights. One researcher, however, found that hand weights could significantly enhance a workout—even for people in excellent aerobic condition—depending on how high the weights are pumped.[2] The problem with hand weights is that they can strain elbows, while ankle weights increase the risk of tripping by throwing you off balance, and may strain knees.

Your Workout

Warm-up. Walk slowly and pump your arms gently.

Stretches. The objective is to stretch the hips, thighs, calves, and arms—the muscles used for walking. See Chapter 4, Focus on Fitness, for some suggested stretches for the major muscle groups. Feel free to add your own. Do what feels best for you. Remember:

TABLE 6.1

....

Walking Schedule For Fitness*

	Pace**	Daily Mileage	Weekly Mileage
Weeks 1–4			
Beginner	30	½	2½
Beginner Plus	20	1	5
Fitness Walker	17	3	15
Fitness Walker Plus	15	4	20
Race Walker	11	5	25
Weeks 2–6			
Beginner	27	1	5
Beginner Plus	20	2	10
Fitness Walker	17	3½	17½
Fitness Walker Plus	15	4½	22½
Race Walker	11	5½	27½
Weeks 3–7			
Beginner	24	1	5
Beginner Plus	18	2	10
Fitness Walker	16	3½	17½
Fitness Walker Plus	14	4½	22½
Race Walker	10	6	30

• Hold your stretch for 10 to 15 seconds or so.
• Do not bounce. Bouncing tends to overextend the muscles and increase the likelihood of strain.
• Go gently and slowly.

Walking Routine: How Far, How Fast, How Soon?: No one can tell you exactly how far or how fast to walk at the start, but you can determine the proper pace and distance by experimenting. If you have not exercised for a long time, we recommend that you begin by walking for 20 minutes at least 4 or 5 times a week at a pace that feels comfortable to

Weeks 4–8

Beginner	22	1	5
Beginner Plus	18	2	10
Fitness Walker	15	3½	17½
Fitness Walker Plus	13	4½	22½
Race Walker	9	6½	32½

Weeks 5–9

Beginner	22	1	5
Beginner Plus	17	2¾	13¾
Fitness Walker	14	3½	17½
Fitness Walker Plus	12	4½	22½
Race Walker	8	6½	32½

Weeks 6 and On

Beginner	20	1½	7½
Beginner Plus	15	3	15
Fitness Walker	13	4	20
Fitness Walker Plus	12	5	25
Race Walker	8	7	35

*This schedule is based on five days a week. All numbers are suggested goals. Stay at each week and/or level until you have attained your goal.

**Pace is in minutes per mile. If you walk 1 mile in 30 minutes you will be walking 2 miles per hour.

you. If that is too tiring or too easy, reduce or lengthen your time. The "talk test" may be useful in determining your pace at the beginning. If you are breathless and can't carry on a conversation while walking, you're going too fast.

If at first you have difficulty in meeting the schedule suggested here, don't be discouraged. You will systematically be building your stamina and strength. Patience is the key to success. Five furious days of activity will not correct five years of inactivity. Folk wisdom has it that it takes a month of reconditioning to make up for each year of physical inactivity.

You should gradually increase your time and pace. For example, as a beginner, after you have been walking for 20 minutes several days a week for one month, start walking 30 minutes each time. Eventually your goal should be to comfortably walk 3 miles in 45 minutes.

Table 6.1 provides some suggested walking schedules. It includes five variations, from beginner to advanced. To use the chart, choose your level by measuring how long it takes you to walk a mile. For example, if you walk a mile in 20 minutes, you should use the Beginner Plus walking program. Start at that level in the chart and continue to build your mileage and pace. Recognize that the table serves as a reference and that your routine has to be individualized. For example, as a "beginner," you may walk for two weeks or so and feel that you can move up to the beginner plus schedule. That's okay!

Cooldown. Walk slowly until you feel comfortable stopping. Stretch if necessary.

Race Walking

I started running sporadically in the mid '60s, inspired by Kenneth Cooper's book on aerobic exercise. Knees started giving out in the mid '80s. Switched from running to walking in 1989. I now compete as a race walker. —Helen, age 55

If you are tired of fitness walking but are not willing to pound the pavement running, try race walking. Because one foot stays on the ground at all times, race walking is less jarring on the body and results in fewer injuries than running. To the small but growing number of adherents, race walking is an ideal way to pursue fitness.

Race walkers have to follow two rules: They must not lose contact with the ground, and the knee of the supporting leg must be straight. The latter rule was added to make the distinction between race walking and running more clear cut. It also keeps the race walker from getting potential energy, whereas in running the bent knee serves to store energy for the next step's propulsion.

It is the straight knee on the supporting leg that gives race walkers their distinctive hip waggle. The race walker's hip rotation also allows for increased hyperextension, which helps increase stride length. While many people who watch race walkers think that the hip action is forced, it's not. It occurs naturally as you pick up speed while trying to maintain a straight knee.

Race walkers use the bent, pumping arm motion (described under fitness walking) to help increase their speed. The combination of the increased stride length and quicker leg and arm rate allows the racer to walk faster than five miles per hour. While this pace may seem to be an uncomfortably fast walk, race walkers claim that the changes in their gait actually make it easier.

For those of us who want the high level of fitness gained by race walking (comparable to the levels found in distance runners), but don't want to compete, take heart. Recreational race walking (where you use the technique to train but don't compete in organized events) is an up-and-coming activity.

Why Race Walk? Race walking is an activity that is challenging, aerobic, and low-impact (unlike running, where with each step the runner lands with the force of three to five times her body weight). It should be especially attractive to the woman who is chronically suffering from running injuries, or for the woman who does not want to run but is not sufficiently challenged by fitness walking. Race walkers regularly beat large numbers of joggers in road races.

Why Don't More Women Race Walk? People stare at race walkers. The gait is sufficiently different that it encourages double takes, and none of us wants to be gawked at. Combine that with a technique that requires some instruction and practice, and you have an activity that is not yet realizing its potential. However, once you learn to do the gait properly, it is no longer awkward; and once you are comfortable with the gait, you may take pride in your accomplishment so that a few stares from onlookers won't bother you at all.

Problems from Race Walking. The majority of race walking injuries happen because of the "too much too soon" phenomenon—that is, increasing mileage too rapidly in too short a time. Shin splints, however, are one problem common to race walkers. In order to keep the foot off the ground during the forward swing, you must dorsiflex (bring your toe towards your body). This extreme angle requires overuse of the muscles in the front of the lower leg, so beginning race walkers often experience soreness or other problems in their shins.

Two other potential problem areas for race walkers stem from poor technique and improper footwear. Overstriding could cause low back pain, while running shoes with thick heel wedges can act to lever the foot forward, thereby putting too much strain on leg muscles. Unlike the shoe requirements for fitness walking, proper footwear for racewalkers is running shoes. (See Chapter 8, Dressing for the Job, for more information on selecting shoes.) **Recommendation:** Try a lightweight training shoe or racing flat.

Race Walking Technique

The technique is similar to fitness walking, with a few adjustments:

1. The arms, bent at the elbow to about 90 degrees, swing freely and just slightly cross in front of the body. In the backswing, your hands should not rise above your waist.
2. Keep the knee of the supporting leg straight. By keeping your hips loose, you will allow for both a natural shift over the straight leg, and a side-to-side rotation. This will increase your stride length. *Note:* Foot placement is in a straight line. (See diagram on page 114.)

Practice Makes Perfect

To get the feel of this new movement you might try the following exercises:

1. Stand in place with both knees straight. Bend one knee slightly, then alternate. Feel the hip adjust.
2. Drawing a line and "walking it" should provide you with practice in foot placement. To loosen the hips further, try crossing over the line, that is, place the right foot to the left of the line and vice-versa.
3. Shoulder rolls are a good exercise to loosen the shoulders. To do a shoulder roll, bring both shoulders upwards toward the ears, keep the jaw free, and breathe freely—don't hold your breath. Push your shoulders back while raised and then drop them. The whole maneuver should take 3 to 4 seconds. The slower the raise and backward movement, the better the stretch and release.

Advice for a Jogger/Runner Who Wants to Switch

If you are a fit jogger/runner and switch to race walking, don't expect to do as much at the beginning as you would running. If you do, you will most likely experience localized fatigue. This is due to the phenomenon of **muscle specificity**, which refers to the fact that each bodily movement or activity uses a specific set of muscles. One suggestion for making the transition easier is to alternate walking, race walking, and jogging/running—doing no more than 5 minutes of each. Gradually reduce the walking and jogging/running segments until within several weeks you are able to race walk the full distance.

Jog / Run

> *The trouble with jogging is that, by the time you realize you're not in shape for it, you've gone too far to easily walk back.* —Marlene, age 48

Jogging and running are relatively simple, inexpensive activities that can be done almost anywhere. It's estimated by American Sports Data, Inc. that in 1996, 31.5 million people over the age of six participated in some form of jog/run activity. Many non-runners believe that joggers and runners must be different from everyone else. After all, they pound the pavement throughout the year, measuring the seasons by their workouts in the snow, rain, cold, and heat. They run at night and at dawn, dodge traffic and irritable dogs, revise schedules and neglect families and friends as they measure their lives in miles per week and running shoes per year.

Yet sports research has neither confirmed nor denied the myth (or the impression) that runners are different. While some research has shown that even the elite long-distance runner seems to have a personality profile similar to the non-runner,[3] other research pinpoints some differences. In one study, runners were found to be more experimental, self-sufficient, unconventional, self-involved, socially reserved, reticent, and shy.[4]

While personalities may or may not be different between runners and non-runners, one area where there seems to be growing agreement is that running (as well as some other activities) can alter one's mood and alleviate some of the symptoms associated with depression, anxiety, and stress. Runners are quick to talk about how running makes them feel. Terms like "happier," "more relaxed," and "less stressed," were commonly expressed by the women runners in our study. Women run because it makes them feel better—a good enough reason in and of itself!

Beginner Start-up.   If you are a beginner, it's important not to leap from your sofa and head for the track to run a mile. As a beginning runner, your overriding philosophy should be achieving peak performance while doing yourself no harm. That means start slowly and build gradually. Think of your plan as having two stages: the **initial conditioning stage**, which typically lasts 4 to 6 weeks, followed by the **improvement conditioning stage**, which can last 12 to 20 weeks and where progression is more rapid. At the end of this time you should have achieved your desired level of conditioning. Then your options become maintenance at this level or an elevation of your fitness goals and a more intensive training regimen.

Don't Be a Dropout. Planning a four- to six-week-long "phase in" will help prevent the "drop-out" syndrome. That syndrome occurs when you enthusiastically begin a program at too high a level for untrained muscles and abruptly end the program due to muscle strain. Remember, even if you could run two miles nonstop several years ago, you should not attempt to start your new program at that level if you have not run much in the interim. The severe muscle soreness that will develop may cause abandonment of your exercise program.

If you are not accustomed to exercise, don't get discouraged during the initial conditioning stage. It's better to do some running, even if it's not as much as you think you want to do, than to do nothing. Do as much as you feel comfortable with and remember every little bit helps enhance your body and health. By starting at a reasonable level, you will allow your body to adapt, so that during the improvement conditioning stage, you can slowly increase either intensity, duration, or frequency.

Note: For those involved in some other type of physical activity and who now wish to try running, remember the phenomenon known as **muscle specificity** described earlier. Despite your current level of conditioning, a new activity may use different muscle groups and it will be almost as if you are starting from scratch. Don't be surprised if soreness develops in those newly used muscle groups.

CHART 6.2A

A Beginning Jogging Program
Using a Timed Approach

WEEK 1
Walk (nonstop) 10 minutes

WEEK 2
Walk 5 minutes, jog 1 minute,
walk 5 minutes, jog 1 minute

WEEK 3
Walk 5 minutes, jog 3 minutes,
walk 5 minutes, jog 3 minutes

WEEK 4
Walk 5 minutes, jog 4 minutes,
walk 5 minutes, jog 4 minutes

WEEK 5
Walk 4 minutes, jog 5 minutes,
walk 4 minutes, jog 5 minutes

WEEK 6
Walk 4 minutes, jog 6 minutes,
walk 4 minutes, jog 6 minutes

WEEK 7
Walk 4 minutes, jog 7 minutes,
walk 4 minutes, jog 7 minutes

WEEK 8
Walk 4 minutes, jog 8 minutes,
walk 4 minutes, jog 8 minutes

WEEK 9
Walk 4 minutes, jog 9 minutes,
walk 4 minutes, jog 9 minutes

WEEK 10
Walk 4 minutes, jog 13 minutes

WEEK 11
Walk 4 minutes, jog 15 minutes

WEEK 12
Walk 4 minutes, jog 17 minutes

WEEK 13
Walk 2 minutes, jog 19 minutes

WEEK 14
Walk 1 minute, jog 20 minutes

WEEK 15
Jog 20 minutes

Notes: Your weekly activity should include at least 3 to 5 sessions per week. Monitor your progress and don't hesitate to back down or speed up. This chart just describes the activity portion of the workout. Each session should consist of a warm-up, stretch, activity, and cool-down.

Source: Adapted from U.S. Department of Health and Human Services, cited in M. H. Williams, *Lifetime Fitness and Wellness*, 2nd ed. Dubuque IA: William C. Brown, 1990.

CHART 6.2B

. . . .

A Beginning Jogging Program
Using Distance as a Guide

WEEKS 1 AND 2
Walk and jog 1 mile.
Jog easy and walk when needed,
or alternate every 100 yards.

WEEKS 3 AND 4
Same distance (1 mile total)
but increase jogging and
decrease walking.

WEEKS 5 AND 6
Jog the entire mile.

WEEKS 7 AND 8
Use these 2 weeks to build up
gradually to 2 miles (lap by lap).

WEEKS 9 AND 10
Jog 2 miles for these weeks.

WEEKS 11 AND 12
Jog 2 miles, but increase your
pace a little each session.

WEEKS 13 TO 15
Use these 3 weeks to gradually
build up to 3 miles.

. . . .

Notes: Your weekly activity should include at least 3 to 5 sessions per week. Monitor your progress and don't hesitate to back down or speed up. This chart just describes the activity portion of the workout. Each session should consist of a warm-up, stretch, activity, and cooldown.

Prepared by Louise Mead Tricard

The nitty-gritty. For the completely sedentary woman who wants to jog or run, a good way of beginning is to start by walking. Aim first for at least one mile of walking, and then gradually increase your walking pace over that mile. Once you've achieved that, consider jogging. When you do your first jog, slip it in within your one-mile walk. Start by walking, do a short stretch of jogging, then walk again.

Two sample running programs for beginners can be found in Charts 6.2A and 6.2B. One is based on time (and provides a slower approach), while the other uses distance. The distance approach was created by Louise Mead Tricard, the author of *American Women's Track and Field: A History*. Ms. Tricard has been a track coach and competitive runner for many years. Remember from Chapter 4 (Focus on Fitness), your activity should begin with a warm-up, end with a cooldown, and include stretches (these parts of the workout are not included in the chart).

What to Do

Going uphill, lean forward, swing your arms (bent at a 90-degree angle) forcefully forward to chest height and back down to your sides. Your stride length will either be normal or slightly shorter, and will be accompanied by faster foot movements.

On the downhill, try to relax your entire body as your speed naturally increases. You might experiment with decreasing the height of your arm swing, while keeping your shoulders loose. Lean forward into the hill and enjoy gravity's pull. Try to avoid landing on your heel.

Escalating Goals

When I was young, I never participated in any physical activity. Since my husband got me out and running two years ago, a whole new world has opened up for me.
—Kate, age 26

You're hooked on jogging/running and now you want to improve. To do so means working on speed, strength, and endurance.

Speed Acquisition. Interval and fartlek training are the nuts and bolts of your speed-work program (see Chapter 5, Routines: The Stars Are the Limit, for more information). They can also be the toughest part. Remember, intervals are done by specifically focusing on doing a specified distance for speed and then resting. When you do a fartlek workout, you combine a long, slow distance run for endurance with interval's speed-building effects.

Strength Builders. If the area where you normally run is predominantly level, you should include hill training as part of your workout. This is especially important if you are going to compete in events where the course, most likely, includes hills. After a thorough warm-up, run up the hill at a brisk pace. It's guaranteed you'll be out of breath when you reach the top, but you can use the downhill jog to recover. Repeat this 4 to 6 times. *Note:* While uphill is tough on respiration, downhill pounding is hard on the legs, and the knees in particular.

Endurance Enhancers. Long, slow distances are the best way to increase your mileage.

TABLE 6.3

....

12-Week Training Schedule for 10-Kilometer Race[*]

Week	Day 1 Miles	Day 2 Miles	Day 3 Miles	Day 4 Miles	Day 5 Miles
1	4	2	4	3	4
2	4	2	4	3	4
3	4	2	1A	2	5
4	4	2	1A	2	5
5	5	2	1B	2	5
6	5	2	1B	2	5
7	5	3	1C	3	6
8	5	3	1C	3	6
9	6	1A	3	1A	6
10	6	1A	3	1A	6
11	7	1B	2	1B	7
12	4	3			Race

....

Legend:
Intervals
1A. 3–4 × 880 yds at comfortable pace—timed for initial (base) time
1B. 6–8 × 440 yds at comfortable pace—timed for initial (base) time
1C. 3–4 × 880 yds at 10K race pace with a 2-minute recovery and 2–3 × 440 yds at slightly faster than 10K pace with a 2-minute recovery
* This assumes that you have trained and run in a 5K race
Prepared by Louise Mead Tricard

While typical daily mileage can range from two to ten or more miles, you should always be aware that when you do the longer distances, you should run at a relaxed pace.

Putting It Together

Chart 6.3 has a sample three-month schedule for a 10-kilometer race that incorporates the various methods just described. It was created by Louise Mead Tricard, a noted expert on women's track and field.

Technical Tips

1. Use easy fartlek runs in order to gently coax your body into running faster.
2. The long run, slightly longer than your daily distance, will add endurance and strength.
3. Hills will develop leg strength and form.
4. Intervals are added only after you've established a good base.
5. Go slowly: Add mileage and intensity gradually to avoid overuse injury.
6. Run hard no more than one or two days a week—your body needs time to recover from intense workouts.

Reminders

1. Give yourself a break and enjoy the rest days. Remember that rest is part of training.
2. Listen to your body and heed its advice. If you feel sore and stiff, rest an extra day or change the schedule and run more slowly than planned.
3. Resume training gradually if an injury or illness causes you to lose a few days. Jumping back where you left off can be harmful.

Stretching Advice for Runners

Running builds strong leg muscles. But as a muscle strengthens from the constant repetitive motion, it also tightens and becomes less flexible, especially if runners neglect to develop opposing muscle groups. Runners tend to suffer from lack of flexibility in the calves, hamstrings, buttocks, hips, and back. Consider the following in creating a stretching program that can work for you (and also see Chapter 4, Focus on Fitness, for more information).

Degree of flexibility. If your hands can't reach past your shins when you're sitting with legs extended on the floor, you probably need to add some hamstring-specific stretches to your routine.

When to stretch. While the newest advice says to stretch after a brief warm-up, some runners have a hard time doing it then. Psychologically, for them, once running starts, it feels like they need to keep going. Avoid that temptation. A few stretches at that point may be helpful. Stretch after your workout as well.

What to stretch. Runners should concentrate on the lower extremities. *Note:* Some experts suggest not stretching the muscles on the inside of the leg (the adductors) because of possible injury.

Other Training Strategies

Training at Altitude: Toil Above to Excel Below. Those of us who dwell at sea level and vacation at higher altitudes are often caught by surprise when we go out to exercise at altitude. Whether it's a jog, swim, ski, or hike, the first few workouts are harder than expected. The workouts are slower, the heart beats faster, and concentration is missing.

The reason is less oxygen. As the altitude increases, the amount of oxygen in the atmosphere declines. But the body's need for oxygen remains the same. Which means that when you exercise at altitude, you must breathe faster to bring a greater amount of air into your lungs in order to get the equivalent amount of oxygen as would be available at sea level.

Within a few days you usually become more or less acclimatized to the effects of altitude. Your lungs are able to breathe in increased amounts of air, your blood will carry more oxygen because the number of red blood cells has increased, and the heart pumps less. In one study, acclimatization resulted in a 19 percent increase in the amount of oxygen in arterial blood at the same time that the volume of blood pumped through the heart had declined 9 percent.[5] Putting all these changes together results in a steady performance improvement in a person who exercises regularly at altitude.

Boulder, Colorado has become a mecca for many top American and international marathoners because of its altitude of more than 5,000 feet and nearby mountain trails of up to 10,000 feet. Some intrepid world class runners, however, are now trekking to Mexico. Here they run 14 miles up dirt paths to the crater of Xinantecatl, an extinct volcano, rising more than two and a half miles above sea level.[6]

Mental Work.   Exercise physiologists are the silent partners of runners. Working in the lab, they have produced research highlighting the influence of psychological states on physiological processes. Of particular interest to endurance athletes is whether cardiorespiratory efficiency can be influenced during performance by psychological strategies such as paying attention to bodily responses, or the reverse, attending to thoughts other than bodily responses.

Recent studies have examined the effect of a runner's psychological state on running economy—the amount of oxygen consumed at a given running speed. A runner who consumes less oxygen at a given speed is working at a lower relative intensity than other runners and therefore is at an advantage. In one study, runners who had stress management training—which included cognitive coping strategies and relaxation techniques—had decreased oxygen consumption.[7]

Extending that research, several studies found that runners benefited from using biofeedback techniques that direct one's attention to bodily states.[8] Because biofeedback is difficult to use during actual racing, researchers have turned their attention to more practical psychological means that runners could use to improve their physiological responses.

A 1995 study found that the most efficient runners reported more use of relaxation—consciously focusing on relaxing muscles during racing—while at the same time not ignoring any muscular tension or discomfort they might be experiencing.[9] Chapter 7, The Competitive Edge, describes other mental techniques that can be used to enhance your performance.

Running Beyond

Marathons and Ultramarathons. The first New York City marathon in 1970 attracted 126 participants, and there were no female finishers. In contrast, almost 50,000 men and women sent in entries for the privilege of being one of the 32,224 people to run in the 1996 New York City Marathon. The 8,673 women represented 27 percent of the participants, and 85 percent of them finished the marathon.

Marathons have come of age. The marathon's phenomenal growth in numbers of contestants makes sense because it is the logical extension of training routines that have increased individual mileage. It has become the ultimate challenge of body and mind for many fitness and recreational runners.

Although marathons have become a mass participation sport, the loneliness of the long-distance runner still exists. In one survey, 59 percent of runners training for the marathon said they train alone, although women were less inclined to do so.[10] Preparing for a 26.2-mile race also tends to isolate individuals from other sports, and increasing weekly mileage leaves little time for other activities.

> *If only Phidippides had made a longer journey to report news of victory, ultramarathons would be on the Olympic program.* —Stephanie, age 36

If you find it hard to comprehend the "ordinary" runner's single-minded devotion to that pursuit, visualize runners who go the extra miles and run not 26.2-mile marathons but 50- to 100-mile ultramarathons. The expectation that ultramarathoners routinely run more than marathoners is not correct. They both typically log 95 to 100 miles weekly; however, they do train differently.[11] The "ultras" do less interval training and longer daily runs. Elite marathoners, on the other hand, seldom exceed 22 to 23 miles on a training run, and place greater emphasis on high-intensity interval sessions, either on the track or during road runs.[11]

Training for Your First Marathon. Runners, novices especially, often prepare to meet the marathon challenge too aggressively. This tends to result in injury and lost motivation.[12] A *New York Times* 1983 survey of marathoners reported 64 percent of the respon-

TABLE 6.4

....

12-Week Training Schedule for a Marathon[*]

Week	Day 1 Miles	Day 2 Miles	Day 3 Miles	Day 4 Miles	Day 5 Miles	Day 6 Miles	Total Miles
1	2	6	2	4	6		20
2	2	6	2	6	6		22
3	4	6	4	8	12**		34
4	4	6	4	8	12**		34
5	8	5	8	5	15**		41
6	5	10**	5	15**			35
7	5	8	5	20**			38
8	4	8	4	15**			31
9	4	10**	5	8	20**		47
10	5	10**	5	5	3	15**	43
11	6	10**	6	3	6		31
12	5	3				Marathon	8 + 26.2

....

[*] This schedule assumes that you are already "a runner"
** Vary rest days as needed—especially after long runs
Prepared by Louise Mead Tricard

dents answered that they had a running injury that made them stop running for at least a week, with knee problems leading the list of injuries.[13]

While opinions vary as to how to train for a marathon, common elements may be found in many of the recommendations. One such element is the emphasis on the long, slow distance method of training, particularly for initiates.[14] Under this method, you would train at a moderate intensity of exercise (60 to 70 percent of maximal oxygen uptake) for a prolonged period (for more information on long, slow distances, see Chapter 5). Another common element is the required longer run once a week.

In a recent study designed to determine the minimal amount of training that would provide adequate preparation to complete a marathon, the authors found that there was no difference between a group that trained four days per week (Group 4) and one (Group 6) that trained six days per week.[15] In this study, both groups had a three- to four-week phase-in designed to progressively condition runners to prevent injuries from the more intense training regimen to follow. Phase 2 was a 15-week regimen that culminated in a marathon. Both groups did training runs based on time rather than mileage, with one 13.1-mile run the exception in Week 10. Both groups followed a monitored training schedule with Group 4 missing two days of short runs a week. However, both groups performed the four longer runs each week.

Over the course of Phase 2, the average training distance for Group 6 progressively increased from approximately 23 miles per week during Week 1 to approximately 48 miles per week during Weeks 11 to 13. For Group 4, it increased from approximately 18 miles per week to 39 miles.

The results confirmed that the single most critical aspect of marathon training is the long training run. At the end of the experiment, there were no differences between the two groups even though Group 4 ran 20 percent fewer training miles. Interestingly, even though the total volume of training was greater for Group 6, it was apparently not enough to cause a greater incidence of injury.

Chart 6.4, also created by Louise Mead Tricard, provides a sample training schedule for a marathon. It is assumed in this chart that you have been building your mileage prior to beginning this schedule. In no case should you increase your long run by more than 3 miles over what you are used to.

Duathlons and Triathlons.   Triathlons will be one of the Olympic competitive events, for the first time, in Sydney, Australia in the year 2000. Triathlons are usually a combination of running, biking, and swimming, while duathlons are usually a combination of biking and running events. The term duathlon is used to distinguish these races from the Winter Olympic cross-country skiing and shooting combination called the biathlon. (*Note:* The majority of biking and running events currently taking place in the U.S. are called biathlons.) Duathlons and triathlons became hot phenomena in the 1980s. Whether the new audience was attracted as an outgrowth of interest in cross-training or the reverse—it generated the interest in pursuing cross-training—isn't clear; however, the two events are continuing to grow in popularity.

To the average recreational athlete, du- and triathlons might conjure up images of iron men and women who can swim 2.4 miles, bike 112 miles, and run the 26.2 miles necessary to compete in the famous Hawaiian Ironman Triathlon. In actuality those extreme combinations account for less than 1 percent of all duathlons and triathlons, while less formidable events are held across the U.S. on any given weekend in the year.

For example, the New York City Central Park Triathlon consists of a 1/4-mile pool swim, a 12-mile bicycle race, and a 5-mile run. That race, held for the first time in 1985, is organized by the New York Triathlon Club (NYTC). Its founder and president, Daniel Honig, has estimated that at least 20 percent of competitors in shorter course duathlons and triathlons are first-timers. Honig has said that "it's a lot easier on the body to do a two-hour triathlon than to do two hours of either running, biking, or swimming."[16] According to Honig, approximately 20 percent of all participants in the events are women.

The advantage of preparing to compete in duathlons and triathlons is the benefit derived from cross-training—it helps prevent overuse problems connected with concentrated training in only one sport. The addition of training for one or two other events relieves the body of the constant pounding that comes from running five to six days a week. This relief is especially important as you age. Thus, it is not surprising to find that the average age for women in Honig's NYTC is 32 (for men it's 34), and that 75 percent of the competitors in NYTC events first competed in running races. While some athletes equally enjoy the three events of the triathlon, many prefer the duathlon because it has no swimming. Those individuals may not be able to swim, don't enjoy it, or are unable to find places to practice. Combine those problems with a limited season (in many geographic areas) for swimming, and duathlons become an acceptable alternative.

If you plan on entering your first duathlon or triathlon, here are some tips:

1. Condition your body to cope with two or three activities, one after another. Chart 6.5 has a 12-week training schedule for both events, prepared by Daniel Honig.

2. Seek advice and the company of experienced duathletes and triathletes. Many informal groups meet to train and sometimes go to races together. Having company makes training more pleasant and allows for encouragement and advice. Good places to find out about these groups are bike shops, athletic supply stores, and gyms. Bike shops also can often provide information on good local cycling routes.

3. As a beginner, you don't need to immediately spend a lot of money for a high-tech racing bike. Honig recommends training and doing your first duathlon or triathlon on whatever equipment you have available. If you find you enjoy the sport, go out and buy a good bike.[16]

4. Choose your first event carefully. The distances of the event should bring out your strengths. For example, if you are a runner, choose a duathlon or triathlon that emphasizes running.

TABLE 6.5A

....

Training Schedule for a Duathlon / Biathlon   A 12-Week Program (in Miles)
Run—3 miles • Bike—20 miles • Run—3 miles

Week	Sun.	Mon.	Tues.	Wed.	Thurs.	Fri.	Sat.	Total
1.	R-6/LSD	Rest	R-6/LSD	B-15/LSD	Rest	Rest	R-6/LSD B-20/LSD	B-35 R-18
2.	B-20/LSD R-6/LSD	Rest	R-6/LSD	B-15/HIT	R-8/LSD	Rest	R-6/HIT B-20/LSD	B-55 R-26
3.	R-6/LSD	B-6/INT R-8/LSD	Rest	B-25/LSD	B-15/HIT	Rest	R-6/HIT	B-46 R-20
4.	B-20/LSD R-6/LSD	Rest	R-6/LSD	B-6/INT	R-4/HIT	Rest	B-15/HIT R-6/LSD	B-41 R-22
5.	B-25/LSD R-6/HIT	Rest	B-15/HIT	B-8/INT R-6/LSD	R-3/INT	Rest	R-8/LSD	B-48 R-23
6.	R-4/HIT B-20/HIT	Rest	R-4/INT	B-10/INT	R-8/LSD	Rest	R-8/LSD B-25/LSD	B-55 R-24
7.	R-8/LSD B-20/HIT	Rest	R-6/HIT	B-30/LSD	R-4/INT	Rest	R-8/LSD	B-50 R-26
8.	R-6/HIT	Rest	B-20/HIT R-4/INT	B-25/LSD	B-10/INT R-6/LSD	Rest	R-10/LSD	B-55 R-26
9.	B-10/INT R-8/LSD	Rest	R-4/HIT	B-20/HIT	R-4/INT	Rest	R-10/LSD B-30/LSD	B-60 R-26
10.	R-10/LSD	Rest	R-4/INT B-20/HIT	B-10/INT	R-6/HIT	Rest	B-30/LSD R-8/LSD	B-60 R-28
11.	R-10/LSD B-8/INT	R-4/HIT	Rest	B-30/LSD	R-4/INT	Rest	B-20/HIT R-10/LSD	B-58 R-28
12.	R-6/LSD	B-20/LSD R-3/LSD	Rest	B-15/LSD	R-3/LSD	Rest	Race Day	Run 3 miles Bike 20 miles Run 3 miles

R—Running
B—Biking
LSD—Long, slow distance
INT—Interval workout

HIT—High intensity training: pace should be between LSD and INT at about 85 percent of maximum heart rate.

Prepared by Daniel Honig, NYTC

TABLE 6.5B

Training Schedule for a Triathlon   A 12-Week Program (in Miles)
Swim—1 mile • Bike—25 miles • Run—6 miles

Week	Sun.	Mon.	Tues.	Wed.	Thurs.	Fri.	Sat.	Total
1.	S-0.5/LSD R-3/LSD	Rest	R-6/LSD	B-15/LSD	S-0.5/LSD R-3/LSD	Rest	B-20/LSD R-6/LSD	S-1.0 R-18 B-35
2.	S-0.5/LSD B-20/LSD	Rest	S-0.5/LSD R-6/LSD	B-15/LSD	S-0.5/LSD R-8/LSD	Rest	R-6/LSD	S-1.5 R-20 B-35
3.	S-0.75/LSD R-6/LSD	B-6/HIT R-8/LSD	Rest	S-0.25/INT B-25/LSD	B-15/LSD	Rest	S-1.0/LSD R-6/INT	S-2.0 R-20 B-46
4.	S-0.75/LSD B-20/LSD	Rest	S-1.0/LSD R-6/LSD	B-6/INT R-4/INT	S-0.25/INT R-6/LSD	Rest	B-15/HIT R-6/LSD	S-2.0 R-22 B-41
5.	B-25/LSD R-6/HIT	S-1.0/LSD B-15/HIT	Rest	B-8/INT	S-1.0/LSD R-6/HIT	Rest	S-.25/INT R-8/LSD	S-2.25 R-20 B-48
6.	S-1.5/LSD R-4/HIT	B-20/HIT R-4/INT	Rest	S-1.0/INT B-10/INT	S-0.5/INT R-8/LSD	Rest	B-25/LSD R-8/LSD	S-3.0 R-24 B-55
7.	S-1.0/LSD B-20/HIT R-8/LSD	Rest	S-0.25/INT R-6/HIT	B-30/LSD	S-1.25/LSD R-4/INT	Rest	R-8/LSD	S-2.5 R-26 B-50
8.	S-.05/HIT R-6/HIT	Rest	B-20/HIT R-6/HIT	B-25/LSD	S-1.5/LSD B-10/INT	Rest	S-1.0/LSD R-10/LSD	S-3.0 R-22 B-55
9.	S-1.0/LSD B-10/INT R-8/LSD	Rest	S-0.25/INT R-4/HIT	B-20/HIT	S-1.5/LSD R-4/INT	Rest	B-30/LSD R-10/LSD	S-2.75 B-60 R-26
10.	S-1.5/LSD R-10/LSD	Rest	B-20/HIT R-4/INT	S-0.5/INT R-4/HIT	R-6/HIT	Rest	S-1.5/LSD B-30/LSD R-8/LSD	S-3.5 B-50 R-26
11.	B-6/INT R-10/LSD	S-1.5/LSD R-4/HIT	Rest	S-0.5/INT B-30/LSD	R-4/HIT	Rest	S-1.5/LSD B-20/HIT R-10/LSD	S-3.5 B-56 R-28
12.	R-6/LSD	S-0.75/LSD B-20/LSD R-3/LSD	Rest	B-15/LSD	S-0.5/LSD R-3/LSD	Rest	Race Day	Swim 1 mile Bike 25 miles Run 6 miles

S—Swimming
B—Biking
R—Running
LSD—Long, slow distance

INT—Interval workout
HIT—High intensity training: pace should be between LSD and INT at about 85 percent of maximum heart rate.
Prepared by Daniel Honig, NYTC

5. Go into your first race with a sound attitude. Don't get discouraged. Enjoy the atmosphere, the physical activity, the spirit of competition, the camaraderie of the athletes, and the fruits of your many months of training. With that attitude, you'll find that there will be a lifetime of other races in which to win medals.

And for Variety . . .

Walking or Running Backwards. It may never catch on as a fitness craze, but walking or running backwards, a technique used by boxers for years, has recently been incorporated into some workouts. Walking or running backwards has been shown to burn more calories and make the cardiovascular system work harder. (Even if it hadn't been documented, it certainly feels like your body is working harder.)[17] Using high-speed cinematography to film volunteers running backwards on a treadmill, researchers found that the stress and displacement is completely different when you run in reverse.[18] Whether or not it goes further than being a novelty fitness activity, some physical therapists have been using it to heal running injuries.[19] If you decide to try backwards walking or running, you should:

- choose a flat, smooth surface, for example, a running track if available.
- begin slowly. Remember, even if you're fit from walking or running, muscle specificity will cause soreness, particularly in your calf muscles.
- increase the distance slowly—perhaps start with 25 to 50 yards at a time.
- turn your head to alternate sides when you look to see where you're going. This will help prevent neck cramping on one side.

Running in Water. Scott Willett, the 1992 winner of the SOS (Survival of the Shawangunks) triathlon (held in New York's mid-Hudson valley), which has an 18.7-mile run, a 30-mile bike ride, and a 2.1-mile swim, trained for the running segment with only two 4- to 5-mile outdoor runs per week. The rest of his time was spent running in the water (and working out on a Nordic Track).[20]

Water running provides the training of land running with virtually no impact. Jogging/running on land subjects joints to a force three times the body's weight. Water, however, is a very forgiving medium. It reduces body weight to only 10 percent of what it is on land, and by its natural buoyancy takes the sting out of landing. At the same time, water offers four times the resistance of air, making for an effective training alternative. Researchers compared running on a treadmill and in water, and found that while heart rate and maximal oxygen usage were lower during water running, breathing was the same. However, the experiment's subjects perceived the exertion for their legs and breathing as higher during water running.[21] A 1996 research study confirmed findings that although

What to Do

- To run in the water, it's best to put on a flotation device such as a vest or water-ski belt. This will make it easier to stay upright. Don't lean too far forward—you'll be dog paddling, nor too far back— you'll be "bicycling." Simply lift your knee and then push the foot straight down behind you.

- A water workout can even include interval training. Use water walking as the interval workout for 30 to 90 seconds and water running for the recovery phase, also for 30 to 90 seconds.

- If you feel uncomfortable in deep water, you may prefer shallow-water running/walking in chest-deep water. Both deep and shallow water activity will foster strength, speed, and endurance.

exercising on land expended more calories than the same exercises performed in the water, moving in chest-deep water decreased ground-reaction forces, making it particularly beneficial for those suffering from orthopedic problems.[22] While seriously overweight women may want to begin their exercise routines with water running, a drawback is that you burn fewer calories, so it is less helpful in losing weight compared to land running. Even using an exercise belt—which supplies additional resistance—in the water does not significantly increase the effectiveness of water walking as measured in caloric cost.[22]

Note: Athletes, fitness enthusiasts, and dancers are using water workouts to fight their training fatigue, and to keep in shape while healing their injuries. Once healed, many continue to cross train in water to prevent staleness and new injuries. Equipment like in-water treadmills as well as pools with built-in currents for additional resistance are becoming available as water exercise becomes more popular.

Water walking. Water walking is more difficult than water running. Water reverses the normal land progression of escalating difficulty as you go from walking to jogging and then to running. By straightening your arms and your legs (lock them so they don't bend) when you water walk, you cause them to act like long levers, thus creating more water resistance. Try both exercises, and you will immediately see the difference—walking is harder.

BEYOND RUNNING

Backpacking

While it's been said that backpacking is a perfect way to ruin a hike, it is a form of recreation for many Americans—although currently it's two and one half times more popular among men than women.[23] Backpacking combines intensive physical activity with an appreciation of nature, and while possible year-round, the most favored times are spring through fall. Backpacking involves hoisting from 35 to 60 pounds on your back and walking several miles a day for a series of days. While a backpacking trip can be as short as overnight, there are many individuals who stay out for extended periods. When the walk is from beginning to end on a major hiking trail, for example, the 2,100-mile Appalachian Trail or Vermont's 270-mile Long Trail, participants are known as "thru-hikers." In a study of thru-hikers on the Appalachian Trail, one of the authors of this book found them to be thoughtful, energetic, and enthusiastic individuals who are strongly motivated to bring about some changes in their lives.[24] These intrepid souls have stepped off life's treadmill and have set aside long periods of time (sometimes as much as six months) to "just" walk with nothing but the possessions they carry on their backs.

To some, blisters and aching muscles are just as much a part of backpacking as panoramic views and songs by the campfire—but they needn't be. To minimize problems and maximize enjoyment, hikers need to prepare their bodies and pack their first-aid kits before setting foot on the trail.

Fit to Hit the Trail

The most important prevention you can do before a hike is to condition yourself physically. The best way to do this is with exercises that simulate hiking. Climbing stairs and, particularly, descending stairs two steps at a time are excellent ways to get your legs and knees in hiking shape. Walking up and down hills also conditions the proper muscle groups. Bicycling can strengthen thigh muscles, which may help prevent knee pain from spoiling your trip. In addition, you can augment your stair-climbing and walking regimen by lifting weights: biceps curls, squats, and seated knee straightening and bending all can be useful.

After a week or two of conditioning exercises, wear a backpack with about 30 pounds (several 5-pound bags of flour, potatoes, books, or sugar) in it while climbing stairs or walking hills. Wearing your backpack before your big trip will also help you identify which parts of your body might rub against the pack. To avoid sore spots, you can pad those areas or adjust your shoulder and hip straps. This pre-hike conditioning time is also a good chance to break in your hiking boots.

A Pack of Potential Problems

Backpackers are vulnerable to a wide range of health problems, from blisters to Lyme disease.[25] Farsighted prevention such as packing a first-aid kit and taking a first-aid course can reduce your risk.[26] Also, choose a hike best suited to your experience and abilities. If you're a novice, warm up with a weekend trip before trying a longer trek.

The following excerpts from *The Physician and Sportsmedicine*, reprinted here with permission, provide useful information about trail first aid.[27]

"**Blisters.** By far the most bothersome problem is blisters. They usually develop within the first few days of the trip. The best safeguard is to wear a lightweight pair of hiking boots that are thoroughly broken in. Two pairs of socks may also help. Next to your skin wear socks made of a material, such as polypropylene, that wicks moisture away from your skin. Wear wool socks over those. Foot powder can also reduce friction.

During rest stops, immediately identify any tender, inflamed areas that will eventually form blisters, and cover these with adhesive bandages or moleskin. If a blister does develop, a ring of moleskin surrounding the raised area can alleviate discomfort.

Don't tear the top off an intact blister, but if it swells considerably, opening it will promote faster skin reattachment. You should puncture the blister three times within the first 24 hours to drain the fluid. But first, sterilize a needle or pin by placing it in a flame until its tip is red hot; then allow it to cool. Apply an antibiotic ointment and sterile bandage after each puncture. If the blister is torn open, apply an antibiotic ointment and a bandage or a hydrogel dressing.

Leg and Foot Pain. Because hiking stresses the bones and muscles of the legs and feet, leg and foot pain is common. Rest or anti-inflammatory drugs can alleviate such pain. Another option is to carry a lighter load; if possible, try to keep your pack between 30 and 40 pounds.

Days off can help ease a multitude of maladies, including leg and foot pain. At least 1 day off during a week's hike is recommended.

Toenail Loss. Many backpackers develop blackened toenails or lose one or more toenails. This is caused by repeated pressure, such as when the toes are jammed to the front of the boot during steep descents. Depending on the length of the trip, hikers can lose toenails during the trip, or after they get back home. To decrease toenail damage, kick your heel to the back of your boot before snugly lacing it, keep your toenails trimmed, and avoid undersized boots.

Chafing. Not surprisingly, repeated rubbing against the backpack produces chafing. To prevent this, adjust the contents of the pack so that the weight rests on your hips and the small of your back. If a tender area does develop, treat it immediately by realigning the pack, padding the irritated skin, and applying petroleum jelly to your skin.

Some hikers' thighs will rub against each other. If this is a problem, wear long pants or bikers' shorts, and use talcum powder or corn starch to keep the area dry.

Scrapes, Scratches, and Sunburn. Any time you're in the wild you are prone to scrapes, scratches, and minor cuts from branches or from falling. Even the best-maintained trail has plenty of natural obstacles. Long-sleeved shirts and long pants protect your skin from the sun and decrease the chance of insect bites, plant irritations, and abrasions. For further sunburn protection, wear a wide-brimmed hat and a sunscreen with a sun protection factor of at least 15. Apply plenty of sunscreen to your nose and lips.

Eating Problems. Some backpackers don't get the right nutrition because they skimp on food to make their pack lighter. The average backpacker needs about 4,000 calories a day from a balanced, nutritious diet high in carbohydrates from starchy foods, such as rice, noodles, and potatoes. You may want to supplement your hiking diet with a daily multivitamin pill. Some backpackers suffer from constipation, even though exercise can improve intestinal function. To keep your digestive system working well and to avoid dehydration, drink plenty of water.

Parasites. Giardia lamblia, a microscopic water-borne parasite, can be a significant problem in some areas. To avoid this parasite, which may cause diarrhea, abdominal pain, and general misery, boil your water for 3 minutes or use a good quality water filter.

A major infectious health problem that was not a concern until recent years is Lyme disease, which is transmitted by a tiny deer tick and is most prevalent in the Northeast, Midwest, and West Coast states. Wear long light-colored clothing with your pants tucked into your socks to help deter ticks.

If you find a tick embedded in your skin, use small pointed tweezers to grasp the tick as close to your skin as possible. Then gently pull straight up without twisting."

Hiking into the Sunset

Don't let potential problems deter you. The physical and emotional benefits of backpacking far outweigh the drawbacks. Adequate preparation and conditioning will help ensure a safe and healthy hike.

OFF THE BEATEN TRACK

Ride and Tie

Although equestrian sports have many virtues, physical and aerobic conditioning for the rider is not one of them. However, one format—Ride and Tie—challenges both horse and rider. It involves running, riding, endurance, and strategy for the team, composed of two runners and one horse. The objective of this internationally recognized sport is to complete a cross-country course (anywhere from 10 to 40 miles) by utilizing teamwork and tactics to maximize each individual's running and riding ability.

The sport traces its origins to a long-ago means of transportation whereby two people with only one horse could travel great distances without wearing down their horse. It became a sport in 1971 when the first competitive Ride and Tie race was held.

In a race, the gun starts everybody off—one partner from each team riding and the other running. The riders go as far as they think their teammates can run. At that point they dismount, tie their horses to trees (or other secure places), and start running. The horses rest until the trailing teammates reach them, mount, and ride to catch up to their partners. A quick exchange of words or signals with their partners lets the second riders know whether to trade places, or continue riding to some distant point on the trail, tie the horses, and start to run again. The teammates alternate running and riding in "leap-frog" fashion. While the minimum number of exchanges permitted is six, strategies can differ. For example, some teammates may switch up to 100 times during a 30- or 40-mile race.

The horses are protected—possibly more so than the humans. Before the event they must first pass a strict veterinary exam. During the race, the teams pass through many "vet checks," check points where the horses are inspected by veterinarians. For more information about this unique sport, contact the Ride and Tie Association, 11735 Wolf Road, Grass Valley, California 95949 (916-268-8474).

Horse Riding

If Ride and Tie is not for you, and yet you want to be more than a passenger on your horse, consider trying to incorporate fitness and physical activity as part of your equestrian endeavors. Unfortunately, a great many riders see no irony in trying to perform when they are unfit or too weak in key muscle groups to ride with finesse. You should be as much of an athlete as is your horse. You need well-developed leg, lower back, side, and abdominal muscles for achieving balance and control atop your horse. Those muscles also help maintain "your seat," and guide your horse in propulsion and directional changes. Exercises designed to increase muscular tone as well as relax joints in these areas are helpful. Because correct posture is also fundamental to maintaining your seat, emphasis should be placed on exercises that help correct alignment. In addition to many of the exercises described in Chapter 4 (Focus on Fitness), exercise videos are now available that demonstrate strengthening and stretching maneuvers useful in preparing for riding. Articles about physical conditioning for the rider also appear periodically in the various horse journals. Some have even been directed to the new mother, providing suggestions on how to get back into shape for riding after the baby has arrived.[28] These exercises should be done at home on a regular basis.

Getting Ready.   As any student of horsemanship knows, a rider doesn't go to the barn, tack up her horse, and start out riding at a canter without warming up her horse. If she does, her horse may pull a muscle and go lame. But riders need to warm up as well. Even the most physical of labors does not prepare the human body for the muscle specificity required for riding. If anything, they may limit it. A proper warm-up can prepare the muscles and joints for the ride ahead.

There are two types of warm-up. One prepares the body physically for the muscle-specific actions necessary for riding. The other coordinates the mind and body, so the rider can develop harmony with the horse, imperative for a good ride. Unfortunately, riders usually don't warm up, although both types can be included in a session without appreciably cutting into real riding time.

Muscle Specifics. As unusual as it may seem, riders can incorporate a warm-up into the grooming and tacking procedure if they take the time to consciously direct attention to their muscles and joints as much as to their horse's needs. For example, in grooming, the rider should use the standard body positions, bending and flexing both sides of the body. Switching hands may not seem like much, but bilateral usage can make a difference if you are one-sided and stiff.

Brushing strokes that traverse the horse's length and use suitable muscular pressure translate to upper body exercise. Toe rises (to reach the top and across to the other side of the horse) and bending (either at the hips or knees) to brush the horse's legs can be used to stimulate lower leg circulation and musculature. Cleaning the horse's hoofs while in a crouched position serves as isometric exercise for the quadriceps, especially because it should be done bilaterally. Here again standard position calls for a change of hand and body flexion as you work on each side.

Saddling the horse can also turn into an exercise because the saddle serves as a weight (western saddles can weigh more than 40 pounds), and the act of carrying and hoisting it onto the horse involves upper body musculature. *Note:* It is a good idea to warm-up your back muscles before grabbing and lifting a saddle.

Your warm-up can continue if you opt to begin the horse's warm-up with a lunge (a form of ground training). While lunging doesn't serve as exercise for the rider if done in the traditional way—with the lunger standing dead center and the horse revolving around the circumference of the enclosure—there is nothing to stop the lunger from moving with the horse rather than standing in the middle.

You are now ready to mount, and even that procedure can be used to best physical advantage. Concentrate on improving your mounting technique so that it looks effortless and graceful. This is no small muscular feat and worth pursuing on both the right and left sides.

Horseback Exercise.   The physical activity of your warm-up need not cease, as it so often does, once you're mounted. Before starting your lesson or trail ride, exercises can be done that stress balance, coordination, and relaxation. While they are ostensibly for the upper body, they do involve bending and leg stretching, and reinforce muscular synchronization and control. The following exercises were recommended by Bonnie Perreault, a Rhode Island-based trainer.[29]

Beginning. The warm-up should start at the walk, either on the trail, around the field, or in the ring. According to Ms. Perreault, the walk is something of a forgotten gait. It takes time to develop a good walk, and it is time well spent for any riding discipline. The walk is the foundation of all future work.

The walk should be carried out on a loose rein, so that the horse has a chance to slowly move into weight bearing. It will also allow you the time to work on your exercises.

Stretch It Out. At the walk, **shoulder rotations** can be the first warm-up exercise. Shoulder rotations (described earlier in this chapter) are simple and easy but highly beneficial in relaxing the upper torso and aiding in postural realignment. This suppling warm-up can also be reversed by bringing the shoulders forward in raised position. This will increase shoulder range of motion and release the chest as well as raise the upper back.

Note: If you believe your horse may "spook" during your initial stretching exercises, ask a friend to help you, either by staying near the horse's head or controlling the horse on a lunge line.

Adding Arms. After shoulder rotation, you can perform a series of easy stretches. In the first stretch, you raise one arm overhead with thumb facing back and palm toward your ear. The **arm lift** is done while you sit evenly in the saddle, with the reins held in one hand. Do not use excessive force or stretch. Undue force will cause imbalance of your seat, and will pull muscles instead of relaxing them. The hand of the upraised arm should be open and soft and not clenched into a fist, as this would cause the muscles to tense. The actual time for the arm lift should be between 15 to 20 seconds per arm, but if cramping or fatigue sets in, cut back the time. Stay aware of your sitting position—try for evenness in both stirrups and no sideward displacement.

This is a moderately safe and simple movement that accomplishes an overall lengthening and straightening of the upper torso. This simple arm lifting stretch, when done with an attempt to gently expand the chest and align the shoulders, calls upon the broad back muscles and stretches the all-important riding muscles in the front of your body (namely the external oblique, internal oblique, and rectus abdominis).

And Now the Legs. The arm lift can be combined with a gentle leg stretch across the diagonal of the body. This exercise, the **diagonal body stretch**, uses opposite leg and arm to accomplish a relaxation of the muscle groups of the upper torso as well as an increased loosening of those muscles in the lower lumbar area. The lower extremities are also activated into a gentle stretch with some lengthening of the inner thigh adductor (commonly known as the "grippers"), as well as relaxation through the hip, knee, and ankle joints.

The diagonal body stretch should follow the same time framework as for the arm lift. In this exercise, however, the raised arm should be angled to produce a diagonal line with your opposite leg, which has been removed from the stirrup. You should remain even through the seat but try to push your foot and hand away from each other, across the diagonal of your body. According to Ms. Perreault, this stretch has proven effective for riders who suffer from low back pain.

Last But Not Least, the Pelvis. The simplest way to stretch this area is to do several **pelvic waist turns.** Twist your entire upper body toward the rear, but only as far as your pelvis will rotate. Don't leave your pelvis locked as you continue to rotate with your upper body but rather move your body as a unit, with the pelvis dictating the extent of the rotation (when it stops, you stop twisting). Return to your starting position and then twist to the opposite side.

The next exercise, the **backward leg stretch,** is ideal because it will relax your hip muscles, drop your legs into position, and put you deep into the saddle. *Note:* Because your movements in this particular exercise have the potential for "spooking" your horse, proceed with caution and do not assume that your horse is going to remain placid. Both this and the next exercise should first be practiced while your horse is not moving; when you and your horse are comfortable, do them at a walk.

Take one foot out of the stirrup, lean slightly forward into your crotch, bend your leg, and bring your foot up and behind the saddle, as far up as you can without causing pain. Don't grab hold of the foot, because this will only force the position and also will disrupt your even seat in the saddle. Once your leg is up as high as you can bring it, sit back slowly onto your buttocks and remain in this position for 5 to 10 seconds. Then drop your leg back down to the horse's side. Let your leg drop quickly and completely instead of lowering it back into place. Repeat the exercise on the same leg 2 more times and then do the other leg 3 times. Finally, try to bring both legs up and behind the saddle at the same time; sit back onto your buttocks and hold for 5 to 10 seconds, then bring both legs back to the starting position.

This exercise can be combined with a **forward leg stretch** to the horse's shoulder. In this exercise, you raise your entire leg forward, following the guidelines for time and repetition previously described for the backward leg stretch. This forward and back combination should significantly release your hips, giving you a larger range of motion.

Mental Conditioning. Many equestrians are nine-to-five workers who push themselves all day at work, accumulating a good deal of intellectual and emotional stress in addition to eight hours' worth of muscle-shortening inactivity. After a busy day, they rush to catch a few hours of relaxation with their horses. However, many times, the reverse occurs and there is more tension and physical strain for both parties involved. The tense rider can, often unknowingly, cause a loss of cooperation by the horse; the resulting disharmony causes further tension. Some things can be done to prevent this from happening. Before you start working with your horse, make an assessment of the mental attitude of the horse and yourself. If the horse is a bundle of energy, having spent the last two days in the stall, it is not fair to expect a quiet performance. If you are in a bad mood,

What to Do

These basic maneuvers can help relieve tension in your upper torso and lower extremities. They should be done routinely, as standard operating procedure before any lesson or trail ride. They can also be done at any time during the ride to maintain what was obtained at the ride's start—relaxed muscles and joints, which contribute to a pleasurable riding experience. A relaxed and supple horse and rider are the smoothest of partners.

riding may not produce any great change (outside of possibly the mood getting worse), especially if the horse is affected by your mood and reacts accordingly.

You should be in a mental condition that will allow for patience, for yourself as well as your horse. Tempers and impatience can spell doom in a horse's training. Your horse may benefit more, for example, from a trail ride, an in-hand training session (such as on long lines or lunging), or even a two-hour grooming, instead of the ring work that you had planned.

Putting It Together

The above are just preliminary suggestions; the potential exists for warm-ups that provide for meaningful physical activity for you as well as for your horse. The restructuring of the pre-ride routine will maximize the opportunities for exercises that will benefit you, will not harm your horse, and will lead to a more physically pleasant ride, not to mention a harmonious and efficient preparation for competition.

Protect Your Head

Over 60 percent of all horse-related deaths involve head injury. Experience, training, and the quietest horse are no guarantee of safety. If you fall, your unprotected head can receive over 1,000 G's of force. Helmets are a **must** every time you ride. Whether you do English, Western, driving, cutting, dressage, jumping, or pleasure riding, wearing an SEI (Safety Equipment Institute) certified helmet is one way to minimize or prevent injury. An excellent and effective 20-minute educational video (Every Time. . . . Every Ride) is available from Washington State 4-H Foundation (7612 Pioneer Way, Puyallup, WA 98371-4998, 206-840-4570). Every member of the horse community should be required to see this video.

In addition to riding helmets, protective vests that absorb impact during a fall, and "quick release" stirrups are available. Unfortunately, riders too often prove the old saw about horses: you can lead them to water but you can't make them drink. Riders have been slow to accept and use any of this tested and demonstrably worthwhile safety equipment.[30]

THE BALL IS IN YOUR COURT

Life is not a spectator sport; use your body or lose it! —Sara, age 42

From on foot to atop a horse, women are on the go, pursuing an active life. Don't be left holding the ball—move on out.

ENDNOTES

1. van Mechelen, W. Running injuries: A review of the epidemiological literature. *Sports Medicine*, 1992, 14(5), 320–335.

2. Auble, T. E., & Schwartz, R. E. Physiological effects of exercising with handweights. *Sports Medicine*, 1991, 11(4), 244–256.

3. Morgan, D. W., Kohrt, W. M., Bates, F. J., et al. Effects of respiratory muscle endurance training on ventilatory and endurance performance of moderately trained cyclists. *International Journal of Sports Medicine*, 1987, 8(2), 88–93.

4. Nieman, D. C., & George, D. M. Personality traits that correlate with success in distance running. *Journal of Sports Medicine and Physical Fitness*, 1987, 27(3), 345–356.

5. Stockton, W. Exercising at high altitude. *New York Times*, August 22, 1988, c13.

6. Longman, J. 13,800 ft up, runners toil to excel below. *New York Times*, October 22, 1995, a1.

7. Ziegler, S. G., Klinzing, J., & Williamson, K. The effects of two stress management training programs on cardiorespiratory efficiency. *Journal of Sports Psychology*, 1982, 4, 280–289.

8. Hatfield, B. D., Spalding, W., Mahon, A. D., et al. The effect of psychological strategies on cardiorespiratory and muscular activity during treadmill running. *Medicine and Science in Sports and Exercise*, 1992, 24(2), 218–225.

9. Smith, A. L., Gill, D. L., Crews, D. J., et al. Attentional strategy use by experienced distance runners: Physiological and psychological effects. *Research Quarterly for Exercise and Sport*, 1985, 66(2), 142–150.

10. Amdur, N. Marathon runners tell poll benefits outweigh problems. *New York Times*, October 21, 1983, a1, 30.

11. Martin, D. E. Marathoners vs ultramarathoners. *The Physician and Sportsmedicine*, 1982, 10(9), 11–12.

12. Dolgener, F. A., Kolkhorst, F. W., & Whitsett, D. A. Long slow distance training in novice marathoners. *Research Quarterly for Exercise and Sport*, 1994, 65(4), 339–346.

13. Amdur, N. Marathon runners tell poll benefits outweigh problems. *New York Times*, October 21, 1983, a1, 30.

14. Higdon, H. *Marathon: The Ultimate Training and Racing Guide*. Emmaus, PA: Rodale Press, 1993.

15. Dolgener, F. A., Kolkhorst, F. W., & Whitsett, D. A. Long slow distance training in novice marathoners. *Research Quarterly for Exercise and Sport*, 1994, 65(4), 339–346.

16. Daniel Honig, personal communication.

17. Capriani, D. J., Armstrong D. J., & Gaul, S. Backward walking at three levels of treadmill inclination. *Journal of Orthopaedic and Sports Physical Therapy*, 1995, 22(3), 95–102.

18. Fitzhenry, A. And now, running backwards. *Staten Island Advance*, October 27, 1986, B6.

    The Walking Magazine. Put your best foot backward. *The Walking Magazine*, 1991, 6(3), 10–12.

19. Morton, C. Running backward may help athletes move forward. *The Physician and Sportsmedicine*, 1986, 14, 149–152.

20. Scott Willett, personal communication.

21. Svedenhag, J., & Seger, J. Running on land and in water: Comparative exercise physiology. *Medicine and Science in Sports and Exercise*, 1992, October, 24(10), 1155–1160.

22. Robert, J. J., Jones, L., & Bobo, M. The physiologic response of exercising in the water and on land with and without the X1000 Walk 'N Tone exercise belt. *Research Quarterly for Exercise and Sport*, 1996, 67(3), 310–315.

23. Puretz, S. Appalachian trail thru-hikers tell all. *American Hiker*, Summer, 1990, 26–27.

    Puretz, S. Trail notes. *Backpacker*, September, 1991, 19(6), 79.

24. Puretz, S. L. Profile of the Long Distance Hiker on the Appalachian Trail. In L. Vander Velden, L. Chalip, & J. Humphrey (eds.). *Psychology and Sociology of Sport: Current Selected Research: Volume III*. New York: AMS Press, 1998.

25. Puretz, S. L. Health problems of the long-distance backpacker. *Australian Journal of Science and Medicine in Sport*, 1992, 24(2), 55–59.

26. Puretz, S. L. First-aid supplies for backpacking. *British Journal of Sports Medicine*, 1992, 26(1), 48–50.

27. Puretz, S. L. Backpacking: Preparing—and repairing—your body. *Physician and Sportsmedicine*, 1992, 20(4), 183–184.

28. Perreault, B. J., & Puretz, S. L. After

the baby: Getting back in shape. *The Sentinel*, 22(23), 1994, 14–15.

29. Puretz, S. L., & Perreault, B. J. A rider's sound and practical warm-up: Part I. *Horse Illustrated*, May, 1993, 17(5), 92–95.

Puretz, S. L., & Perreault, B. J. A rider's sound and practical warm-up: Part II. *Horse Illustrated*, June, 1993, 17(6), 48–50.

30. Campagna, D. Riders not embracing safety equipment. *Albany Times Union*, August 29, 1995, c1,3.

7 The Competitive Edge

ADELAIDE HAAS, PH.D.

My boyfriend thought our women's softball game was kind of funny. He couldn't get over the women complimenting the other team when they had a good play. "Guys just don't do that," he said. —Barbara, age 21, college student

THE WINNING WOMAN

The women playing softball with Barbara generally viewed their game as fun and friendly. Having a good time was more important than winning. Many team members admitted to "not being very good," and others said that "anyone who wanted to play was welcome." This contrasts with many local-level male teams where men who are aging and slowing down feel compelled to drop out so as not to be a handicap for the other players.

Women, as well as men, exercise and engage in sports for various reasons. We want to feel healthy, stay trim, and enjoy the camaraderie. Sometimes, we really want to win. About one-third (31 percent) of the women in our survey reported that they competed, actively strove to win, in some of their physical activities. Games such as tennis, and team sports like softball, appear to be competitive by their very nature. However, we found that it was the attitude, as seen in Barbara's example, more than the activity which defined competition.

About the same number of women in our survey indicated that they ran for exercise as indicated that they swam. While both activities can easily be performed without a thought to winning, about half the runners competed, while only 1 percent of the swimmers did.

On the other hand, every game of tennis, softball, and soccer has a winner and a loser. Yet of the women who played tennis, only 13 percent indicated that they "competed." About 42 percent of the softball players considered their game competitive, compared to

60 percent of the soccer players. Our data strongly suggest that it is motivation more than the actual activity which determines competitiveness.

Attitudes

The Competitive Personality.   What makes people want to compete? Coaches know that "mind-set" is almost as important for winners as physical readiness. James Gavin, a researcher at Concordia University in Montreal, devised a simple scale that can be used to assess your competitive nature.[1] You can test yourself on it using Table 7-1.

Non-competitive people tend to prefer to simply go out and hit tennis balls or rally rather than play a game and keep score. Competitors who enjoy running want to know who in their age/sex category is participating in a particular race so that they can predict their chances of bringing home a ribbon. Non-competitors may keep track of their own times or accomplishments, and if they are competitive it is only with themselves. However, as "non-competitors" begin to excel, they may want to compare themselves with others and enter the competitive arena.

"The Iceberg Profile." Successful athletes, especially elite ones, have been described as having "the iceberg profile." This does not mean that they are cold or pointed. The iceberg profile is based on psychological mood characteristics. According to several research studies, top competitors tend to be below average in these traits: tension, depression, anger, fatigue, and confusion. However, they score higher than normal in vigor. When all characteristics are graphed they resemble an iceberg, with vigor at the peak.[2]

Over-doers. Some competitive people go overboard in their desire to win. At an extreme is the infamous Nancy Kerrigan incident. In 1994, three men (including the bodyguard of Olympic ice-skating contender Tonya Harding) were arrested for assaulting competitor Nancy Kerrigan. Harding's role in this attack was never made explicit, but she, at the least, knew about the planned violence and did not attempt to stop it. In Cinderella fashion and with much media attention, Nancy Kerrigan went on to win the Olympic silver medal.[3]

Not all overly competitive individuals are involved in aggressive behavior toward others. Some direct their competitiveness inward. Athletes who train too much, lose too much weight, or otherwise abuse their own health and welfare are also over-doers. The female triad (eating disorders, amenorrhea, and eventually osteoporosis) is the price some women athletes pay for striving too hard.[4] This is discussed in more detail in Chapter 18, Beware of the Danger Zones and Chapter 11, Menstrual Matters.

Being "Feminine."   The traditional female role may conflict with the competitive personality. Researchers have identified some traits as being particularly masculine and others as

TABLE 7.1

....

Competitive / Noncompetitive Style Inventory

For each question, circle the word that best describes you.

Mostly – I am this way most of the time.　　　　**Sometimes** – I am sometimes or occasionally this way.
Often – I am often or frequently this way.　　　　**Rarely** – I am rarely or never this way.

	Mostly	Often	Sometimes	Rarely
1. I enjoy competitive games and sports.	4	3	2	1
2. I perform better when I am competing against someone equally skilled.	4	3	2	1
3. I avoid situations where there are winners & losers.	1	2	3	4
4. I get anxious or upset when friends start acting competitively.	1	2	3	4
5. I find competitive situations very stressful.	1	2	3	4
6. I like to challenge friends when we play social games.	4	3	2	1
7. Competition bothers me.	1	2	3	4
8. It bothers me to watch people fighting each other to get ahead.	1	2	3	4

Scoring
Add up the points from each of your answers. Then, write your total score in the space provided. Identify your competitive/noncompetitive style in the list below.

Category	Style	Score Range
1	Highly competitive	28–32
2	Moderately competitive	23–27
3	Intermediate	18–22
4	Moderately noncompetitive	13–17
5	Highly noncompetitive	8–12

Your Total Score _____　　Your Rating Category _____

....

Adapted from *Psychosocial Activity Dimension Scales*: used with permission of James Gavin, Ph.D., Dept. of Applied Social Sciences, Concordia University, Montreal, Canada

being more feminine. For example, "independence" and "willingness to take risks" are considered masculine, while "sensitivity to the needs of others" and "affection" have been labeled as more feminine. Although both women and men are a composite of these traits, some leanings toward the "feminine" may result in noncompetitive urges.[5]

The Caring Woman. In her book *In a Different Voice*,[6] psychologist Carol Gilligan pioneered the analysis of some important psychological differences between the sexes. Gilligan and later researchers suggest that most women engage in tasks with a strong "ethic of care" and empathy. So even when a woman may want to win, she also is deeply sensitive to the feelings of others.[7] This may help to explain Barbara's softball game, described at the beginning of this chapter. Members of opposing teams can care about and encourage one another.

Lucky Me. **Attribution theory** is a psychological view of how events are perceived. According to several studies, more females than males attribute the outcome of an athletic contest to factors outside of themselves. That is: Girls and women are more likely to say that they performed well because they were lucky, it was a good day, the other team was not in their usual top form, etc. Boys and men more often acknowledge that winning comes from their own internal factors such as skill and hard work.[8]

The Impostor Syndrome. Related to this is the **"impostor syndrome,"** in which successful people believe that it is just a fluke or luck that they have achieved a particular accomplishment. These people believe that they are masquerading as winners and are not actually who others believe them to be. While both truly successful men and women may believe they are impostors, this incorrect assessment is found more often among women.[9]

Fear of Success. Winning may be viewed as a two-sided accomplishment. On the one hand, if you win, you have succeeded. You are better than your opponent, and you can bask in your victory. On the other hand, however, you may fear that others will like you less if you have demonstrated better skill. This goes beyond the "caring" described earlier, where you do not want to hurt another's feelings. The attitude we are now considering is self-protective, trying to guard oneself against the negative aspects of success.

Consider the following situation, reported to us by one of our college students:

My boyfriend, Harry, and I used to run together at least three times a week. He's been running for years and I just started several months ago, although I've always been athletic. Lately I've noticed that I can go faster than he can. I think this bothers him, because he's started to make excuses about not being able to meet me to run.

I'm afraid that I've injured his ego, and he may not like me anymore. I've considered quitting running and going back to other types of exercise, running slower, or dumping Harry. At this point I'm kind of in limbo.

—SallyAnn, age 22, college student

The concept of "fear of success" was first described by psychologist Matina Horner. Its cornerstones are: (1) high achievement is inconsistent with femininity, and (2) female success carries with it the threat of social rejection. Horner based her theory on responses of men and women to a hypothetical situation:

"After first-term finals, Anne (or John in half the stories) finds her/himself at the top of her/his medical school class."

Horner found that the majority of women predicted negative outcomes for Anne but a happy future for John. On the other hand, the men who participated in the study did not generally predict problems associated with success.[10]

Thinking Your Way to Victory.   To become really good at anything, you have to develop the right mind-set. You need to develop self-confidence, set goals, engage in mental rehearsal, manage anxiety, and learn to flow.[11] We discuss each of these in turn.

Developing Self-Confidence. Often we decide that we do not even want to try various tasks because we are afraid that we will not be able to succeed. It is easier to say "Oh, I can't do that," rather than tackle the task. Lack of confidence may come from having experienced criticism in the past. Sometimes friends or family members, in an attempt to be helpful, can be so critical as to impair your self-confidence.

Lack of confidence may also be the result of unrealistic comparisons. For example, if you decide that you want to learn to ski and your first attempt is with a friend who is an expert, you are likely to come away with feelings of inadequacy. Similarly, many women are discouraged by commercial exercise/aerobics video tapes that show dancers engaging in difficult movements. These women would be better served by a very elementary approach and models who are more within reach. Expertise in most things takes a long time to accomplish. *Hint:* To develop self-confidence, set realistic goals that take you forward from where you are now.

Setting Goals. Whatever type of athletic endeavor interests you, you will progress best if you set appropriate goals.

• **Make your goals personal.** It does not matter what someone else has accomplished; you are working toward your own personal best. Your goal may simply be to go out and run or walk for half an hour five times a week without regard to speed.

• **Set goals that are appropriate to your current level.** Do not expect to complete a marathon if you have not successfully run shorter distances. Don't ski down "double diamonds" before you have mastered "green" and "blue" slopes. Goals that are beyond your current skill will only lead to frustration and loss of self-confidence.

• **Set specific goals.** It is better to say you will walk/run a mile or walk/run for X number of minutes than to say you'll walk/run for a while.

> **Good goal:** In tennis, hit five backhands in a row down the line.
>
> **Poor goal:** Play as hard as you can.

• **Set short-term goals that lead toward long-term goals.** In the tennis example above, short-term goals would be: try to hit one good backhand on day one, two on day three, three on day five, four on day seven, and five on day ten.

• **Keep track of your accomplishments.** Write down your time, distance, hits, or scores on a regular basis. This way you can monitor your improvement.

• **Recognize that progress is slow.** Don't expect overnight miracles. While your objectives should be challenging, they should also be realistic.

• **Don't be depressed by setbacks.** Progress is not only slow, it is erratic. Some weeks you may find that you are moving forward; other weeks you may feel nothing is happening, or worse, that you are slipping back. This is normal. Be patient, stay with it, and the tide will turn.

Mental Imaging. Dr. Jerry Lynch, sports psychologist and marathoner, writes in *Runner's World*,[12] "Visualization is the foundation from which your greatest dreams can be realized." In most spheres of life, accomplishment occurs by first setting goals (having a dream) and then imagining them happening.

To use mental imaging in athletics, you must set aside a time when you are likely to be free of interruptions. In a comfortable sitting or lying position, breathe deeply and slowly for about one minute. Then picture yourself in your physical activity. Engage all your senses. Every part of your body is relaxed, yet focused and strong. If your game is tennis, try to visualize exactly how you would hit the ball if you did everything exactly right. If you are a swimmer, imagine yourself cutting through the water with smooth, efficient, powerful strokes.

Another way to utilize mental imagery is to watch others who are very accomplished. By closely observing the pros on television or in actual competition, and participating with them in your mind's eye, you will enhance your own skills.[13]

Managing Anxiety

I wake up early the morning of a race, and I feel raring to go. But I also tend to have a queasiness in my stomach and sometimes a touch of diarrhea. When I get to the stadium, I feel a rush of excitement. I feel my body's adrenaline pumping me up and making me ready to go go go. However, my palms are also sweating with nervousness. —Tahisha, age 27, local running competitor

Anxiety before any competition is normal, but does it help or hinder performance? Scientists have tried to measure anxiety and understand its role in competitive athletics.

• **The Case for the Inverted U.** The "inverted U" hypothesis suggests that a certain degree of psychological arousal (including anxiety) is necessary for peak performance. Coaches work to pep up their team members so that they will give their best. On the other hand, too much anxiety will be detrimental to success. The inverted U pattern, which depicts the general relationship between arousal and performance, was first described by theorists Yerkes and Dodson in 1908. It has been evaluated since in numerous studies.[14] Some researchers claim that it is too simplistic and not quite accurate. Newer ideas such as "**catastrophe theory**" and "**zones of optimal function**" have received considerable scientific attention.

• **Catastrophe Theory.** In brief, catastrophe theory predicts that once a person is overly aroused, that individual's performance deteriorates dramatically (or catastrophically), unlike the gradual decline depicted in the inverted U.

• **Zones of Optimal Function.** Zones of optimal function refer to the individuality of athletes. This theory suggests that no single explanation of arousal and anxiety holds for all. Some people can function well with a very high level of arousal, while others would fall apart in a similar emotional state.[15]

According to research studies, the more skilled the athlete, the higher the level of arousal or anxiety that is needed to obtain optimum performance. Beginners do better with lower levels. In addition, arousal tends to be greatest when the competition is perceived to be most intense.[16]

Finding Your Zone of Optimal Function

Scientists have used questionnaires that probe athletes' level of anxiety. They have compared performance in specific events with reported anxiety levels. While instruments such as the Sport Competition Anxiety Test (SCAT)[17] may be impractical for most of us to use, you might attempt to note your arousal level on a scale of one to five prior to a competition and then afterward record your performance and the conditions.

Once you have a feeling for the amount of pre-event arousal that works best for you, you can try to increase or decrease it for optimum performance. To increase your arousal, give yourself a mental pep talk and try to "psych yourself up" prior to an event. Reducing arousal may be more difficult. Techniques such as attempting to relax body parts through mental focus, visualizing calming scenes, and preparing yourself to "flow" (described below) may all be helpful.[18]

Learn to "Flow."   Lorraine Moller, a New Zealand elite runner, commented on the women racers from Kenya who placed first and second in a recent mini-marathon. Moller suggested, "In our Western culture, I think we get too bogged down with time and place and strategies." When asked how to catch up to the Kenyans, she responded, "I think just throw away your watches."[19]

Susan Jackson, a professor of Human Movement Studies and Psychology at the University of Queensland in Australia, has studied the "flow" experience in elite athletes.[20] One aspect of flow is described as "transformation of time." You are in the moment. As Lorraine Moller advised, you've thrown away your watch.

Flow also involves enjoyment and concentration. An elite athlete interviewed by Jackson described the feeling this way:

"Where I've been happiest with my performance, and I've felt sort of one with the water, and my stroke, and everything . . . I was really tuned into what I was doing. I knew exactly how I was going to swim the race, and I just knew I had it all under control, and I got in and ah, I was really aware of what the whole, of what everyone in the race was doing . . . and I was just totally absorbed in my stroke, and I knew I was passing them all but I didn't care. I mean it's not that I didn't care. I was going, 'Oh, this is cool!' And just swam and won, and I was totally in control of the situation. It was really cool."[20]

How Is Flow Achieved? Top athletes experience flow when they are performing at their best. But how do **you** do it? The following suggestions may help:

• **Focus**. Try to pay attention to what you are doing. Concentrate on your movements and your form. This is your time to exercise and/or compete. You are putting all your mental energy into your activity.

• **Relax**. While this may sound like the opposite of focus, it is not. Rather than forcing yourself to run or swim faster or hit harder or stronger, think of relaxing into your movements and keeping your body focused yet loose.

• **Dance**. Perhaps dancers know this best. The most graceful movements occur when the body is relaxed yet fully concentrated. Think "I'm dancing to success." (Sometimes music helps!)

• **Enjoy**. Your exercise or competition should be fun. This is your time. During practice, vary what you do. Remind yourself of the pleasure, and enjoy![21]

The Safety Bonus.   We have been talking about mental attitudes that can help you

What We Know

Women can be very successful athletic competitors. For many, however, characteristically traditional female traits can hold them back.

What to Do

If you want to compete, strive to develop self-confidence, set realistic goals, manage your anxiety, recognize that it is okay to win, and learn to flow.

become a better athlete. But your mind can not only permit you to be faster and stronger, it can also keep you from injury.

Researchers at the University of Arizona have found that "athletes able to attain higher positive states of mind are less at risk for injury."[22] These states of mind permit athletes to focus on their task and enjoy the event. These are the very features that we described in the previous section as important for developing the feeling of "flow."

The researchers noted that the most common reason for injuries reported by elite gymnasts was "lack of concentration," which is the opposite of focus. If you are a runner, it is easy to see how distraction by a passing sight might cause you to not pay attention to footing, thereby causing a fall. Similarly, ball players must "keep their eye on the ball," not only to play well, but to play safely.

The Physical Self

Until the last several decades, it was widely believed that women could not and should not engage in vigorous athletics.

A Brief Chronology. The first "modern" Olympics, held in Athens in 1896, was a male-only competition. "The common wisdom held that a woman was not physiologically capable of running mile after mile; that she wouldn't be able to bear children; that her uterus would fall out; that she might grow a mustache; that she was a man or wanted to be one."[23] In 1928, women competed in the 800-meter race, but the event was ruled "too great a call on feminine strength" and was not included in the Olympics again until 1960. It took until 1984 for women marathon runners to be part of the games. And the 1996 Olympics were the first ones to include women's softball and the women's triple jump.[24]

The past restrictions may have been partly attributable to genuine concern that women would injure themselves. It was thought that because women's bodies are softer, they are more easily hurt. However, in addition to concern for women's physical well-being, it was often considered "unladylike" and simply not socially acceptable for women to participate in activities requiring competition, physical contact and aggression, or strength and power.[25]

Not all physical activity for women has been restricted. Hard work in the home and in the fields has long been accepted. Some recreational activity was also permitted. For example, historically, women have been encouraged to dance and to engage in ice-skating, gymnastics, golf, tennis, and swimming. The misdirected concern for women may seem contradictory since the "accepted" female activities demand considerable strength and some require aggressiveness as well. For example, most dance requires power as well as agility, house and field work are very physically demanding, and, to win a tennis game, aggressive moves are clearly needed.

Fortunately, today women can strive for physical fitness and enter sporting arenas of all types. Top female athletes are applauded, and countless amateurs regularly participate in races, play soccer, and engage in other once taboo physical activities. In the previous section, we described psychological preparation for successful athletics and competition. We now turn our attention to physical demands.

Built to Win.   Are there physical types that tend to excel at different sports? Does it take long legs to be a top runner and a broad upper body to win at swimming? Are athletic stars born or made? While intuitively we might believe that athletic prowess is in the genes, training may be equally important. Researcher Jackie Hudson expounds on this position: "People who expend meaningful effort improve and perhaps become excellent; people who do not expend meaningful effort can expect to deteriorate in performance and remain estranged from ability."[26]

As coaches are fond of saying, "It's the attitude, not the aptitude, that carries you to the altitude."[27]

When the physiological attributes of top athletes are examined, it is often difficult to separate the effects of training from natural endowment.

A Look at Some Top Performers

Champion Long-Distance Runners. Thomas Pipes, of the National Athletic Health Institute in Inglewood, California, summarized research studies that compiled data on the body build of elite women runners. The findings were clear: Champion women long-distance runners had "ectomorphic (tall and thin) body builds and little body fat" compared to "average" women. But, Pipes concludes, "while there would seem to be a predisposition of body type that would influence the individual's ability to perform in an event, . . . (success) would appear to be a combination of both genetic(s) and training regimens."[28]

Other studies of endurance athletes focus on metabolism as measured by such things as VO_2max, maximum heart rate, and lactate profiles. While considerable variation has been found in these factors among athletes, it is clear again that both biology and conditioning play a role.[29]

Elite Female Basketball Players. Researchers at the University of Toronto Sport Sciences Centre examined the physiological components that were considered important to game performance in members of Canadian national women's basketball teams. Elite players were found to excel in aerobic power, endurance, and sprinting ability. These skills can all be enhanced through training. On the other hand, current athletes were generally taller and heavier than elite players of ten years ago; at the least, the former characteristic is a biological one.[30]

Top Volleyball Players. Speed, coordination, and height might be considered necessary to excel in volleyball. Researchers have found that college tournament players tend to be slightly taller and heavier and have broader shoulders and narrower hips than other college women.[31] Another study suggested that the characteristics of elite volleyball players are such that coaches should work to "reduce percentage of body fat" along with "increasing the vertical jumping ability" of their team members.[32]

Working with What You Have. In Chapter 5, Routines: The Stars Are the Limit, we describe ways to help you gain endurance and become stronger and more agile. While it may be harder to become a star basketball player if you are five feet tall, you can certainly work to improve your game. You can also look at your body type and gauge what activity might best take advantage of how you are built. It is easier to work with your assets than to fight them.

> *My older sister loved tennis, golf, and softball. In fact, she enjoyed and excelled in any game that involved a ball. Since I always admired her and wanted to be like her, I decided I would become a ballplayer, too. Those were frustrating times for me. I simply didn't seem to be able to develop the strength, speed, or coordination. Fortunately I had a friend who was a member of our local "Y." She talked me into joining a yoga class when I was a junior in high school. That changed my life. I loved the gentle stretches. To my surprise I became quite good. I still do yoga regularly.*
>
> —Mary, age 30, psychotherapist

What to Do

Don't be afraid to try an athletic activity that appeals to you. You can shape your body by discipline and carefully planned workouts. But if you feel frustrated, just relax, and go with what comes easier to you.

Body Image. Many women are dissatisfied with their bodies. The most common self-perception is that we are overweight. A classic study by researchers Strunkard, Sorenson, and Schulsinger asked college women and men to look at line drawings of different body types and (a) pick the figure that they felt was most like their own and (b) select the figure that they considered ideal.[33] The study showed that while men are generally satisfied with their body shape, women tend to believe that they are too heavy. Recent investigations confirm that female college athletes are no different from nonathletes in believing that they should slim down, although athletes in general believe that they are closer to their "ideal" and so don't have as far to go.[34]

Most sporting events that have been traditionally encouraged for women focus on slimness. It has only been in the past decade or so that body building and muscular development have gained some social acceptance. *New York Times Magazine* style editor Holly Brubach writes, ". . . recently, we have discovered elegance in the swell of a woman's quads, in the tapering form of her lats, in the way her delts square the line of her shoulders. Women, as they have gradually come into their own, have at last begun to feel at home in their bodies . . . ."[35]

Can You Handle the Pain? While the old locker room adage "no pain, no gain" has been disproved, competitive athletics are not painless. (See Chapter 16, Understanding Aches & Pains.) From simple muscle fatigue to torn ligaments and broken bones, the aches and pains of working out and competing are well known. If you are going to be a winner, it is certain that you will experience some physical pain along the way. Sports history, including the 1996 Olympics, has many examples of players who have continued to compete despite broken bones and other injuries.[36]

The perception of pain is a very personal thing. No one can actually tell how much something hurts someone else. In fact, the concept of pain is best viewed as involving at least two factors: (1) intensity, that is, from feeling nothing to feeling something excruciating, and (2) ability to tolerate, or the degree of pain that you can withstand.

Several investigators have studied pain in athletes and nonathletes. Researchers Evelyn Hall and Simon Davies[36] utilized a procedure that measured subjects' reactions to placing their right arm in a bucket of ice water for a maximum of five minutes. The volunteers were asked to respond to the sensation by indicating on a continuum their perception of the intensity of this experience from "no sensation" to "the strongest sensation I can imagine." They also indicated on a separate continuum their emotional response from "not bad at all" to "the most intense bad feeling for me." Female athletes viewed the pain as less severe and more tolerable than female nonathletes. These women athletes were similar to male athletes in their perception and tolerance of pain, and significantly more accepting of pain than male nonathletes.

Professional ballet dancers were also subjects in an ice water pain experiment.[37] The dancers, just as the other athletes, had higher pain sensation and pain tolerance thresholds than nonathletes of their age. Bleeding toes, muscle aches, and exhaustion are well known to dancers. Those who make the grade have learned to accept these problems.

Endorphins: Natural Pain-Killers. Everyone who exercises vigorously owes some of their pain tolerance to hormones (composed of amino acids) called **endorphins,** which are produced by the body's pituitary gland. Endorphins are released into the bloodstream during and after strenuous physical activity. They are released at other times as well and in differing quantities in different people. They serve two major functions. They provide us with that glow of well-being, often thought of as the "exercise high," and they permit us to withstand pain for several hours after their release. While endorphins may allow all of us to withstand minor workout-related pain, it is possible that highly competitive athletes may produce larger amounts of these chemicals, and may therefore be able to bear pain others might find intolerable.[38]

Sports Inventory for Pain. Pain has also been studied from a purely psychological standpoint. Without actually subjecting people to any discomfort, researchers have

FIGURE 7.1

....

*The items below are similar to ones found in the "Sports Inventory for Pain."
The lower your score, the more able you are to tolerate pain.*

Rate yourself 1 to 5 as follows, then add up your total score.

1 = Definitely True	4 = Generally Not True
2 = Generally True	5 = Definitely Not True
3 = Undecided	

1. Pain is a challenge, and I don't let it bother me.
2. I do not think about being injured.
3. Pain is just part of the game.
4. I try to ignore pain and simply go on.
5. When I am hurt, I tell myself to be brave.
6. I don't even notice minor injuries.
7. When I'm in an event, I won't let pain into my consciousness.
8. When I get injured, I tell myself not to think about it.
9. Pain is not something I worry about.
10. Competition is more important than trying to stop pain.

....

Adapted from Meyers M. C., Bourgeois, A. E., Stewart, S., & LeUnes, A. Predicting pain response in athletes: development and assessment of the sports inventory for pain. *Journal of Sport and Exercise Psychology*, 1992, 14, 249–261.

developed a paper and pencil test to gauge how we psychologically cope with pain. The *Sports Inventory for Pain* (*SIP*) consists of 25 items and calls for a response of one through five, from definitely not true to definitely true.[39] Figure 7-1 contains items similar to those in this inventory.

A Feminist Perspective. Mary Duquin, a professor at the University of Pittsburgh, suggests that competitive athletes are often expected to be willing to "sacrifice bodily health and well-being for victory." She maintains that this is counter to the "valued integrity of the body . . . (which) is a consistent theme in feminist psychology."[40] Women are taught to care for their own bodies and nurture others. In sports, you may not only injure yourself, but you also may physically hurt someone else.

What We Know

Women athletes and professional dancers can tolerate more pain than nonathletes and nondancers. We don't know whether this is because of an "inborn" ability to cope with pain, perhaps related to higher levels of endorphins, or because they have learned this as part of their training.

What to Do

If a competitive activity appeals to you, recognize that pain may accompany it. You must be your own judge as to whether the experience risks more discomfort or pain than you are willing to accept. You are not a "wimp" if you don't chose competitive soccer or downhill skiing. If you want to compete, you have many other options. If you don't want to compete, but just "work out," that's okay too.

In her book, *Are We Winning Yet*, Mariah B. Nelson puts forth a feminist way of viewing pain and violence in competitive sports:

"We seem to have come full circle, from the days when men said, 'Our games are too dangerous for you,' and women argued, 'No, they're not,' to an era in which some women are saying, 'We've tried your games, and you know what? They are too dangerous. From the looks of your mutilated bodies, they're too dangerous for you too. We're going to make up our own games, or alter your games so we can take care of ourselves.'"[41]

THE VIEW FROM WITHOUT

Women athletes do not live in a world apart. They are influenced by families, friends, neighbors, institutions, the law, and the media. We talk more about parental and other individual types of influence in Chapter 13, Starting Early: A Family Affair. In the next few pages we consider legal constraints and support for women athletes and the role of journalists and radio/television broadcasters.

Permission to Play

Title IX.   Until recently, American women were excluded from most competitive and professional sports. A major breakthrough occurred when the United States Congress passed Title IX of the 1972 Education Amendments.

Born in the 1970s. Stimulated by the civil rights movement of the 1960s, and using language similar to that of Title VI of the Civil Rights Act of 1964, Title IX intends to provide equality for females:

"No person in the United States shall, on the basis of sex, be excluded from participation in, be denied the benefits of, or be subjected to discrimination under any education program or activity receiving federal financial assistance."[42]

Although Title IX was not directed specifically at physical education, it had a major impact on women and sports. In effect, Title IX assured that women in educational settings would have equal access to physical education courses and teams. Some critics were afraid that this would impair the profitable nature of high school and college sports such as basketball and football. Others were titillated with visions of coed wrestling and unisex locker rooms. But the actual result of Title IX was to offer many new sports, activities, and athletic scholarships to females where once these had been denied. In addition, girls were exposed to competitive athletics at younger ages and so developed both interest and ability.

Refined in the 1980s. The original Department of Health, Education, and Welfare guidelines stipulated that all programs were subject to Title IX regulations if the umbrella institution received any federal funds. However, those opposed to Title IX in college athletics stated that only specific programs receiving federal funding should have to comply with the law. In other words, if intercollegiate sports did not receive any direct U.S. government support, they should not be required to provide equal opportunity for women.

The Title IX controversy came to a head in the 1984 *Grove City College v Bell* case. Although this small, private Pennsylvania college had not been involved in gender discrimination, its administration did not want to succumb to federal examination and therefore refused to sign a statement saying that it complied with Title IX. Because of this, the U.S. government withheld student grant funds. Grove City College, on behalf of the students, sued for reinstatement of their grants. Taken to the Supreme Court, the decision was that only those specific programs that receive federal monies must adhere to Title IX. Since it was the students who were given federal support in order to pursue their education through a financial aid program, the college did not have to provide equal athletics and physical education to women and men. This was a major setback for women in sports and athletics.[42]

The Grove City decision was turned around in 1988 when Congress passed the Civil Rights Restoration Act (CRRA) over the veto of then President Reagan. CRRA reversed the Grove City decision and clarified that an entire institution had to comply with the Title IX regulations if any part of that institution was to receive federal funding. High school and college physical education and competitive sports were again legally required to be equally available to females and males.

Challenged in the 1990s. In the early 1990s, Brown University, forced to cut back on expenditures, stopped funding the women's gymnastics and volleyball teams and also reduced support to men's water polo and golf. Brown administrators believed that since the cuts involved both male and female sports, their action was not a discriminatory one. The judge's ruling, however, was that Brown did not offer varsity sports opportunities for women and men in proportional numbers to the student enrollments, nor did it expand sports programs for women to meet demand. Brown was required to find a way to allocate more resources to women's teams.[43]

Partly to force clarification on issues such as those raised by the Brown University case, the U.S. Education Department published a set of rules requiring that colleges and universities annually issue a report specifying expenditures and participation in women's and men's intercollegiate athletics. A public budget and enrollment figures would make it easier to verify compliance with or violation of Title IX.[44]

What Price Equality? While nearly all educational facilities now support the goal of equal opportunity in sports and athletics for women and men, controversy surrounding Title IX remains.

Looking for the Women. Some school and college officials have complained that there simply is not as strong an interest in athletics among women as there is among men. A recent survey of high school juniors and seniors reported that 47 percent of boys were interested in athletics, compared to 29 percent of girls.[45] If this is the case, isn't it unrealistic to expect equal representation of the sexes on sports teams?

Athletic directors of programs at community colleges in New York state have commented on the complexity of the mandates of Title IX. One college canceled women's tennis, basketball, and soccer due to lack of interest. Another school reported only three players showing up for the first week of basketball, resulting in termination of that intercollegiate program. Dr. D. David Conklin, president of Dutchess County Community College, offered the following perspective: "We're trying to find those women's sports that are attractive to our students. But we are finding that there are sports that aren't as attractive to female students as in the past."[45]

Are Feminist Ideals Lost in the Male Sports Model? Perhaps part of the problem in attracting females to some sports can be explained by the following feminist perspective. Traditionally, the focus of athletics for women has not been competition. The National Section for Girls' and Women's Sports, in its 1953 *Standards*, emphasized that sports should be for everyone. The *Standards* stated, "The goal of sports is not to find the 'best' team or player but to give opportunity and pleasure to all participating."[46]

Mary Boutelier and Lucinda SanGiovani of Seton Hall University suggest, "women's alienation from sport, their indifference to it, and their reluctance to enter it stem in large measure from the fact that, as it has existed historically, what sport celebrated, what sport offered, what sport demanded, what sport rewarded do not reflect much of women's experience of the world."[47] See the discussion of feminine "handicaps" earlier in this chapter.

For Title IX to be truly effective, the broadest range of opportunities for both competitive and noncompetitive physical activity must be made available to members of both sexes from an early age.

Media Messages

From Invisibility to Center Stage. In the 1970s, when a surge of research into women's issues began, investigators documented that women received less publicity than men. This held true for women in the arts, politics, and athletics. Those few women who made "the news" were often referred to by their husband's name (e.g. Mrs. John Jones) or by their first name alone. This limited and slanted media coverage diminished women's activities in many spheres. Attention to current newspapers and television programming reveals how much progress has been made toward equal media treatment of the sexes—but we still have a way to go.

"Symbolic Annihilation." The term "symbolic annihilation" was coined by media researcher George Gerbner to indicate that when women's activities are not brought to public view, it is as if they never happened. A study of sports reporting in major newspapers in 1980 revealed that only 2 percent was devoted to women's sport. In 1984, that figure went down to 1.3 percent.[48] Slight progress was reported in a 1991 study, which determined that 4 percent of sports stories were about female athletes.

Not only was little mention made of women's athletic activities, references to it tended to trivialize the accomplishments. Coverage of women athletes often focused as much on their attractiveness and personal lives as on their physical performance.

Even the words used to describe excellence are often quite different depending on the gender of the player. For example, researchers note that when comparing sports reporting of women's and men's basketball and volleyball, terms such as "brilliant shot," "strategic placement," and "analytic ability" are more often used in reference to men, while "graceful," "smooth," "easy to watch," and "beautiful" are more typical descriptors for women.[49]

"You Mean There Are Men Also Competing in Atlanta?" The headline above by sports writer George Vecsey appeared in *The New York Times* just prior to the 1996 Olympics.[50] Two out of five Olympic competitors were female, and the publicity surrounding their participation was impressive.

The *New York Times Magazine* ran a special issue devoted exclusively to women Olympians, and television devoted approximately equal air time to women's events. Female athletic stars have become household words. Basketball guard Sheryl Swoopes has a Nike shoe named for her. One marketing executive commented, "Women athletes from the Olympics seem to have a bigger draw than any other celebrity we've ever used. Maybe it's because they are more universally known."[51]

The Word Is Out. Today, so many women athletes are well known that it is impossible to talk about them all. Few informed Americans have not heard of Joan Benoit, Chris Evert, Steffi Graf, Dorothy Hamill, Sonja Henie, Florence Griffith Joyner, Jackie Joyner-Kersee, Billie Jean King, Olga Korbut, Martina Navratilova, or Grete Waitz. These women and many others serve as inspiration to females of all ages who want to engage in competitive athletics.[52]

The word is out! If you have the drive to compete, the opportunity is yours.

ENDNOTES

1. Douthitt, V. L., & Harvey, M. L. Exercise counseling—How physical educators can help. *Journal of Physical Education Research & Development*, May–June 1995, 31–34.
2. Morgan, W. P. Test of champions. *Psychology Today*, July 1980, 14, 92–102, 108.
   Patten, C. A., Harris, W., & Leatherman, D. Psychological characteristics of elite wheelchair athletes: the iceberg profile. *Perceptual and Motor Skills*, 1994, 79, 1390.
3. Swift, E. M. On thin ice. *Sports Illustrated.* January 24, 1994, 80 (3), 16.
4. Putukian, M. The female triad: eating disorders, amenorrhea, and osteoporosis. *Medical Clinics of North America*, March 1994, 78 (2), 345–356.
5. Gill, D. L. Psychological perspectives on women in sport and exercise. In Costa, D. M., & Guthrie, S. R. (Eds.). *Women and sport: interdisciplinary perspectives.* Champaign, IL: Human Kinetics, 1994, 341–359.
6. Gilligan, C. *In a different voice: psychological theory and women's development.* Cambridge, MA: Harvard University Press, 1982.
7. Duquin, M. E. She flies through the air with the greatest of ease: The contributions of feminist psychology. In Costa, D. M. & Guthrie, S. R. (Eds.). *Women and sport: interdisciplinary perspectives.* Champaign, IL: Human Kinetics, 1994, 296.
8. Le Unes, A., & Nation, J. *Sport psychology*, 2nd edition. Chicago: Nelson Hall, 1996, 419.
9. Holmes, S. W., Kertay, L., Adamson, L. B., Holland, C. L., & Clance, P. R.

Measuring the Impostor Phenomenon: a comparison of Clance's IP Scale and Arvey's I-P Scale. *Journal of Personality Assessment*, 1993, 60 (1), 48.
10. Horner, M. S. Toward an undertanding of achievement-related conflicts in women. *Journal of Social Issues*, 1972, 28, 157–176.
11. Meyers, A. W., Whelan, J. P., & Murphy, S. M. Cognitive behavioral strategies in athletic performance enhancement. *Progress in Behavior Modification*, 1996, 30, 137–164.
12. Lynch, J. Mind over miles. *Runner's World.* May 1996, 31, 80–94.
13. White, A., & Hardy, L. Use of different imagery perspectives on the learning and performance of different motor skills. *British Journal of Psychology*, May 1995, 86 (part 2), 169–80.
14. Le Unes, A., & Nation, J. *Sport psychology*, 2nd edition. Chicago: Nelson Hall, 1996, 121.
15. Gould, D., & Udry, E. Psychological skills for enhancing performance: arousal regulation strategies. *Medical Science, Sports & Exercise.* April 1994, 26 (4), 478–485.
16. Raglin, J. S., & Morris, M. J. Precompetition anxiety in women volleyball players: a test of ZOF in a team sport. *British Journal of Sports Medicine*, March 1994, 28 (1), 47– 51.
17. Martens, R., Vealey, R. S., & Burton, D. *Competitive anxiety in sport.* Champaign, IL: Human Kinetics, 1990.
18. Meyers, A. W., Whelan, J. P., & Murphy, S. M. Cognitive behavioral strategies in athletic performance enhancement. *Progress in Behavior Modification*, 1996, 30, 137–164.

19. Demasio, N. F. Race for 7,500 ends up duel of 2 Kenyan villages. *The New York Times,* Sunday, June 11, 1995.
20. Jackson, S. A. Toward a conceptual understanding of the flow experience in elite athletes. *Research Quarterly for Exercise and Sport*, 1996, 67 (1), 83.
21. Lynch, J. Mind over miles. *Runner's World.* May 1996, 31, 80–94.
22. Williams, J. M., Hogan, T. D., & Andersen, M. B. Positive states of mind and athletic injury risk. *Psychosomatic Medicine*, 1993, 55, 468–472.
23. Longman, J. How the women won. *The New York Times Magazine*, June 23, 1996, 23.
24. Longman, J. How the women won. *The New York Times Magazine*, June 23, 1996, 23–27.
   Colliton, J. Keeping pace with today's active women. *The Physician and Sportsmedicine*, July 1996, 24 (7), 29.
25. Guthrie, S. R., & Castelnuovo, S. The significance of body image in psychosocial development and in embodying feminist perspectives. In Costa, D. M. & Guthrie, S. R. (Eds.). *Women and sport: interdisciplinary perspectives.* Champaign, IL: Human Kinetics, 1994, 307–322.
26. Hudson, J. L. It's mostly a matter of metric. In Costa, D. M,. & Guthrie, S. R. (Eds.). *Women and sport: interdisciplinary perspectives.* Champaign, IL: Human Kinetics, 1994, 150.
27. Le Unes, A., & Nation, J. *Sport psychology*, 2nd edition. Chicago: Nelson Hall, 1996, 512.
28. Pipes, T. V. Body composition char-

acteristics of male and female track and field athletes. *Research Quarterly*, March 1977, 48 (1), 244–247.

29. Roalstad, M. S. Physiological testing of the ultraendurance triathlete. *Medical Science Sports & Exercise*, 1989, 21 (5 Suppl), S200–204.

30. Smith, H. K., & Thomas, S. G. Physiological characteristics of elite female basketball players. *Canadian Journal of Sports Science*, 1991, 16 (4), 289–295.

31. Hosler, W. W., Morrow, Jr., J. R., & Jackson, A. S. Strength, anthropometric, and speed characteristics of women volleyball players. *Research Quarterly*, 1978, 49 (3), 385–388.

32. Fleck, S. J., Case, S., Puhl, J., et al. Physical and physiological characteristics of elite women volleyball players. *Canadian Journal of Applied Sport Science*, 1985, 10 (3), 122–126.

33. Hallinan, C. J., Pierce, E. F., Evans, J. E., et al. Perceptions of current and ideal body shape of athletes and nonathletes. *Perceptual and Motor Skills*, 1991, 72, 123–130.

34. Hallinan, C. J., Pierce, E. F., Evans, J. E., et al. Perceptions of current and ideal body shape of athletes and nonathletes. *Perceptual and Motor Skills*, 1991, 72, 123–130.

DiNucci, J. M., Finkenberg, M. E., McCune, S. L., et al. Analysis of body esteem of female collegiate athletes. *Perceptual and Motor Skills*, 1994, 78, 315–319.

35. Brubach, H. The athletic esthetic. *The New York Times Magazine*, June 23, 1996, 51.

36. Hall, E. G., & Davies, S. Gender differences in perceived intensity and effect of pain between athletes and nonathletes. *Perceptual and Motor Skills*, 1991, 73, 779–786.

37. Tajet-Foxell, B., & Rose, F. D. Pain and pain tolerance in professional ballet dancers. *British Journal of Sports Medicine*, 1995, 29 (1), 31–34.

38. Anderson, K. N., & Anderson, L. E. *Mosby's pocket dictionary of medicine, nursing, & allied health*, 2nd edition. St. Louis: Mosby, 1994.

Cooper, K. H., & Cooper, M. *The new aerobics for women*. Toronto: Bantam Books, 1988.

39. Meyers, M. C., Bourgeois, A. E., Stewart, S., & LeUnes, A. Predicting pain response in athletes: development and assessment of the sport inventory for pain. *Journal of Sport and Exercise Psychology*, 1992, 14, 249–261.

40. Duquin, M. E. She flies through the air with the greatest of ease: The contributions of feminist psychology. In Costa, D. M. & Guthrie, S. R. (Eds.). *Women and sport: interdisciplinary perspectives*. Champaign, IL: Human Kinetics, 1994, 285–306.

41. Nelson, M. *Are we winning yet?* New York: Random House, 1991, 185.

42. Carpenter, L. J. Letters home: my life with Title IX. In Cohen, G. L. (Ed.). *Women in sport: issues and controversies*. Newbury Park, CA: Sage, 1993, 82.

43. *New York Times*. The bias against women's sports. *New York Times*, Editorial, April 5, 1995, a24.

Thomaselli, R. Schools are struggling to field women's teams. *Poughkeepsie Journal*, January 21, 1996, 66.

44. New York Times. Colleges told to publish sports costs. *New York Times*, National Section, December 3, 1995, 37.

Cohen, G. L. *Women in sport: issues and controversies*. Newbury Park, CA: Sage, 1993.

45. Thomaselli, R. Schools are struggling to field women's teams. *Poughkeepsie Journal*, January 21, 1996, 66.

46. Welch, P. Governance: the first half century. In Cohen, G. L. (Ed.) *Women in sport: issues and controversies*. Newbury Park, CA: Sage, 1993, 74–75.

47. Boutilier, M. A., & SanGiovanni, L. F. Politics, public policy, and Title IX. In Birrell, S., & Cole, C. L., (Eds.). *Women, sport, and culture*. Champaign, IL: Human Kinetics, 1994, 107.

48. Birrell, S., & Theberge, N. Ideological control of women in sport. In Costa, D. M., & Guthrie, S. R. (Eds.). *Women and sport: interdisciplinary perspectives*. Champaign, IL: Human Kinetics, 1994, 341–359.

49. Cohen, G. L. Media portrayal of the female athlete. In Cohen, G. L. (Ed.). *Women in sport: issues and controversies*. Newbury Park, CA: Sage, 1993, 174.

50. Vecsey, G. You mean there are men also competing in Atlanta? *The New York Times*, July 14, 1996, Section 8, Special Pullout Section, 2.

51. Longman, J. How the women won. *The New York Times Magazine*, June 23, 1996, 27.

52. Woolum, J. *Outstanding women athletes: who they are and how they influenced sports in America.* Phoenix, AZ: Oryx Press, 1992.

8

Dressing for the Job

DONNA I. MELTZER, M.D.

Unisex clothing is great . . . or is it? The term "unisex" implies suitability for both men and women. Historically, the purchase of unisex sporting clothing has meant that a woman is simply buying the smaller size range in clothing designed for a man's body. In Chapter 2, we reviewed many of the skeletal and physiological differences between women and men. Needless to say, unisex clothing may not fit or be comfortable for all women.

Fortunately, over the last decade some clothing outfitters have recognized that women's needs are different. We are now seeing more and more women's running shoes and shorts, bike shorts and tights, and other apparel designed specifically for females. No longer will women have to squeeze their hips into men's shorts that gape in the crotch!

This chapter will review some clothing particulars. It is not meant to be exhaustive. Despite our body differences, some women may find that men's or unisex clothing provides a better or more comfortable fit. Others will not. One area unique to women, however, is the selection of bras.

SPORTS BRAS

The size and consistency of breast tissue varies among individuals and within the same individual at different times of the menstrual cycle. As noted in Chapter 2, breasts are composed mostly of fatty tissue, and this determines your breast size. Heredity also plays a role in your ultimate breast size and shape.

Just as clothing comes in different sizes to fit different bodies, so do bras. One thing is for sure—in sports bras, one size does not fit all! In fact, a single size may not even be appropriate for you on every day of your cycle. The nature of your activities may also influence your choice of a bra. If you cross-train, you may want to own an assortment of different bras.

Be Fit: Choosing the Right Sports Bra for You

One of my biggest problems is finding a sports bra that fits me. I am five feet, seven inches tall, weigh about 148 pounds, and wear a 38D bra. Many of the sports bra companies do not manufacture a bra that fits me. Extra-large for them seems to be a C cup. The designers should realize that not every athlete is flat-chested.

—Nancy, age 30

With body movement, breasts swing in a pendulum-like motion. A properly fitted bra should help to minimize extreme up and down motion and also limit side to side movement.[1] You may want to test this by running in place in front of a mirror—with and without your bra. Alternatively, you may cup your hands on your breasts or bra and see how you can further limit the swing. This may help you determine the degree of support you should be looking for in a sports bra. As a rule, large-breasted women notice more motion and hence require more support than small-breasted women. Therefore, a rigidly constructed bra may provide a better fit for the former, while a more stretchy bra may be more appropriate for the latter. Large-breasted women also often do better with a sports bra that holds each breast firmly and separately in a cup instead of compressing them against the chest wall.

Once you decide that you want to invest in a sports bra, you will need to consider torso and cup size to ensure a proper fit. Remember, one size or style does not fit all. Watch out for sports bras that are manufactured in just three sizes: small, medium, and large. These may not be sufficient if you have a large torso and small bust or vice versa. You may want to look for a manufacturer that separates the sizes into torso and cup. When you shop for a sports bra, make sure you take the time to try it on for size and comfort. A sports bra that fits well should feel snug, but not constricting.

Consider Your Sporting Activity. Different exercise routines require varying amounts of arm movement. A bra with elastic straps may be more suitable for activities that involve a great deal of arm and shoulder stretching, such as basketball and volleyball, whereas a bra outfitted with nonelastic straps may provide a better fit for sports requiring less upper extremity motion, such as jogging and running. Some women find that bra straps must be wide and stretchable, so they don't slip down the shoulders. Most of us know there is nothing more annoying than having bra straps constantly slip down or cut into our shoulders. Before you purchase a sports bra, try jumping in place and swinging and stretching your arms to check that you are getting good support. Make sure you do this simple exercise before you cut off the price tags!

Some women athletes prefer bras that have a hook or clasp in the front as opposed to the back to avoid trauma when rolling or diving onto hard surfaces.[2] Think about this if you are a gymnast or perform mat exercises. Several types of sports bra have no fasteners or hooks; however, you should be very careful about ensuring proper fit. Also, watch out for bras that have crisscross straps in the back, which may not provide adequate support for the well-endowed woman. If you engage in contact sports, a bra with extra padding may afford some additional protection.

Fiber and Fabric. Choice of fiber and fabric weight should be influenced by personal preference, sensitivity, climate, and seasonal conditions. For example, if you are exercising in the outdoors in the middle of winter, you may want to wear a sports bra that is made of a heavyweight fabric. While some women wear padded bras for protection during contact sports, this is also an option for women engaged in cold-weather sports.

Other quality features to search for in bras include absorbent and nonallergenic materials that are durable and easy to launder. Fabrics that are designed to wick away perspiration are especially useful for hikers or other athletes who are active for extended periods of time. You may want to look for stretchy fabrics that breathe and wick moisture from the skin, such as *Coolmax* and *Lycra*.

Although it may be tempting to buy new sports bras in bulk, it is probably wiser to buy just one and test it out. Check one bra out and see if the interfacing or seams chafe your skin. During and after a vigorous workout, note whether there is decreased support when the bra is saturated with perspiration. Remember, your bra should always be comfortable, both at rest and during exercise.

Tips for Buying a Sports Bra
- Carefully evaluate the bra's fabric and overall fit.
- Practice exercise movements (jumping and twisting) in the bra you intend to purchase.
- Make sure the bra's design is compatible with your chosen sporting activity.

Protecting Against Jogger's Nipples. Both women and men runners may complain of "jogger's nipples," an irritation of the nipples that is produced by chafing against a shirt or bra.[3] This condition has also been seen in bicyclists and appropriately dubbed "bicyclist's nipples." Using a lubricant such as petroleum jelly or talcum powder, as well as gently applying a piece of adhesive tape, may help to decrease friction on the nipple. This chafing problem may also be minimized by carefully selecting undergarments. While women

What We Know

- *A bra is not an essential undergarment for every athlete.*
- *A comfortable bra that provides good support is best.*
- *The ideal fit for a sports bra is not too tight and not too loose.*

have the option of donning or removing a bra, both sexes may remedy the problem by wearing silk or synthetic undergarments. If you do wear a bra, you should avoid purchasing a sports bra that has seams or ridges in the nipple area that could be a source of chafing.

What If I Don't Wear a Bra?

For many years I ran without wearing a bra. My mother used to warn me that my breasts would sag if I didn't wear a good-fitting one. My bust seems pretty flabby these days—I wonder if she was right. —Betty, age 47

Some women may choose not to wear a bra with daily activities or when they exercise and may wonder if there are any long-term consequences to this. It is a myth that your breasts will sag and droop if you exercise without the support of a bra. As you age, the percentage of breast fatty tissue increases, while the amount of glandular tissue diminishes, which might explain why breasts seem less firm at age 60 than they were when you were 21 years old. A bra will not prevent the normal breast relaxation that comes with aging.

What about breast soreness or the risk of cancer? While breast soreness after exercise has been reported by some female athletes, the likelihood that this will be a problem is not known because so little research has been conducted in this area. Large-breasted women may suffer more discomfort than small-breasted women when they vigorously exercise without support.

There are also a lot of concerns today about developing breast cancer. You need to be reassured that there is no known association between breast trauma and a predilection toward the later diagnosis of breast cancer. Hence, your reason for wearing a bra should be based primarily on comfort.

BICYCLING

In the 1890s the bicycle was introduced to America. At that time a skirt lifter (a stick-like device) was invented to help women pick up their petticoats and skirts in order to facilitate mounting a bicycle.[4] Over the years, as fashions have changed, so has cycling apparel and equipment. We've come a long way!

Shorts for Cycling

Two years ago I decided to take a bicycling vacation in Mexico. In the last decade I had traveled thousands of miles on my road bike and never experienced saddle soreness even when I wore regular running shorts. I had a rude awakening on the back roads of Mexico on my mountain bike. On the second day of the trip I unpacked my well-padded bike shorts—a day too late. The constant bouncing around on rough terrain brought tears to my eyes and would have been worse had I not had cycling shorts. Fortunately, we switched to riding on asphalt, and I was able to continue and even had some terrific cycling days. I will never forget that painful saddle soreness.

—Iris, age 36

The resolution to add cycling shorts to your wardrobe is an individual one. Some cyclists swear by them, while others are comfortable riding in any old pair of shorts. Your anatomy, type of bicycle and seat, and riding terrain may help the decision-making process.

Fit for a Female.   A common theme in this book has been that women are not built like men. Needless to say, unisex clothing may not provide the best fit for women cyclists. Compared to men's shorts, the women's model should have a higher waist that is cut lower in the front than in the back to better accommodate the riding position. It should be roomier in the hips, narrower in the waist and have shorter, fuller legs. The legs in women's shorts should be just long enough to prevent your thighs from rubbing directly against the saddle seat.

The overall construction of your bike shorts is also crucial for your comfort. Make certain that your cycling shorts or tights do not have panel seams that could be irritating and chafe your thighs. If the bike shorts are not comfortable at rest or while sitting on a bike seat, just think how uncomfortable you will be after pedaling for a few hours. Do not be afraid to go and try on a pair of shorts and sit on a bike seat before making a final purchase.

Seek and You Shall Find. You may have to go from store to store before finding the right pair of cycling shorts. Don't be fooled by tags that advertise the "ladies'" model—go beyond the label and look at the design and construction. Some bikers have questioned why women are often forced to wear men's clothing when 46 percent of the U.S. cycling population is female.[5] When riders were informally polled about manufacturers of women's cycling apparel, only five companies came to mind. However, with research, 22 companies were found to make women's bike clothing. Perhaps we just have to shop around more.

Undies or Not

Every summer I join my sisters for a family reunion. We bike ride and camp outdoors. To this day, my older sister is appalled that I prefer to cycle with my padded shorts but without any underwear. Am I out to lunch? —Lynne, age 37

Since some biking shorts have liners shaped with the female anatomy in mind, you may opt not to wear underwear. Newer bike shorts have liners made of three layers: a soft, comfortable layer next to the skin; a middle layer made of shock-absorbing gel or foam; and an outer layer made of fleece or terrycloth that wicks moisture away.[6]

You may find with repeated wear and washing that terrycloth or similar fabric of the outer layer tends to "pill" and cause discomfort. A liner or crotch pad made of chamois is a favorite of some riders. The next time you are in a bike or sporting goods store, compare the liners in the men's and ladies' bike shorts. The men's and ladies' liners should have different shapes and curves. The stitching and seams of the women's liner should also be distinct, and should not have a center seam, which can be very uncomfortable.

Tips

- Try to find liners made of chamois cloth.
- Check out the stitching and seams for irritating interfaces.

Washing Instructions.   Repeated washing and drying can take their toll on your clothing. Anyone who has invested in cycling shorts has done just that—invested money. If you want your investment to last, you need to take proper care of it. One authority has recommended warm (not cold) water for washing bike shorts made of *Lycra*, in spite of the manufacturers' recommendations. Cold water washing may lead to stretching of the fabric, while warm water keeps the material firm and elastic.[6]

Taking the Chill Off

In temperate areas where snowfall is light or nonexistent, avid cyclists can pedal all year round. Over the last few years, innovative apparel constructed of high-tech fabrics has been introduced so that cyclists do not freeze their buns off. Unfortunately many of these thermal "hot pants" employ unisex sizing, which may not provide a comfortable fit for all women.

Here are some features to consider when you shop for winter cycling bottoms. Buy tights that are snug but not restrictive. Many models are sold as bib tights, which provide extra protection to shield the waist and lower back from wind and chill. However, some women may find the bib straps uncomfortable on their chest and too restrictive around their upper torsos.

Keep in mind that if you choose bib tights, you will need to remove your jacket at rest stops (men have the option of purchasing bib tights with zippers). Men, on the other hand, have been known to suffer from "frozen genitals" during winter cycling rides, which is a problem women riders don't have to worry about.[7] If you are one of those people who require frequent bathroom breaks, think about the layers you will be removing at each pit stop. And if it's cold outdoors, the last thing you'll want to do is take off your top as you lower the bottoms!

If you head out cycling on overcast days or after a rain shower, you should choose a fabric that is water resistant. Staying dry is just as important as staying warm. You may want to consider materials that offer wind protection as well. Also, look for fabrics that are durable and easy to launder.

Gloves

Cycling gloves may be thought of as protective or safety equipment. A supplement to the foam padding on the handlebars, these fingerless gloves come with varying degrees of padding and can serve as shock absorbers; they also provide protection from blisters. In case of a fall, gloves can also protect the hands of the rider from serious abrasions.

Not surprising, most cycling gloves have not been designed for women. (Remember that we tend to have smaller hands and wrists than men.) There are some companies that now make this distinction and actually manufacture gloves for women in small, medium, and large sizes. Although a man's small glove may seem to fit, pay attention to the sizing around the wrist. Many of our cycling friends have agreed that it's definitely worth the effort to locate a pair of gloves that truly fit.

Footwear

I am a runner and avid cyclist who rides several days a week. I also have rather wide feet. For years, I have searched for a pair of cycling shoes that can accommodate my wide width. I have not encountered too much difficulty in finding shoes for running and aerobics, but bicycle shoes are a different story. —Latisha, age 29

Re-"Cycling" Shoes. If you are a recreational rider, you probably do not need to go to the trouble and expense of purchasing a pair of cycling shoes. Many women cyclists have found that a pair of old running shoes does the trick for them. If you chose this route, make sure that the soles are flat and stiff so that they fit into the pedal or toeclip easily and do not flex each time you put weight on the pedal. One advantage of using old running shoes, aside from the recycling and cost factors, is that we assume the shoes fit you in the first place and were comfortable.

Shoe Shopping. If you cycle regularly and want to improve your form, however, consider adding a pair of cycling shoes to your wardrobe. Most cycling shoes come in unisex sizes, which may not offer you a perfect fit. If you take the unisex or men's shoe route, be careful to avoid shoes with a heel that is too wide and a forefoot that is too narrow. The toebox should fit comfortably and not make your toes feel like sardines in a can. When shopping, wear the type of socks that you are most likely to wear while cycling to ensure a more ideal fit. Also, if the shop has a stationary bike, don't be afraid to get on and pedal to make sure you will be comfortable while riding.

Complete with Cleats. Many cycling shoes come with cleats and have stiff soles that attach to the pedal for more efficient pedaling. It takes time to get accustomed to wearing cleated shoes and also some expertise to make certain they are aligned appropriately. Remember that the cleats may need several adjustments before the right fit is found. The last thing you want is to have a pair of new bike shoes that force your feet and knees into an awkward riding position. This is not only uncomfortable and inefficient, but will ultimately cause undue stress on the lower extremities.

Using Your Head: Helmets

An entire chapter could be devoted to one of the most important bicycle safety devices—the helmet. Helmets are now required or recommended in many sports and should not be thought of as interchangeable from sport to sport. Although bicycle helmet safety standards have been set, they are not yet mandatory. Two private organizations, the American National Standards Institute (ANSI) and the Snell Memorial Foundation, have established some guidelines to provide the consumer with information on the protection provided by different helmets.[8] You should ask your bike shop salesperson to point out the brands that meet the most stringent safety standards.

Buying a Helmet. A common complaint voiced by women cyclists is ill-fitting helmets; that is, they frequently slide down over the eyes. A government-commissioned research study finally recognized this complaint as valid. After measuring over 100,000 heads, the researchers found that women's heads are smaller, more rounded, and wider across the temples. This finding prompted one helmet company manager to design a bike helmet specifically for women—one in which the wearer does not have to tip the helmet back for a comfortable fit. On this model, the chin strap and buckle are made smaller and curved for a more acceptable fit on the jaw.[9]

Not every brand of helmet fits every rider, male or female. Once you decide on a brand, try it on and find the smallest helmet size that fits you comfortably. You may use sizing pads to fine-tune the fit. The helmet should not slide down over your eyes, and the straps should be adjusted so that they are equally tight.[10]

A few models are made especially for those who have long hair and tend to wear their hair in ponytails. When trying on helmets, try to remember to style your hair in the way you will most often be wearing it when you cycle. However, you can always use sizing pads to make minor adjustments.

Tips
- Prior to finalizing your clothing purchases, try wearing the shorts or tights and shoes while sitting on a bicycle.
- When buying a helmet, wear your hair as you would when cycling.

RUNNING

When I started running during college two decades ago, I remember all running clothes seemed to be designed for men. Gradually, more running shoes and things like shorts were marketed for women. Why did it take so long?

—Becky, age 48

To put it simply, clothing must fit comfortably. Several companies make running clothing with the female figure in mind so that your top need not slip off your shoulders and your shorts need not chafe as they ride up and down. These companies now design clothing specifically for women—that is, they no longer just downsize men's models and feminize the colors, but they make these garments fit the female figure: wider in the hips and buttocks, etc.

Many women's models also come with an inner liner so underpants need not be worn. Some women prefer these models so as to avoid underpants, which can be a source of chafing and may be too warm in the summer. The bottom line, so to speak, is that your shorts should feel comfortable and not restrict movement.

Carrying Keys

When I run in the summer, I have no place to put my house key. In the winter months, I can attach it to my mittens or gloves. In the summer when I wear shorts, the key pocket is so small I cannot use my keychain. I often resort to wearing men's unisex shorts because they have convenient back patch pockets. I feel safer having it accessible and then do not have to be bothered with concerns that I may lose it.

—Bobbi, age 32

Unfortunately, many women's shorts do not have back patch pockets like the men's models. Keys or money may be placed in a special belt or a carrier designed to attach to your running shoes. Some runners simply attach a single critical key (for example, your front door key) and thread it through their shoe laces. If you do this, be sure to thread the key carefully in a few places so you won't lose it should your laces come untied.

If the Shoe Fits

I didn't begin to run with regularity until I graduated from college. I still remember my first pair of (women's) running shoes. They were stiff and cushionless and had painful hot spots. At that time, I thought they were the best thing that happened to women's sporting equipment. I could never run in them today. In fact, I often wonder why I didn't suffer any injuries with the mileage I put in . . . maybe I was just young and healthy. —Wendy, age 44

Running shoes are the one piece of equipment I always pay close attention to. I do not own any fancy Gore-tex running suits; instead I spend my money on well-constructed shoes, even if they are expensive. It's also interesting that I always purchase the same name-brand shoes because they seem to fit my feet and running style well.

—Karen, age 33

The saying "if the shoe fits, wear it" is just one aspect of running shoes that needs consideration. Any shoes, whether they are athletic or dress shoes, should fit the wearer and not be uncomfortable. Just think about the number of times and the amount of force generated each time your feet hit the ground when you run a mile. This is reason enough to select the proper shoe and pamper your feet.

Consumer health advocate Jane E. Brody notes that you should not purchase shoes by size, but for fit. She correctly points out that foot size tends to get bigger with advancing age, weight gain, and even throughout the day.[11] In fact, in one recent study of 356 healthy women with an average age of 42 years, 60 percent noted that their shoe size had increased since they were 20 years old, but 75 percent had not had their feet measured in more than five years. Also, in 66 percent of these women, one foot was larger than the other (the right in 36 percent, and the left in 30 percent.)[12]

Some women may notice that their feet tend to swell throughout the day, especially when standing in one place for prolonged periods, so a shoe that fits well in the morning may be a bit snug by the evening. If you fit this profile and you exercise in the afternoon or evening, you may want to purchase new shoes late in the day.

One of the biggest mistakes you can make is to purchase a pair of running shoes because they are the hottest shoes on the market. Aside from purchasing shoes that are sports specific—tennis shoes for playing tennis, running shoes for running—there are other factors to consider. To find the best running shoe for yourself, you will need to consider several characteristics, including: your gait, your body weight and foot size, your weekly mileage, and the surfaces on which you run.[13]

Innies or Outies?   Much has been written about "pronators" and "supinators." These terms simply refer to an inward or outward rolling of the foot. A normal foot lands on the outside of the heel and then rolls inward (pronates) slightly, which helps to absorb shock. Many companies market shoes for these different traits; hence, it pays to know if you pronate (roll in) or supinate (roll out) or if you have a neutral gait. You can identify your gait by watching yourself in a mirror as you walk. It may also be helpful to have someone stand behind you as you either walk or run. You should instruct them to pay close attention to how your foot lands on the ground. You will want your running shoe to neutralize or balance the way your foot strikes the ground. If in doubt, you may ask your local retailer to suggest a running shoe appropriate for your gait.

"Last" But Not Least.   You may have heard the sales associates in the local running shop talk about lasts. They probably weren't referring to their race finishing times, but to shoe construction. The last is the foot-shaped form around which a shoe is constructed. There are three basic types of lasts: straight, semi-curved, and curved. We mention lasts here not to confuse you, but to help you select a running shoe that is best for you. Shoes with a straight last have the heel and forefoot in pretty much the same line. The forefoot bends inward in curved-lasted shoes. Shoes with a semi-curved last fall between the two extremes.

Straight-lasted shoes offer the most medial support and are best for runners who overpronate. Most shoes have a semi-curved last because this shape accommodates a large variety of foot types. Even pronators may find a semi-curved shoe more comfortable than one that is straight. Supinators can compensate for their gait with a curved or slightly curved last. If you have a high arch, you may want to choose a shoe with a curved last. Similarly, runners with a low arch or flat feet should seek out a shoe with a straight or semicurved last. Curved lasts are popular among racing shoes. Shoes with a curved last also tend to be rather flexible, but unfortunately, they are not very supportive.

Other Features.   Other features to look for in running shoes include good cushioning, shock absorption, flexibility near the toes, and overall stability. Make sure that the shoe is well constructed. Look at the soles, check for flexibility, and look at the lacing system.

Some shoes are heavier than others. You may prefer a lightweight shoe for races or for fast-paced training and wear a heavier shoe for routine workouts. It is usually difficult to judge the weight of the shoe while you are walking up and down the aisle in the sporting goods store. Try picking up one shoe and comparing it with a different brand with your eyes closed. On a long run, a few ounces here and there make a big difference.

Women who have wide feet may consider buying men's or boy's shoes. To figure out your equivalent size in men's shoes, just subtract two from your current shoe size. For example, if you normally wear a woman's size ten but find the width a bit on the narrow side, you may get a better fit in a man's size eight because it is a quarter-inch to half-inch wider.[14] One drawback to this method is that the heels on the men's model may be too wide; while the forefoot width discomfort may be alleviated, a heel problem may have been created. This may be corrected by judicious heel padding by a shoemaker or sometimes even a qualified shoe store salesperson. If you choose a man's model, also make sure that the last isn't too stiff compared to the woman's version.

Designer Shoes

I have been buying my running shoes at the same shop for the last couple of years. The sales people are all runners and seem to know all the details about the women's running shoes. Last summer when I was indecisive about the fit of a shoe, they told me to take the shoe home and wear it for an hour or so on carpeting. I really appreciated the personal touch and the fact that they did not want me to feel pressured.
—Kate, age 39

The best-selling shoe may not always be the best shoe for you. Hence, you may want to "test run" the shoe in the store. As Kate noted above, some specialized shops will let you take the sneaker home to make sure it fits and feels good. While the late 1970s and early '80s focused on outsoles, durability, traction-waffle designs, flared heels, and blown rubber soles, the mid '80s shifted the focus to the midsoles and cushioning features such as gel and air. In the '90s, emphasis is being placed on the fit.[15] Technology has come to the stage that it is rare to have running shoes that need a break-in period or have the "hot spots" that were so prevalent in years past.

As with other equipment, your running shoes should feel good. Running shoes for women have come a long way, but women still need to be informed consumers and not tolerate ill-fitting shoes at any time! As the market for women's athletic shoes continues to skyrocket, we must remember that our feet are different from men's and we deserve just that—different shoes. Equality in the shoe store should not mean the same shoes.

Hints for Achieving a Proper Fit

I bought my first pair of women's running shoes in 1976 when I started running. I was new to the sport and thought they were great. In fact, I remember going back six

What to Do

- *Purchase shoes for fit, not by size.*

- *Have your gait analyzed prior to making a shoe purchase.*

- *The most trendy shoes may not be the right ones for you.*

months later and buying the same exact style and brand. In looking back, I can't believe I wore such poorly cushioned shoes and did not suffer any serious injuries.

—Wilma, age 43

If you walk into any sporting goods store, you will more than likely encounter rows and rows of shoes—shoes for all different sports and separate areas for men's and women's styles. Unfortunately, there are usually more men's than women's models, which is a bit baffling since women play many sports and probably buy just as many, if not more, shoes.

Selecting a pair of athletic shoes is in many ways easier today than it was a decade ago, when shoes were not available for specific sporting activities. One good rule of thumb for running gear is to purchase a good pair of shoes that will provide you with optimal comfort, support, and cushioning.

Whether you are an avid runner or new to the sport, you may want to ask a knowledgeable salesperson for help when purchasing a pair of running shoes. Just as the auto companies come out with new model cars, so do the shoe manufacturers. Many of us find it hard to keep up with the latest innovations and styles.

Do not be afraid to try on several pairs of shoes and to run up and down the aisle before you make a final purchase. When you walk or run, your feet elongate and spread out as they hit the ground. The shoe you purchase should feel comfortable and give you a degree of cushioning and support specific to your needs. The same holds true for athletic shoes for other sports, such as tennis, aerobics, etc.

Shoe sizes will vary by style and according to manufacturer. Have your feet measured regularly, especially as you grow older. Make sure you have both feet measured and select a shoe to fit the larger one. Don't purchase shoes that are too tight with the expectation that they will loosen up with time. Test "run" new shoes for comfort.

Tips: Footwear

- When trying on shoes, wear the same socks that you wear while exercising.
- Buy shoes during the same time of day that you plan to exercise.
- Take time when shopping for shoes. If you can't find the right shoe, try shopping elsewhere.
- Foot size is not static—have your feet measured annually.

Staying Warm

I have been running and cycling regularly for the last 15 years. Although I prefer the summer months, I must admit that it is refreshing to don a pair of running shorts and heavy sweatshirt and run in freshly fallen snow. People often stop and ask if I am cold when I run in shorts in the middle of the winter—but as long as it's not too windy, I am usually quite content. —Elisse, age 44

Layering clothing has proven to be one of the best ways to stay warm in cold weather, whether you are exercising or not. Air tends to get trapped between the various layers of clothing and thereby retains body heat and insulates you from the cold external elements. Most cold weather sports call for three layers: inner or base layer; a middle insulator; and an outer layer or protective shell to fend off air, wind, and moisture.

The last thing a runner wants is bulk. Layering need not add bulk, and in fact can be lighter than one heavy garment. Another advantage to layering is that you can always remove a layer without entering a deep freeze.

New Fabrics Keep You Drier.   To keep warm in the cold winter months, both women and men athletes must try to stay dry. While exercising, the body generates a lot of heat and sweat, which is why the inner or base layer of clothing is so important. If your base layer can't manage moisture, it won't matter how many layers you wear over it. Many fabrics are available nowadays that are capable of wicking moisture away from your body. Polypropylene materials are much softer than they were a decade ago, and while they may be better at getting rid of moisture, they have a tendency to retain body odors. Many of the newer fabrics are chemically treated to solve this problem. Some brand name fabrics that are suitable for an inner layer include: *Thermastat, Capilene, Thermax, Coolmax,* and *Lifa.* These brands offer both tops and bottoms.

Proper Layering.   The inner or base layer should fit you snugly to maximize moisture management. If there is an air space between your skin and the base layer, sweat will stay on your skin and cold air will find its way in.

Your middle layer of clothing should continue to transport moisture outward but also capture body heat. Wool is a good insulator, but it is also heavy when wet and has a tendency to be itchy. Synthetic fleeces such as *Polartec, Synchilla,* and *Therma Fleece* are lighter weight, easy to launder, and insulate just as well.

The outer layer or shell must fend off the elements and thus should be wind and water resistant or waterproof. Various microfibers are available to give protection against the elements, yet still allow breathability. You should make sure that the shell is not too tight, especially if it is to be worn with a bulky middle layer. Pay attention to the design of the shell, whether it is a jacket, pants, or coverage for your hands, head, or feet. A layering arrangement is recommended for your hands, head, and feet as well as your trunk and legs. When purchasing mittens, hats, and socks, follow the same principles of an absorbent inner layer, warm middle layer, and weather resistant outer layer.

Keeping Your Cool

Running in June through August takes just as much planning as December through March. While I needn't worry about layers of clothing, I find that on very hot and humid days I need to pay close attention to the fabrics in order to avoid materials that retain wetness and then chafe my skin. —Jenny, age 27

Summer running is not as simple as putting on any pair of shorts and a top and lacing up running shoes. If you run all year round, you know how much heat and sweat your body generates during the summer months. Some runners try to avoid cotton fabrics because cotton holds moisture and can get very heavy when wet. *Coolmax* is one brand name polyester fabric that has become very popular for summer running shorts, liners, and tops. Apparently, its fiber structure offers 20 percent more surface area than other fibers, resulting in faster moisture transport and evaporation. Another fiber made by *Nike, Dri-F.I.T.*, is said to be made of tiny bundles of fibers that can transport moisture—perhaps more efficiently.

TENNIS

Although you do need to find a court, relatively little gear is required for tennis: a racket, some balls, and a good pair of tennis shoes. Your foot type, body build, and style of play will be the determinants for shoe selection. For example, if you are concerned about speed and agility, a lightweight tennis shoe may be the best option. On the other hand, if you are overweight, a well-cushioned, heavier shoe may be the better alternative.

Some women tennis players who are unable to find comfortable shoes that are wide enough in the toe area resort to wearing men's shoes. However, as noted earlier, a better fit for your toes may be offset by the fact that men's shoes also have wider heels and a last that may be too stiff for some women athletes. Make sure that you can wiggle your toes and that the heel is a bit snug, but not tight. There should be a space approximately the width of your thumbnail between the end of the shoe and your longest toe.

The side-to-side movement in tennis mandates that you look for a shoe that offers stability. A firm heel counter may help to minimize rear foot motion, and external support straps may offer added protection during sudden stops. Make certain that your tennis shoes will cushion your feet adequately and that there is reinforcement in the toe area.

SKIING

The Layered Look and Other Alternatives

Staying warm in the winter months is much easier these days than it was when

I was growing up. I remember learning to ski in blue jeans and a heavy ski jacket and being very uncomfortable. Today, even though I spend more time on my skis and less time picking myself up, I have learned to use layers of clothing to stay warm and dry.

—Liz, age 49

Layered clothing seems to be the buzzword of the last decade. In addition, many new fabrics have been developed that can help keep you warmer and more comfortable. Choosing the right layers is as important as layering itself.

Think of cold as the absence of heat. In other words, to stay warm while skiing, you must keep the heat produced by your body in rather than just keeping the cold out. It is equally important to try to stay dry. Your comfort and safety level will depend on your body's heat production and the environment in which you are skiing. We've all read of unfortunate souls who have gotten drenched, developed hypothermia, and froze to death in cold weather. Proper layering can help to avert these potential disasters!

Effective Layering.   Start with a pair of long underwear against your skin to keep you warm and transport moisture to the outside. You may want to consider synthetics such as polypropylene, as they tend to wick moisture away faster than natural fabrics like wool and silk. *Thermax* (manufactured under the Dupont label) and *Capilene* tend to be softer and less odor retentive.[16] Most of these fabrics come in lightweight, midweight, and heavy or expedition weight. If you are performing aerobic work such as cross-country skiing, you will probably find the lightweight styles more to your liking. Midweight fabrics are well suited to Alpine or backcountry skiing. The heavier weight fabrics can be lifesaving in subarctic conditions.

The next layer of clothing should serve to slow down heat loss. Some skiers use this layer while warming up and later peel it off. Several options exist for this middle layer, including the very popular polyester fleece pullovers and wool sweaters. Some downhill skiers use down or synthetic fill jackets as a middle layer. Middle layers that are outfitted with zippers may enable you to cool off a bit without having to abandon the middle layer altogether.

The outer layer should be windproof, waterproof, and breathable. It is just as important to keep the wetness out as it is to expel any moisture the body generates. Two-way zippers and zip-up underarms are added conveniences on jackets.

Ski Pants

Women's pants tend to be higher waisted and cut fuller in the hips than pants designed for men. Pants with long zippers often help with ventilation and are certainly easier to slip over boots. If you like to carry gear such as sunscreen or your keys, be sure to count the number of pockets on your jacket and pants to be sure you'll have enough space to stow everything.

An alternative to pants is the one-piece ski suit. Women may find that they stay warmer in one-piece suits, as there are fewer openings to let warm air escape or to let cold drafts enter at the back and waist. In addition, these suits tend to be less bulky and thus more comfortable than a traditional two-piece outfit. On the downside, it is often difficult for women to obtain a proper fit so that the crotch does not ride up. In addition, one-piece suits tend to be less conducive to layering. They may also be a bit inconvenient when nature calls.[17] The last thing you want is for the rest room to be a dressing room!

Hats and Gloves

Since body heat is also lost from the head and extremities, it is important not to overlook hats and mittens or gloves. Mittens are usually warmer than gloves, because the fingers huddle together to conserve heat. The same layering principles apply here. Whatever ski outfits you select, warmth and comfort must reign. Before purchasing a garment, try it on and bend and stretch in it to make sure it will be comfortable. Don't forget—you are buying active wear because you will be active.

WATERWEAR

I am a white water enthusiast and often paddle on weekends with a mixed singles group. It is always a toss-up as to whether to wear a one- or two-piece swimsuit—if I wear a one-piece suit, I don't have to worry about losing a top or bottom when I get tossed into the white water; however, it's always a big to-do when it comes to something as simple as taking a wee. —Annie, age 29

Swimsuits are not just for swimming. In fact, swimwear has come a long way in 90 years. While many women wear swimsuits for swimming, they are also worn by water skiers, surfers, triathletes, and beach volleyball players—not to mention the casual beach lounger. As with any athletic equipment, it is important to have clothes that fit properly so you can concentrate on your activity and not your outfit.

CHOOSING A SWIMSUIT

Think Comfort

I recently joined a health spa and after building up the courage to go for a swim, I emerged from a dive with my bra piece hanging below my breasts. It took weeks be-fore I could face the swimming pool again; however, when I did, I made sure I wore a one-piece suit with criss-cross straps. —Emily, age 26

The most important factor to consider when purchasing swimwear is comfort. This theme has been emphasized previously and should not be overlooked. If your swimsuit is uncomfortable for whatever reason, you may not perform well, or you may suffer some adverse consequences.

If you are evaluating a swimsuit to use for pool workouts, it should be durable and provide a snug fit. A slightly tight fit may be important to minimize gaps where water can flush through. Water splashing against your chest and underarms adds drag, which ulti-mately makes you swim slower and work harder. That's fine for training, but not suitable for competitive events. Fabrics made of nylon or *Lycra* usually provide a snug fit.[18] While suits made of *Lycra* mold better to body contours, they also lose elasticity with time. On the other hand, nylon tends to be sturdier and outlasts *Lycra* but has the drawback of ab-sorbing more water, which adds an element of resistance. A *Lycra* suit is less abrasive than one constructed of nylon.[19]

Your snug-fitting swimsuit should allow just enough room that it doesn't cut into your underarms, shoulders, thighs, or groin. The bra part of a two-piece suit should not slide up and down. Other features to consider include a higher-cut neck, which is ideal for diving and helps to keep the breasts covered. You may need to experiment with suits that have different designs and widths of straps to find a suit that seems the most com-fortable and the least restrictive. Your choice of a swimsuit design may also be influenced by your predominant type of swimming stroke.

Not Just for Swimming.   If you are wearing your swimsuit for surfing, then aside from a tight fit, look for wide shoulder straps with a T-cut back to help keep the top from riding up. Bottoms with a high cut should provide freedom of movement. Similarly, beach vol-leyball players may want tops that allow ample arm movement and bottoms with high-cut legs that won't ride up.[20]

Suiting Your Body Type.   What about the recreational swimmer who wants physical comfort but also peace of mind that her swimsuit is flattering? After all, not all women who spend time at the beach or pool are elite athletes with trim figures. Plenty of women are now turning to swimming to help promote weight loss, so these hints may be helpful.

Spandex, which is an elastic fiber, may help to shape and give the body a firmer look. Although the average spandex content in swimsuit fabrics is usually about 15 percent, a fabric made of 18 percent or 32 percent spandex will further improve the image. The addition of a side wrap made of elastic interlining can help to reduce tummy bulge.[21]

A woman with wide hips might try a dark-colored suit. To minimize a pear-shaped figure, try a skirted suit with straight lines. Tiny shoulder straps also help to accentuate the shoulders and take the focus away from the fuller bottom. Likewise, if you have heavy thighs, you will want to emphasize details that draw the eyes upward and away from the area you want to minimize. In this case, a bold V-neck top may help. Also, a high-cut leg may give the legs a longer, slimmer appearance. The woman with short legs can also use the trick of wearing a high-cut suit and, in addition, may try horizontal detailing across the midriff to create waist interest. The swimsuit wearer who would like to de-emphasize a large rear can do so by hiding behind a skirt.

Many suits are sold with the option of a cup bra or shelf bra. As a rule, the tops are not sized as one would find with a bra, so it is a matter of trying on and checking for comfort, fit, and support. Large-breasted women may wear two-piece suits and not look ill-proportioned if they select one with a full cut and wide straps. A tank suit with a high neck, armholes, and back and also a built-in bra is a good option for the well-endowed woman. Conversely, the woman who wants to maximize a small bust may try a wide-swept neckline that bares the shoulders and gives the illusion of a fuller look. Many swimsuit manufacturers now have an option of suits that are made for the tall individual with a long torso, so the suit does not cause discomfort in the crotch.

Tips

- Carefully evaluate the pros and cons of all the different fabrics.
- Select a bathing suit style that compliments your best features and fits your body type.
- Look for manufacturers that sell tops and bottoms separately.

Suits and Private Parts.   Ginny, who is in her early thirties, works full time at a desk job and at nights and on weekends labors over a computer keyboard working on her master's thesis. For relaxation and exercise she joined a health club where she rides a stationary bicycle and then swims for 20 minutes. Over the last two years she has had several bouts of vaginal irritation and been diagnosed with yeast and "trich" infections that seem to be recurrent. She reports, "I keep asking the physicians and nurse practitioners at the women's health center whether it is the swimming or not . . . I am still waiting for an answer that makes sense."

While we're on the topic of swimsuits, a few words need to be mentioned about vaginitis. Vaginitis, which is simply an infection or inflammation of the vagina, is a common health problem for women. Vaginitis may have an infectious origin, such as from yeast (or candida), trichomonas, bacteria, or a noninfectious cause such as a chemical irritation. Each condition has different symptoms and treatments, which are beyond the scope of this chapter. For years, the jury has been out as to whether sitting around in a wet bathing suit can cause vaginitis. Some feel that the panty part of a wet swimsuit provides a warm, moist environment that allows organisms to thrive. One infectious disease expert, Jack Sobel, M.D., believes it is the chlorine in swimming pools that is irritating to the vagina, thus allowing a yeast infection to flare up.[22] More research needs to be conducted before we can answer the question of whether bathing suits are the culprits or not. But to possibly minimize the risk, change out of your bathing suit soon after leaving the water and promptly rinse out the chlorine.

Avoiding Bad Hair Days: Swim Caps

Another piece of gear that you may want to have on board is a swim cap. Swim caps made of *Lycra* or silicone, though easier to put on, may not keep your hair as dry as a cap made of latex. If you experience difficulty placing a snug cap on your head, you may consider first applying a small amount of hair conditioner. Not only does it help the cap to slide on, but it also reduces the amount of tangling.

Goggles

Purchasing a comfortable pair of goggles is often a matter of trial and error. Why? Not all women and men look alike—they have different facial features. Just as one pair of glasses does not fit all individuals, the same concept applies to goggles. However, it's getting easier to find goggles manufactured with the female in mind. These goggles are designed to fit a woman's smaller eye sockets and narrower nose bridge.[23]

Although you can have goggles made up with prescription lenses, it may be unnecessary, as many swimmers who wear regular goggles note that their eyesight actually improves due to the refractive effect of water. Aside from improving vision, goggles help to reduce eye irritation caused by swimming for long hours in a chlorinated pool or in open water. However, lens fogging is a common problem. Lenses with anti-fog coatings are available, or you may apply a few drops of a chemical or simply use your saliva to keep the lens clear. Another decision point involves whether you want clear or tinted lenses. The choice may depend on whether you swim indoors or out.

You will probably have to try on various pairs and make adjustments to the nosepiece and strap before you find a comfortable and good fit. Some goggles have a one-piece frame without a nosepiece, which may not be optimal for the swimmer who has a wide nose bridge.[24] Be careful not to keep the head strap too tight as a headache may ensue. Some swimmers find that a model with double straps is more comfortable. This is probably because double or split straps help to redistribute pressure, thus providing a tight but more comfortable fit.[25]

SUN IN

I still remember the first bad sunburn I got when I was a child. In those days, we didn't know much about how damaging the sun could be to our skin. As much as I like the feel of the warm sun, I try to avoid outdoor activities when the sun's rays are strongest. I also always make sure I have sunscreen on. —Joan, age 52, who has been diagnosed with precancerous skin lesions

Whether you are snorkeling in the Caribbean or winter skiing in the Alps, you need to protect your skin and eyes from the dangers of ultraviolet rays. Sunbathers are not the only ones who are at risk for damage to their skin by the sunshine—anyone who is outdoors during daylight hours should take certain precautions. Sunscreen should be in your equipment bag if you engage in outdoor activities. The latest data demonstrate that your sunscreen should be at least SPF 15.[26] You may also want to wear a hat with a large brim and loose long-sleeved clothing if you are going to be in the sun. While goggles are recommended safety equipment for many indoor and outdoor sports, sunglasses may be appropriate for other activities.

ALL DRESSED UP

Over the last two decades or so, many advances in women's sports clothing and gear have been made. This does not imply that there is no room for improvement. Women need to be informed consumers and not just settle for smaller sized men's gear painted in floral or pastel colors with a "women's" label slapped on the tag.

Equipment and clothing manufacturers must study women closely and begin (or continue) to design gear more appropriately. In addition to safety and comfort factors, women who have properly fitted clothing will be better able to enhance their sports performance. Women should not settle for second class clothing and equipment.

ENDNOTES

1. Gehlsen, G., & Albohm, M. Evaluation of sports bras. *Physician Sportsmedicine*, October 1980, 8 (10), 89–96.
2. Hunter, L. Y., & Torgan, C. The bra controversy: Are sports bras a necessity? *The Physician and Sportsmedicine*, November 1982, 10 (11), 75–76.
3. Levit, F. Jogger's Nipples. *New England Journal of Medicine*, 1977, 297 (20), 1127.
4. Stein, Anne. Pedaling to Freedom. *Women's Sports and Fitness*, 17 (8), November/December 1995, 27.
5. Zukowski, Stan. Clothes Call. *Women's Sports and Fitness*, April 1996, 18 (3), 66–67.
6. Ellis, T. H., Streight, D., & Mellion, M. B. Bicycle safety equipment. *Clinics in Sports Medicine*, January 1994, 13 (1), 75–98.
7. Pavelka, E. Hot pants. *Bicycling*, January 1994, 35 (1), 76–79.
8. Ellis, T. H., Streight, D., & Mellion, M. B. Bicycle safety equipment. *Clinics in Sports Medicine*, January 1994, 13 (1), 75–98.
9. Neporent, L. Fit for a woman: The top innovations in sports equipment made just for us. *Women's Sports and Fitness*, Jan–Feb 1994, 16 (1), 76–83.
10. Ellis, T. H., Streight, D., & Mellion, M. B. Bicycle safety equipment. *Clinics in Sports Medicine*, January 1994, 13 (1), 75–98.
11. Brody, J. E. How to select shoes that will not damage your feet. *New York Times*, October 11, 1995.
12. Frey, C. Pain and deformity in women's feet. *The Journal of Musculoskeletal Medicine*, Sept 1995, 12 (9), 27–32.
13. Wischnia, B and Brunick, T. *Runners World*. April 1995, 30 (4), 48–49.
14. Wichmann, S. with Martin, D. R. Athletic shoes: Finding the right fit. *The Physician and Sportsmedicine*, March 1993, 21 (3), 204–211.
15. Kuehls, D. Fit to be Tried. *Runners World*, October 1993, 28 (10), 76–77.
16. Getchell, A. Get layered. (Guide to winter dressing.) *Women's Sports and Fitness*, Nov–Dec 1995, 17 (8), 50–55.
17. Lerman, J. Skiwear: What works. *Skiing*, December 1994, 47 (4), 138–141, 207–210.
18. The best athletic swimsuits (tips on how to purchase a comfortable swimsuit). *Glamour*, May 1993, 91 (5), 226.
19. Cox, L. Seaworthy. *Women's Sports and Fitness*, July/August 1995, 17 (5), 73–75.
20. Lee, J. Swimsuits that work out: How to find the right fit for your sport. *Women's Sports and Fitness*, April 1994, 16 (3), 82–85.
21. Perfectly suited. (Picking the right swimsuit.) *Family Circle*, May 16, 1995, 108 (7), 80–81.
22. Lippert, J. Say good-bye to yeast infections. *Redbook*, June 1993, 181 (2), 46.
23. The lowdown on swim goggles and sports sandals. *Women's Sports and Fitness*, March 1993, 15, (2), 78–79.
24. Eye opener. The University of California, Berkeley *Wellness Letter*, Sept 1993, 9 (12), 7.
25. The lowdown on swim goggles and sports sandals. *Women's Sports and Fitness*, March 1993, 15, (2), 78–79.
26. Wentzell, J. M. Sunscreens: The ounce of prevention. *American Family Physician*, April 1996, 53 (5), 1713–1719.

9 Gearing Up: Making Informed Equipment Decisions

DONNA I. MELTZER, M.D.

A chapter on exercise equipment for women? Yes! Perhaps you are already familiar with many of the sporting goods available for women. If so, we will try to make you a more informed consumer. If you are new to sports or looking to upgrade your current sporting gear, read on. Many women find it enlightening when they finally discover equipment that fits them—be it unisex gear or apparatus designed specifically for active women. We will also share some helpful hints about what to look for in a health club.

WOMEN AND BICYCLES

Bicycling has become one of the most popular sports in the United States. Although the bicycle is simply a means of transportation for some Americans, it is also used to build or maintain cardiovascular fitness or may be prescribed as part of a rehabilitation program. For others, men and women alike, bicycling may just be recreational.

> *I have fond childhood memories of bicycling to and from elementary school with my sisters and friends. I abandoned my bike during high school and did not resume riding until after college—mostly for recreation. As I increased my daily mileage and level of fitness, it became apparent that my 10-speed "boys" touring bike was not that comfortable. On long rides I developed neck strain and saddle soreness. A decade later, I shopped for two months before I found a cycling store that spent a good deal of time measuring and then fitting me with a racing bicycle that was suitable for my shorter torso and smaller hands. Although it was rather expensive, my new bicycle is one of my better investments—it's unbelievable the pleasure I derive from riding a bike that finally fits me! —Wendy, age 44*

Would you ever purchase a pair of shoes that were uncomfortably too wide or too big? Would you ever purchase the first pair of shoes you tried on? Probably not—unless they were the only shoes available. However, many women have this experience when it comes to choosing a bicycle. In the past, the top-quality bicycles were built with the male physique in mind, yet purchased and used by both men and women. In the last decade or so, many advances have been made. Bikes that have been designed by women and for women riders are now available.

Bike Shopping

Not all bikes are created equal. Whether you are a serious rider about to upgrade your bike or new to the sport and looking to purchase a new or used bike, there are things you should think about before you set out shopping. Ask yourself some of the following questions:

- Do I want a man's or woman's frame?
- On what type of terrain will I be traveling—dirt mountain roads, city streets, paved country roads?
- How can I tell if a bike fits me?
- What kind of handlebars do I want?
- How many speeds do I want? 1, 3, 5, 10, 12, 18, or more?

Once you have answered (or tried to answer) some of the above questions, your next decision involves where to shop. If you know your size and exactly what you want, you may consider mail order shops, which may save you a few dollars. While you have the added expense of shipping and handling, it may be offset by a savings in sales tax. However, most women will probably want to be measured and to test ride a stationary bike adjusted to simulate the size bike they are about to purchase. Many shops will also let you take bikes outside for test rides. If you remember our discussion in Chapter 2 about some of the musculoskeletal gender differences, you will recall that women are not just shorter than men, but they also have shorter torsos, wider hips, and smaller hands—all very important when purchasing a bicycle.

About 12 years ago, I purchased my first "good" bicycle—or so I thought. I now think back that my "fitting" consisted of me sitting on the bike while the owner held the front wheel steady. This time, I shopped around and found a store that spent time having me sit on a sizing bike while they adjusted the seat, handlebars, etc. I continued to shop around and then returned to the shop that emphasized having a good-fitting bicycle. Again, they spent nearly an hour re-measuring and having me test ride the adjustable bike. They seemed sensitive to the fact that a woman has to be very careful about getting the proper fit on a man's bicycle. I couldn't be much happier with my new bike. —Marcy, age 40

Bike Anatomy. Most bikes today can be divided into racing, touring (road), mountain (all-terrain), and hybrid bikes. The major differences lie in the frame and the "components," which consist of handlebars, brake sets, and wheels.

Setting the Framework. Bike frames, which can be distinguished by the position of the crossbar, come in three styles: men's, women's, and **mixte**. The typical men's or boy's bike has a diamond-shaped frame with a top tube or crossbar that is parallel to the ground, while the women's bike has a low-slung top tube. In between the two is the diagonally positioned double lateral tubes found in the mixte frame. The mixte frame is considered to be stronger than the ladies' frame, but not as solid as the diamond-shaped man's version. With the advent of all-terrain bikes, the mixte frames have taken a back seat. Consequently, you may have to shop around to find a suitable mixte frame.

If you are planning on wearing a skirt while riding, have trouble lifting and swinging your legs around, or want to be able to dismount easily, a women's or mixte bicycle frame may be appropriate. Several years ago, most of the top-quality bicycles were built on a men's frame. Today, women have more options—including better components and lighter weight frames—without having to purchase a bike with a parallel crossbar.

In 1985, a woman engineer named Georgena Terry decided to design a bike specifically for women, whether they were under five feet or close to six feet tall. You might say that she reinvented the wheel, because she ended up designing a line of bikes where the front wheel is smaller than the rear so that short-torsoed women do not have to reach a great distance to the handlebars. (A smaller front wheel was necessary to keep the pedals from bumping into it when the top tube was shortened.) If you are having difficulty finding a well-fitting bicycle, you may want to investigate Terry's company, Terry Precision Cycling for Women, which is celebrating its tenth anniversary of making bikes and apparel exclusively for women.[1]

Scouting Out the Terrain. The type of terrain that you plan on riding will help you to determine which type of bicycle is best for you. If you plan to ride on rough mountainous terrain, you will want a fat-tired mountain bike. Some people who live in urban areas find that these all-terrain mountain bikes are just that—great for dirt roads and pot-holed city streets. On the other hand, if you anticipate riding on well-paved roads, a lightweight racing or touring (road) bike might suit you better.

A cross between road and mountain bikes yields a breed called the **hybrid.** Hybrid bikes have sturdy frames with wheels capable of handling paved or unpaved roads. If you plan on riding on different surfaces and unpredictable terrain, the hybrid may be an ideal bike for you.

Sizing Up the Job.   Once you have decided on a type of bike and frame, it is crucial that you aim toward achieving the proper fit. There are a couple of approaches: you can determine the standover height by measuring your inseam, which is the distance from the floor to your crotch, or you can find a suitable fit by trial and error. The trouble with the latter method is that your bike shop must either have the bikes in stock or be willing to spend time while you try each bike on for size. Hopefully, they will have a stationary bike that can be adjusted to simulate the specifications of your future purchase.

A general rule of thumb is that if you straddle the crossbar of your bike (assuming it is a man's frame), you will want to clear the crossbar by about one to two inches for a road bike and about three to six inches for a mountain bike.[2] Be sure to wear shoes similar to the ones you wear while cycling in order to test for optimum fit.

Once you have calculated the appropriate standover height, your next step is to determine whether you can reach the handlebars without undue stretch and discomfort. If you can't, a shorter stem may bring the handlebars closer. The problem can also be remedied by moving the saddle seat forward (but not far enough to affect your pedaling style). A quick upper body sizing test is to place your elbow against the nose of the saddle and see if the fingers of your outstretched hand reach the handlebar with ease. If the handlebar is well out of your reach, saddle and stem adjustments will probably not completely solve the oversized top tube length problem.

Don't underestimate the importance of a good upper body fit. A common complaint among women who ride bikes made for men is neck strain and an achiness between the shoulder blades. As discussed in Chapter 2, women are not built to the same proportions as men and tend to have shorter torsos and shorter arms. Consequently, on a bike designed for men, women end up having to strain to reach the handlebars and brakes. This is a surprisingly common problem even with the mixte frames. Next time a pack of cyclists passes you on the street, take note of whether the women are riding with outstretched arms and locked elbows compared to the male riders. Hopefully you never fit this description!

Tips
- Select a bicycle that fits your size as well as your riding style.
- Your bicycle should be sized to fit both your lower body and upper torso.
- Be careful—men's bicycles are not designed with women in mind.

Get a Handle on This.   Another component to consider when purchasing a bicycle is the type of handlebar: "drop"-type bars are generally found on racing and touring bikes, while upright handlebars (straight or curved) are often associated with all-terrain and hybrid bikes. More recently, handlebars have even been modified with forward reach attachments to improve aerodynamics and comfort level.

Since we also have narrower shoulders than our male counterparts, handlebar sizing should not be ignored. On a road bike, the handlebar width should be nearly equal to your shoulder width, so your arms aren't spread too far apart. However, racers sometimes find they breathe more easily when their hands are positioned farther apart. Sizing is less of a problem with the flat handlebars of mountain bikes, which can be shortened with a hacksaw until a more ideal fit is achieved.

Get a Good Grip.   If you do a lot of cycling, you will want to pay attention to the padding of the handlebars, not only to get a better grip, but also to avoid any nerve injury to the wrist and hand. (Cycling gloves can also help. Some pointers on selecting cycling gloves were reviewed in the previous chapter, Dressing for the Job.) Pay attention to the way your hands grip the handlebar. Do this before you make any dramatic changes to the handlebars or brake levers. On a road bike, rest your hands on the brake hoods while going at an easy pace. When you exert yourself, you may position your hands on the top of the handlebar, or on the handlebar drops when going fast. On a mountain bike with a flat handlebar, grasp the bar with a firm—but not too tight—grip. You will want to brake with your index and middle fingers while the other fingers maintain a grip on the bar.

Taking a "Brake."   Another component to critically evaluate is the comfort and safety of the brake lever. Since women tend to have smaller hands than men, they often must stretch to reach the brake levers, which may be fatiguing (if not disconcerting) on long rides. If this profile sounds familiar, it may be worthwhile to inquire about short-reach brake levers.

Your brake levers should be within close reach, especially if you are traveling at high speed down an incline. Here are some pointers to help ensure safe braking: On a road bike, you should be able to reach and squeeze the brake levers while your hands rest comfortably on the brake hoods. On a mountain bike, you should be able to reach the brake lever and pull it with at least two fingers while your hands rest on the grips. With both types of bikes, it is crucial that you are able to squeeze the brake levers enough to come to a full stop.

Don't Sit This One Out.   No discussion of bicycling equipment would be complete without a few words about saddle woes. One study of amateur cyclists of both sexes participating in a week-long 500-mile ride demonstrated that 64 percent of the cyclists experienced buttock pain and 33 percent reported groin and crotch discomfort.[3] Another study reported that on a 4,500-mile ride across the U.S., nearly all of the participants experienced at least mild saddle soreness.[4]

To prevent or alleviate the problem of saddle soreness, you should make sure that your bike seat fits you. It has been suggested that if you are constantly shifting on your seat while riding, you should try out a women's saddle, if you have not done so already.[5] Several saddle seats are designed specifically for the female figure. As a general rule, women's saddle seats are wider in the rear and have a shorter nose. Some newer models have a central area cut out to reduce pressure on the vaginal area (especially the labia and clitoris). You might try adjusting the saddle so that the nose points downward, which will diminish pressure in these areas.

If your saddle fits well and you still experience discomfort, you may want to check the padding of the seat and your shorts. Gel and sheepskin paddings are available and can be placed over your bike seat. These products have earned mixed reviews. Another approach would be to invest in a good pair of cycling shorts or tights. (Review the discussion in Chapter 8 for more information.)

One last suggestion for correcting saddle soreness is to adjust the position and height of the seat. You will need someone to stand and hold your bike steady while you determine the correct seat height. With your heels on the pedals, sit on the seat with your pelvis level. Next, pedal backwards and adjust the seat so your knee is fully extended (straight) when the pedal is at its lowest point. Then place your feet on the pedals in a correct riding position so that the balls of your feet are directly over the axle of the pedal. In this foot position, a proper seat height is obtained when the knee is bent 15 to 20 degrees, again with the pedal at the lowest position.[6]

What We Know

Factors to consider when purchasing a bicycle:

- *frame size*
- *handlebar type*
- *ability to reach the brake levers*
- *saddle comfort*
- *number of gears and speeds*

How Many Speeds?   You can nearly date a person by asking them how many speeds their first two-wheeled bicycle sported. Some people may remember only a single speed, while others considered themselves lucky to have owned a three-speed bike, and still others regarded ten speeds as the norm. Today, many bikes come outfitted with more than ten speeds.

Most recreational riders fare well with a wide range of gears to handle all the different terrain and elevations they may encounter on an outing. A narrow range of gears is probably more suitable for the die-hard racer or the recreational cyclist who rides on level terrain.

Americans love trends. It is therefore not surprising that many techniques and styles have developed from the two basic kinds of skiing: Alpine and Nordic. Alpine or downhill skiing is one of the most popular forms of the sport in the United States. Paralleling the pursuit of cardiovascular fitness, however, we've witnessed a growing American interest in Nordic, or cross-country, skiing.

Freestyle skiing is a form of downhill skiing and **telemark** is a technique of downhill skiing accomplished with a particular type of cross-country equipment. Snowboarding, ski jumping, skating (on short, slick skis), and speed skiing have also grown in popularity over the years.

For each of these different types of skiing, there is equipment to match. Ski gear seems to change from season to season. For example, the current trends are shorter skis and those with slightly curved parabolic shapes. All this variety is great, but it can also be overwhelming to recreational downhill and cross-country skiers as well as to first-time buyers.

Whether you are a veteran of the ski slopes and trails or new to the sport, there are things that you should appreciate about ski equipment. While we cannot change the anatomical differences that set us apart from our male counterparts, we can at least look for gear that better suits our different sizes and shapes.

Alpine (Downhill) Ski Equipment

The Skis

Last winter, friends at work talked me into renting a ski lodge with them. I was a novice downhill skier and basically inherited some hand-me-down ski equipment. Midway through the season and after much research, I splurged and bought new boots and skis. That was one of my wisest investments as I immediately began to ski better. —Judy, age 33

Alpine (downhill) skiing, as the name implies, is skiing down a slope. It is a speed sport where the skis are wide and have bindings that fit both the heel and toe of the boot to the ski.

In the early 1980s the first "feminine" skis were marketed; these tended to be low-end models. However, today you can buy high-performance skis made especially for women.[7] You just need to know what to look for in ski gear.

Women who are strong and aggressive skiers and who prefer high speeds may have no problem with "unisex" skis. However, not all beginners and recreational skiers want to give up control in favor of speed. Whatever your skiing style or skill level, it's important to have gear that fits your body type. (Remember all the anatomical differences we pointed out in Chapter 2.) Although women's skis are available, some women may prefer men's or unisex skis.

Aside from sizing, the major difference between women's skis and men's or unisex skis has to do with flex distribution. As a rule, women's skis tend to have a balanced flex, which means the tip and tail of the ski give the same amount under pressure and bend in a more or less even arc. Skis with an even or balanced flex are fine for maintaining control in soft snow or on bumps at slow speeds. However, you may prefer an unbalanced flex pattern with a stiffer tail than tip in order to keep from skidding and losing control at high speeds on icy surfaces.

Changing your equipment can help change your skiing. If you are one of those skiers who finds herself always skidding into turns, you may want to look into the recently developed parabolic, or "shaped," skis. Parabolic skis, which have wider tips and tails for increased stability, are now in the spotlight. These skis have revolutionized skiing for beginners by allowing turns on the slopes to be almost automatic. These skis can be purchased in unisex and women's versions.

Women are often more comfortable with skis made of lighter materials and a looser weave, so that they are better able to edge and carve into turns. Lightweight, softer skis also tend to perform better in powder and are superior shock absorbers on uneven terrain. If you are a strong, relatively heavy skier who likes skiing fast, you may be able to apply enough pressure to a pair of stiff skis to initiate turns without losing control and speed. Advanced skiers who have climbed the learning curve may find that the traditional longer and narrower skis perform better.

Women have a lower center of gravity and carry more weight in their hips and buttocks than men. Consequently, you may want to adjust the ski's binding sites. Otherwise, you may find your ski tips crossing over one another, making them more difficult to control. On unisex or men's skis, try mounting the bindings slightly forward to help redistribute the added seat weight, so that balance is maintained and turns can be negotiated with more ease. This is often done routinely on the women's versions.

Boots.   Several years ago very few alpine ski boots were available specifically for women, but things are changing, albeit slowly. One skier has pointed out that while bootmakers have recognized that women's feet, ankles, and calves are different from men's, they still fail to make shells that match the shape of a woman's foot.[8] She notes that anatomic differences only appear in the liners, and that women who ski frequently may find that the liner eventually molds to the shape of the shell, which is designed for a man's foot. The end result is a sloppy fit.

When buying ski boots, remove the inner boot to ensure that the hard outer plastic shell fits your foot. Be alert to the fact that many of the so-called "women's" shells tend to be scaled-down men's models. In years past, little attention had been paid to the fact that women generally have higher insteps and narrower heels. Fortunately, nowadays many ski gear manufacturers are designing women's ski boot shells that actually fit women. Look carefully at the design and not just the label!

With that achieved, you will need to strive for a liner or inner boot that also fits your foot. Since most women have shorter calves and smaller ankles than men, unisex liners might not do the trick. Women's ski boots should have shorter, flared cuffs because of our lower tapered calves, but should not be so soft that control is forfeited. (The cuff is the part of the shell that surrounds the ankle and lower leg.) Avoid purchasing ski boots with high cuffs, which will pinch your calves and cut off the circulation to your feet.

The top-of-the-line women's ski boots may offer some of the same technical features found in men's ski boots, such as shaft alignment (or cuff canting) that centers the leg in the boot shaft. This is especially important if you, like many women, have knock-knees.[8] Without a cant adjustment or alignment, bowlegged skiers will stand on the outside edges of their boots, and knock-kneed skiers will stand on the inside edges.

For finishing touches, think about adding heel lifts to your ski boots. Heel lifts help to maintain proper balance. They work by moving your center of mass forward and promoting more ankle flex.

Let's face it, ski boots are expensive. Many skiers have discovered that it is often easier to save money on skis than on boots. If you are thinking of purchasing new boots, be realistic about your skiing ability. Buy for fit, not for looks. Some boots allow you to make adjustments as your skiing improves. Look into this before splurging on new boots—especially if you were happy with the fit of your old ones. Some skiers tell women to throw away their men's boots and only consider women's versions, but only you and your pocketbook can make this decision.

Finding ski boots that fit you is not an easy task. It takes research and perseverance. What is a good fit for one person may not be comfortable or safe for you. Don't settle for just any ski boot. And by all means, don't be afraid to shop around.

Tips
- Find a ski outfitter who is interested not just in selling, but also in fitting.
- Beware of ski shops that lack experience in catering to women skiers.
- You want to work with a retailer who can answer your questions.

Nordic (Cross-Country) Equipment

Skis.   Nordic (cross-country) skis are skinnier than alpine varieties and have bindings that leave the heels unattached to the skis. The energy required to maintain motion makes it a sport of endurance that is tops for aerobic conditioning.

Over the years, cross-country skiing has become more and more specialized. The sport is increasingly defined by the type of terrain: track and off-track. Track skiers tend to use prepared trails at a cross-country resort or golf course, or tracks made by snowmobiles. Some folks use the term touring to describe this type of skiing. These skis tend to be lightweight.

Once you leave the trails and head for the backcountry, you are considered an off-track skier. Here, you will frequently encounter irregular terrain, snow drifts, and other natural obstacles. If you are considering off-track skiing, look for skis that are on the heavier side, as they will handle the rugged terrain more effectively. Backcountry skis should be wider than touring or track models. A wider ski will also give better flotation in soft, slushy snow.

One of the latest evolutions in cross-country skiing is skating. Skating is done on a groomed trail (without tracks) and is so named because of the "skating" stride the skier uses to propel herself. It is also one of the more labor-intensive forms of cross-country skiing. Skating skis evolved from racing skis and are usually narrow and light. With the advent of shorter skate skis, this style of skiing became easier to perform. Once you become a polished skater, you may find that longer skis allow you to ski faster because your body weight is distributed over a longer distance. Beginners should start with shorter skis and work their way up because longer skis can seem unwieldy and may deter the novice skier.

Don't make a mistake and attempt to learn to skate well on touring skis. There are differences in the skis, boots, and bindings that distinguish the various forms of skiing.

Although more and more women are taking up cross-country skiing, the equipment does not seem to be made specifically for women.[9] The bottom line for purchasing a pair of skis (whatever the type) is to do plenty of research. Browse through the latest ski magazines, speak to other skiers, and ask lots of questions in the ski shops.

Boots.   Cross-country ski boots need to do more than keep your feet warm and dry. The boots, in conjunction with bindings, should provide support and flexibility. Make sure that your boots fit and feel comfortable. The more boots you try on, the better the odds that you will find a brand and model that matches your foot. Be as selective with your cross-country ski boots as you would with a pair of running shoes.

Most track or touring boots are cut lower in the ankle than their off-track cousin. In the backcountry, your ski boots should also be heavier and warmer than touring boots.

It is now easier to find a compatible match between boots and ski bindings. Assuming that you have found a comfortable boot, let's take a look at the bindings. For touring, the boot/binding system should allow your heel to rise up and down, providing lateral support with minimal resistance. Off-track and skating bindings should be stiffer so that the heels of the boots do not wander too far from the skis.

Poles: Downhill and Cross-Country Skiing

Ski poles should be thought of as extensions of your arms. Because of their simplicity, the importance of ski poles is often overlooked. The four parts of a pole that you need to evaluate are the shaft, basket, tip, and grip. Whether you are a downhill or cross-country skier, you will want the shaft of the ski pole to be strong yet lightweight.

New alloys and space-age materials that are constantly being developed for use in ski poles have revolutionized the gear. Check with a reliable ski store for the latest in materials. Keep in mind that you cannot judge the weight of the pole by the diameter of the shaft. An ultra-skinny "pencil pole" may weigh more than the latest composite wider pole. One of the more recent innovations is a hybrid pole made of both aluminum and composite materials.[10] Some skiers prefer the composite poles because of their shock-absorbing characteristics.

One method of testing the size of an Alpine pole is to turn it upside down and grasp the pole below the basket. This technique helps you achieve a more accurate fit because you will be taller when wearing ski boots. Your arm should form a right angle at the elbow. Alternatively, you could strap into your boots and skis to test out the length of the ski pole. You should note that poles that are too long for you may cause you to lean backwards.

Cross-country ski pole length is dependent on the type of skiing you will be doing. Skating poles should be stiff and reach your chin or nose, while touring ski poles should reach between your armpit and shoulder. A longer length is required for skating because you will be swinging your arms in a greater arc. You will also need a longer pole if you intend to ski in the backcountry because the poles tend to sink into unpacked snow. Telescoping poles are a good choice because they can be adjusted to different lengths according to terrain and snow conditions. Adjustable poles are especially useful if you plan to ski in the backcountry. You can extend them to help with uphill climbs, retract them as you head down hills, and use in two different lengths for traversing.

Poles come with a variety of baskets, from wide ones for powder skiing to small disks for racing. Many factors will influence your choice of a basket. While a large basket may prevent the pole from sinking too deeply into the snow, it may also increase the resistance in the wind and snow. For backcountry and telemark skiing, slightly spiked, carbide-tipped poles are most durable. If you ski mostly on soft powder, less expensive poles with rounded tips are acceptable.

Since most ski equipment is designed for men, women need to seriously look at the fit of the grip. This is especially important due to the anatomical differences in hand size as well as the number of thumb injuries caused by falling onto a hand that is gripping a ski pole. When shopping for a pole, make sure you wear gloves so you have a better idea of the true grip. (Would you shop for running shoes without your socks?)

The fact that ski poles come in matched sets for the right and left hands is often over-looked. Hold your poles upright and note to which side the top strap falls on the handle—left for the left hand and vice versa. The grip should feel comfortable and you should feel in control of the swing. Ultimately, your choice of a ski pole will depend on where and how you ski.

GETTING IN LINE

More and more in-line skates are available for women than ever before. Remember, our feet and ankles are distinct and not just smaller men's versions. Some of the advances seen with in-line skates include lower cuffs to fit women's legs better and easier-to-use braking systems.[11] As with most gear, you get what you pay for. Lower-end skates usually have smaller and cheaper wheels with less durable bearings and flimsy liners. A fitness skate usually has more expensive wheels and bearings that roll smoothly, as well as a good boot. The boot should be well padded and, most of all, comfortable from the onset, whether you are a first-time skater or an accomplished one.

TENNIS, ANYONE?

Rackets

What about selecting the right racket? A tennis racket should be selected according to how its characteristics match your tennis style and technique. Some qualities to consider include head size, power, control, comfort, and string tension.[12] Since several variations of tennis rackets are available, you will also need to consider the construction, materials, flexibility, and weight of the racket.[13]

Most rackets today are made of "composite," a combination of shock-absorbing materials.[14] Composite materials tend to be lighter in weight. This is important for women who may not have the upper body strength to handle a heavy racket.

Another important feature to consider is head size. In the mid-seventies, the first oversized model was manufactured. Instead of the traditional 70-square-inch surface area, oversized heads are 110 square inches. The larger heads give players more stability against off-center shots and more power to the swing, along with the obvious advantage of more surface area with which to hit the ball. On the downside, oversized tennis rackets are harder to maneuver and make it more difficult to angle certain shots. Some people have complained that these oversized, powerful rackets have made the game too fast. Another innovation that has invaded the tennis scene is the racket that is one to two inches longer than the standard racket.[15] Your playing style helps determine if the "extra-long" is for you. It has been reported that extra-longs help to improve serve and give more power and reach. Since women tend to be shorter than men, the extra-long racket is a win-win proposition for the smaller player. While a little extra reach may benefit the person of average height, it is incrementally advantageous for the smaller tennis player.[16]

After deciding on weight, width, and length, other features to evaluate are string gauge and tension. Thicker strings are usually stronger and last longer, but thinner strings can be bouncier and may increase playability.[17] The more inflexible a tennis racket, the more power it will generate. If you have a powerful stroke, you may want to select a racket that has more flexibility. Similarly, those with slower strokes should have a stiffer model to add power. You may also want to experiment with adjusting the tension. If the strings are pulled too tightly, it may be hard on the frame and your elbow. On the other hand, if the strings aren't tight enough, you might have a difficult time controlling your shot.

Getting the Grip Right.   One of the most important features for a woman tennis player to evaluate is the grip. Women have smaller hands than men; therefore, they need to make extra sure that the handle fits properly. A racket handle that is too big may make you grip the racket too tightly, which could cause wrist or arm strain.[18] On the other hand, a larger handle may be easier to control when tennis balls hit the racket head off-center, because there is less twisting of the racket upon ball impact, resulting in less shock and strain on your playing arm.[19] Your grip size should be the largest you can hold with comfort.

Sizing Things Up.   One easy method used to determine proper grip size is to measure the distance from the tip of your ring finger to the crease that crosses the center of your palm. (You may note that there are several long creases on your palm; however, one usually seems more prominent than the others when you flex or bend your hand inward. This is the palmar crease.) When making the measurement, you should measure in between the middle and ring fingers and also make sure you use the dominant hand, which will be holding the racket. This number in inches should correspond to the circumference of the racket handle that best fits your hand.[19]

If you are between sizes, you may wish to opt for the smaller-sized grip because you can always build up the grip with padding and tape. If your tennis racket grip is worn and tattered, it should be replaced, as a worn-out grip does not provide a cushion against shock and vibration. You may want a flat, smooth grip or a raised, contoured surface that makes the grip easier to hold.[20]

Tennis racket handles are now being designed to help limit shock and vibration.[21] If you are plagued with upper extremity injuries that are not corrected with proper racket and grip size or adjustments in string tension, you may want to explore some of the newer innovations in handle design and construction.

JOIN THE CLUB

Golf clubs, whether private, public, or quasi-public, don't truly recognize women golfers, sometimes in subtle ways: not enough toilets in bathrooms, and little encouragement to young girls if they are interested in golf. —Helen, age 49

More and more women play golf these days. Some women find golf is a gentler form of exercise than, say, jogging or cycling; many are intrigued by the challenge of a good golf game, and for others it is love at first swing. Whatever the reason, the number of amateur and professional golfers is on the rise.

There are specific issues for women golfers to consider when it comes to equipment. Much of what has been said earlier about comfort in clothes and shoes applies to golf apparel. For years, manufacturers have produced golf clubs with women golfers in mind. However, be aware that some manufacturers simply put a "women's" label on golf clubs that are really made for men but downsized to fit a women's shorter stature.

Your height, build, and the length of your arms need to be considered when fitting golf clubs. The type of golf club a beginner might select is very different from what a pro would feel comfortable swinging. Do not be led astray by name brands, promotions by the professionals, and recommendations of friends. Choose a club based on size, feel, and stroke mechanics—in other words, your own opinion.

You might want to consider a personalized golf club. While they are more expensive than the basic models, customized clubs can be less expensive than some best-selling name brands. A less expensive route to customization is to get fitted by a pro and then see if you can match the specifications without having a club custom built.

Volumes have been written about the different types of golf clubs: woods, irons, wedges, and putters. The types of clubs you decide to carry in your bag are somewhat arbitrary. Many golfers opt for a set of 14 clubs: a driver for teeing off, two or three woods for the longer shots, a set of irons for approaching the green, two or three wedges for getting out of difficult situations, and a putter.[22] Here are a few pointers to help make your selection of clubs easier.

While many women are tall enough to handle a man's club, other features should also be considered. Look for a golf club that is not too heavy. Compared to men, women have less upper body strength and therefore do not want a club that seems too heavy while swinging. You may want to have your golf swing analyzed by a professional to help determine the best set of clubs for you. All the irons should weigh the same and have a matched center of gravity when you compare a five iron with a nine iron. The same holds true for the other clubs.

Just as properly fitting grips are important, so are the shafts of clubs. Stiff shafts tend to help maintain an accurate swing, while a more flexible shaft will increase swing speed. Not surprisingly, many women need to have more flexibility in the shafts to add speed. On the other hand, if you tend to swing fast, you may want a golf club with a stiffer shaft.

Since putting accounts for 43 percent of all golf shots, you should evaluate this club carefully.[23] The length and shaft angle should complement your physique and posture: The putter should be long enough to allow you to practice without incurring back pain and it should also allow you to position your eyes directly over the putting line with your hands directly under your shoulders. Find the lightest putter that fits. The grip should also fit properly. Lastly, your putter should feel solid and promote confidence.

WEIGHT TRAINING EQUIPMENT

I used to jog on a regular basis until a new job forced me to change my exercise routine. I now travel a few days a week and often find myself checking into hotels in large metropolitan areas. I soon discovered the hotel health clubs. Initially, I exercised on the treadmills, which was really boring. Once I learned some of the ins and outs of the weight training machines I was hooked. —Madeline, age 33

Free Weights vs. Weight Machines

You can build and maintain strength with either free weights or weight machines. Which one is for you?

Free weights have been around for a long time and are not very expensive. Free weights allow for a natural range of motion. They also score high on the "low maintenance" scale. On the downside is the safety factor. Having someone "spot" you helps to reduce the risk of serious injury. As simple as an exercise program involving free weights may seem, novice lifters usually benefit from having someone instruct them in proper form and style.

What We Know
Free Weights vs.
Weight Machines

FREE WEIGHTS
Pro
• *low cost*
• *maintenance-free*
Con
• *spotter may be needed*

WEIGHT MACHINES
Pro
• *safer*
• *easy to use*
Con
• *expensive*
• *space requirements*

Dozens of different weight training machines are available today. As a rule, exercise machines tend to be safer than free weights as there is little risk of dropping a weight on yourself, hence eliminating the need for a spotter. Because machines guide your movement through a set path, there is less chance for injury. Many beginners may find exercise machines appealing as they do not require a tremendous amount of skill to use. But machines usually require more space and are also more expensive than free weights.

Free weights are neither better nor worse than weight training machines; selecting one or the other depends on the individual and that individual's fitness goals.

Combining free weight and machine training is a popular option. By varying your routine, you make exercise anything but routine. In addition to reducing boredom, exercising different muscle groups with different exercises helps to maximize your strength training.

Free Weights: Shopping Tips.   Free weights include dumbbells and barbells, which allow you to perform a variety of exercises. You decide on the movement and the amount of weight. Dumbbells, which can be lifted with one hand, allow you more freedom of movement compared to barbells. Dumbbells come in a variety of weights. The weights you select will depend on the body part you want to strengthen.

Quality features to search for include contoured handles to improve comfort level and hexagonal ends to keep the weights from rolling away. Foam or rubber coatings in bright colors may add to comfort but will also add to the cost. The decorative colors are certainly more attractive than steely gray weights, especially if you are going to store your dumbbells out in the open. If you want to expand your workout and include bench pressing and squatting, barbells are another option. Pay attention to the thickness of the bar to make sure you will be comfortable gripping it.

Weight Machines: Shopping Tips.   As complex as they may seem, most weight machines are simple to operate. These weight machines are also referred to as multi-gyms or multi-station units because of all the different exercises that can be done on a single machine. You will want a home gym with enough features to strengthen your major muscle groups. Make sure your setup allows a full range of motion: You should be able to fully straighten your arms and legs to gain the full benefits of the exercises.

The big question with training equipment is whether a five foot, three inch woman weighing 120 pounds can effectively and safely use the same machine that is designed for a five foot, ten inch man weighing 200 pounds. Dan Baldwin, president and CEO of Nautilus, didn't think women could. So, in 1990, he began marketing Women's Nautilus, strength training machines designed for a woman's smaller frame.[24] The company redesigned the frames, bars, and movement arms and downsized and repositioned other parts so women would not have to sit in unnatural positions to use the equipment. The weights were also modified to make them less intimidating to novice lifters. You may want to investigate this equipment if you find yourself always stretching when you should be resting.

At this point, we assume that you are motivated and the weight machine will not simply gather dust in the corner. Be certain that you have plenty of space, not only in surface area, but also in vertical clearance. The machine should fit your body size and also be sturdy enough so it does not wobble every time you make a move. Lastly, you want not only versatility, but also ease. If it takes a long time to assemble an attachment to exercise a different muscle group, you may lose interest quickly.

EXERCISING AT HOME: THE MACHINES

Now that you have made the decision to try aerobic machines to achieve or maintain fitness, you have some big decisions ahead of you. While exercise equipment for the home gym has become more readily available and affordable, the selection can be mind-boggling. Before buying any equipment, consider how often you plan to use it and why. Stair climbers, treadmills, stationary bikes, cross-country skiing devices, and rowing machines can all be used for warm-up or for a total aerobic workout. While there is no single piece of equipment that will exercise every part of your body, many of these machines will give you a vigorous workout. The more you plan to use a piece of equipment, the more important quality becomes.

Step on It: Stair Machines

Stair machines, also known as stair climbers or steppers, have become very popular with women because the machines are good cardiovascular conditioners that concentrate on toning the hips, thighs, buttocks, and calves. The workout replicates climbing an endless flight of stairs, but without the impact.

Dependent vs. Independent Action.   There are two types of stair machines: those with dependent action and those with steps that work independently. Stair climbers with dependent motion require you to straighten out your leg as you step down before the other pedal can rise. More expensive models usually have an independent stepping motion where the movement of one pedal is not affected by the other. Independent action may be less stressful to the knees because the climbing and stepping movements tend to be more fluid.

Manual vs. Electronic Models.   Stair climbers may be either manually or electronically controlled. Less expensive manual models rely on hydraulics to control the pedals. The electronic versions use cables, chains, and flywheels to supply resistance, which results in smoother climbing. Many computerized versions are now available, and these may be more motivational, as they allow you to change the resistance and the depth of the stepping, in addition to giving you instantaneous feedback on time spent exercising, distance traveled, your pace, and calories expended.

The Cost Hurdle.   Stair climbers for home use usually cost between $200 and $500, whereas the sturdier computerized models typically found in gyms can easily carry a price tag of over $2,000.[25] Look for a machine that is steady and free of wobbles as you step and increase the pace. If you are prone to knee or hip problems or plan to use the stepper as part of a rehab program, make sure you can adjust the height of the steps to mitigate the chances of stressing these joints.

Other features to look for include pedals that are large enough to allow you to step comfortably and that remain parallel to the floor as you step. These properties are important to make sure that you do not lose your footing as you increase the intensity of your workout. Select a stair climber that has sturdy handrails should you require them to maintain your balance. Models without handrails often do not encourage proper body mechanics. (Remember, leaning on the handrails or monitors means less weight gets transferred to the pedals, resulting in an easier workout.)

Stepping Form.   Maintain erect posture throughout the workout. Start with small steps and gradually increase the stepping pace and depth. Do not lean on the control panel. If you are so tired that you must rest your body weight on the rails or monitors, ease up.

Running in Place: Treadmills

A treadmill can offer you all the advantages of walking, jogging, or running without any of the disadvantages of dealing with inclement weather, vehicular traffic, and other hazards. They have been popular in health clubs for years, and are becoming increasingly popular for home use as well. They appeal to many people: senior citizens desiring a low-impact, weight-bearing exercise that can be performed at any pace, baby boomers who work long hours and want to unwind in a safe environment, and young folks interested in cross-training or seeking the challenge of a new routine.

Treadmills can provide a workout at varying speeds and can be adjusted to simulate walking or running uphill. Workouts on a treadmill are great for the cardiovascular system and, although they focus on the lower body, you may consider swinging your arms or using a model with movable handlebars to help condition the upper body as well.

Motorized vs. Nonmotorized.   The decision to invest in an electric motorized treadmill instead of the manual nonmotorized type is really not that difficult. Your pocketbook and intended usage will help settle this issue fairly quickly. If your goal is to bring outdoor running indoors and you want a really vigorous workout, go with the motorized machine—provided you can afford one. Motorized treadmills can cost thousands of dollars (depending on the amount of added gadgetry); a serious runner should expect to spend at least $1,000. The extra dollars spent on a high-quality motorized treadmill may be money well spent, especially if you plan to use the treadmill on a regular basis. On the other hand, the simpler manually operated treadmills (your walking motion will drive the belt) usually cost somewhere in the three-figure range.

   Motorworks. Try to select a treadmill that has a powerful motor—at least 1.5 horsepower. Not only may it last longer, but a motor with a higher horsepower (preferably 2.0 or greater) is important if you want to use the treadmill at maximum speed. If any of the intended users of the treadmill are heavy (whether from muscle bulk or body fat), you should consider the stronger motor. Another feature to inquire about is whether the motor has a "continuous-duty" rating. This simply means that the machine maintains a steady horsepower rating that does not fluctuate when in use.

Belts and Decks.   When shopping for a treadmill, look for one that has a walking or running surface that is wide and long enough for your stride. Manual treadmills usually have a shorter belt and deck that tend not to accommodate a runner's stride. (The deck is the platform upon which the belt moves.) The best surface is neither too hard nor too soft, and acts as a good shock absorber. Search for decks made of layers of material that will be durable and quiet, as opposed to plastic-covered particle board.

   Good treadmills tend to have belts and decks that require very little maintenance. Inquire about this before you purchase a treadmill for home use. Make sure that the belt will require minimal adjustments and that adjustments are easy to make. If possible, look for a model that requires only dusting, not oiling and lubrication.

Speed and Incline.   Before making a purchase, decide what speed range and incline best meet your needs. Treadmills for walking usually go up to only 5 or 6 mph, whereas fit runners may want to go up to a fast 10 or 12 mph (a 6:00- or 5:00-minute mile pace, respectively). No matter what your maximum speed is going to be, make sure the treadmill starts slowly at a safe speed of 0 to 0.5 mph in order to avoid any sudden jerky starts.

The percent of incline can range from a low of 2 to 4 percent to a high of 10 to 15 percent. Test out some models to help determine the degree of incline that will best suit your workout. Make sure that you can vary the grade during your exercise routine.

The Display.   Evaluate all the readouts on the display panel. Will a simple timer do the trick for you, or do you want sophisticated programs that include heart-rate monitoring? Generally speaking, the more whistles and bells adorning the control panel, the more you will pay for the treadmill. Displays of time, speed, and distance traveled are standard on many treadmills today. Some of the high-end models will be fully programmable and capable of determining your heart rate, target heart zone, and estimated number of calories burned during a workout.

It is important that you have easy access to the display panel. You should be able to read the display while walking or running. Be certain that you have easy access to the "pause" or "stop" buttons and that your treadmill is equipped with an emergency shut off should you need to suddenly terminate your workout.

More Purchasing Tips.   Make sure that you test the equipment before you make a final purchase. Evaluate the smoothness of the treadmill belt when you accelerate and decelerate on motorized machines. Don't forget to pay attention to the noise factor and the safety rails. Lastly, read the warranty and service contracts carefully. Some warranties only cover moving parts for a limited period of time. Look for a company that guarantees the deck for an extended period of time.

Stationary Bikes

By pedaling a stationary bike indoors, you can reap the aerobic benefits of cycling without worrying about outdoor hazards. Indoor cycling is also an excellent activity for those concerned about losing balance, especially pregnant women and older people. Some stationary bikes have dual action and are outfitted with movable handlebars to exercise the upper body.

Upright vs. Recumbent.   There are two basic types of stationary bikes: upright and recumbent. You are probably more familiar with the upright version in which you sit on a saddle as if you were riding a regular bicycle. Bikes with recumbent seats allow you to sit with your hips flexed and your legs extended in front of you. You may wish to consider a recumbent bike if you have back or shoulder problems. Some women prefer recumbent models simply because they help users avoid buttock and groin discomforts that are frequently encountered with upright saddle versions.

"Training" Wheels. You may consider turning your own bicycle into an exercise bike with a device called a roller stand, also known as a trainer. They sell for approximately $100 to $200 and are popular among cyclists who want to ride their own bikes all year long. Roller models require the cyclist to keep pedaling and also require some skill to maintain balance. Some exercisers may prefer a stationary trainer that is stable when the rider stops pedaling.

Tips on Buying a Stationary Bicycle. You can purchase an exercise bike for as little as $100 or spend thousands of dollars on one with a programmable computer. Whether you choose a basic bike or one with a lot of high-tech gadgetry, make sure that the bike can be adjusted to fit you (and your family members, if necessary). The frame should be sturdy and the machine should have a smooth pedaling motion. Make sure you can readily mount and dismount the bike. You should be able to easily read and adjust the items on the control panel. You will want the saddle to be well-padded, adjustable, and comfortable. In order to prevent your feet from slipping off the pedals, check out the toe straps. They should allow you to slide your foot in without difficulty.

Cross-Country Ski Machines

You can get an excellent upper and lower body workout with indoor ski machines, which simulate cross-country skiing. The constant scissoring motion of your arms and legs is an excellent low-impact aerobic activity that minimizes the amount of stress to the back, knees, and hips. As your feet glide in their "skis," your arms grasp poles (or handles attached to pulleys) and swing back and forth.

Two types of ski machines are available: dependent and independent. Ski machines with dependent motion allow one ski to travel forward as the other ski moves in reverse. A machine with independent leg motion requires you to push and pull your feet in both directions, which usually results in a more vigorous workout. Beginners using cross-country ski machines where arm and leg motion are independent often require some practice before the skiing movement seems more natural.

Skiing Form. Maintain good posture while skiing; that is, do not droop over and lean on top of the hip padding. In order to avoid back and shoulder strains, try not to over-stretch your arms. Remember, it takes practice to coordinate the arm and leg motions until they are spontaneous.

Buying Tips. Machines can be purchased for less than $200, but be prepared to spend more if you want one with smooth sliding skis. Test out the ski machine to make certain it is sturdy and can accommodate your stride. Adjustable leg and arm resistance adds another dimension to your workout—just make sure that you can adjust the tension while exercising. If your model comes with ski poles, the height and resistance should also be adjustable. While you are skiing, the foot straps should hold your feet securely.

Rowing Machines

The three basic types of rowing machines are: piston machines, oarlock rowers, and flywheels. Hydraulic piston machines, which have two arms that move back and forth in a horizontal plane, offer variable resistance and tend to be less expensive than the other models. They are also more compact and easier to store. Oarlock rowing machines have arms that pivot freely, and often make it harder to perfect your stroke. Pricier models have a cable attached to a flywheel, which provides a more fluid action that simulates actual rowing or sculling.

Rowing is not as simple as you may think. Skill is required to maintain correct form—that is, to keep your back straight and not lean too far forward or backward. This activity may be preferred by those who want a good aerobic workout that will build strength and flexibility while sitting.

Rowing Form.   Start by extending your hips and legs, but do not use your arms and shoulders until the end of each stroke. Try not to bend at the waist, as this can strain your back muscles.

Buying Tips.   Test drive your rower to make sure the frame is sturdy and does not move as you row. The seat should be comfortable and glide smoothly. You should be able to fully extend your legs at the end of each stroke and not have to stretch too far forward at the beginning of a stroke. Make sure that you can get in and out of the rower without too much difficulty and that you can adjust the handles and foot positions.

Tips
Before you buy:
- Research the product.
- Make sure you have enough space.
- Have a budget.
- Test out the equipment.
- Read the warranty.

- *Stair machines offer aerobic conditioning and are easy to use.*

- *Treadmills allow you to design your own indoor walking, jogging, or running program.*

- *Stationary bikes are simple to use and require little coordination.*

- *Cross-country ski machines enable you to simultaneously work your upper and lower body.*

- *Rowing machines build strength and flexibility.*

Tips

Evaluate equipment for:

- noise level
- sturdiness
- types of functions
- comfort and fit
- speed and power
- accessories

WHERE TO TRAIN

Are you one of those exercisers who enjoys group company and competition? If so, a commercial gym may work for you. A gym or club is also a good bet for those who lack the space and finances to set up their own home gym. However, some women may prefer the privacy of home for exercising. In addition to privacy, a home gym affords the exerciser a good deal of control. You determine when and how long you want to exercise. There is no travel time, and you'll never have to wait in line for equipment. To make it worthwhile, you will have to be self-motivated enough to exercise on a regular basis. Although the initial cost of setting up a home gym may be quite an investment, you won't have to pay monthly or annual dues. Some professionals advise testing out machines in a commercial gym before buying your own. This way you can test out your motivation and have a better idea of what types of equipment you want to own.

Health and Fitness Clubs

It's been about sixty years since physical fitness pioneer Jack LaLanne opened up the first exercise gym in the United States. Since that time, health and fitness centers have sprouted up all over the world. Nowadays, these clubs attract a diverse group of exercisers with varying degrees of fitness—men and women of all ages and races can be seen huffing and puffing next to one another.

Is Membership in a Health Club for You? There are lots of reasons to consider enrolling in a health or fitness center—and lots of reasons not to. Let's see if we can help you make the decision. Review your exercise and fitness goals. Do you need access to certain equipment and facilities? Do you need instruction and supervision? Will mingling with other exercisers motivate you? Can you afford the cost of membership? Are you truly committed to exercising? If you have answered "yes" to most, if not all, of these questions, it sounds as if you are ready to join a club.

Selecting a Club: Some Guidelines.   Enrolling in a health club can be a serious financial investment. Often, a club expects you to commit yourself by signing a contract, so it makes sense to do your homework before obligating yourself (and perhaps part of this year's paychecks). Be a wise consumer: Investigate clubs that you are considering with the following thoughts in mind.

Beginning Your Evaluation. Talk to your friends and coworkers who are members of local clubs. Use the yellow pages of your phone book to find out which centers are located nearby. You can call to obtain preliminary information, but don't be surprised if they offer you a free tour along with a sales pitch. Accept the tour, but keep the promotion in perspective. Visit a number of facilities and comparison shop.

Making the Selection. The following pointers highlight some key factors that you should consider before you sign on the dotted line.

• **Location.** Try to select a club that is located near your home or workplace. If you are exhausted after a day in the office, you are more apt to go and work out if you have to drive by the gym on the way home. Make sure there is ample parking in the lot, especially during peak usage times.

• **Hours of Operation.** Consider your schedule and the hours you may want to exercise. If you are likely to visit the club during "rush hour" (between 4 P.M. and 7 P.M. on weekdays), make sure that the equipment is plentiful. Do the club hours vary by the season of the year? Get the specifics on early morning, late evening, and weekend hours.

• **The Equipment.** A well-equipped club should have both strengthening and cardiovascular conditioning equipment. Look at the variety of machines and make sure that they are clean and in good condition—a number of machines with "out of order" signs should be a red flag. Do they offer machines made specifically for women? Keep in mind that you want female-friendly equipment, such as bike seats made for women. If you like gadgetry, make sure that the machines have fancy gizmos to keep you from getting bored during a workout.

• **Other Facilities.** Check out the other facilities, such as swimming pools, tennis courts, and jogging tracks. Extras such as saunas, steam baths, and whirlpools are appealing after a workout, but will they really enhance your fitness goals?

• **Rating the Staff.** Make sure that there are enough qualified staff members available during all hours of operation. Are they friendly, professional, and approachable? Find out if they are trained to handle medical emergencies. Ask yourself if you would want a certified athletic trainer to help you out. If so, are appointments required, or is there a trainer or other qualified personnel available at all times?

- **Cleanliness.** Another important feature to check out is cleanliness. Do the gym and locker room smell unpleasant? Are the showers, bathrooms, and lockers spotless? Unsanitary surroundings are distasteful and can be hazardous to your health.
- **Cost.** Finally, investigate the cost of membership, which varies widely. It often pays to be skeptical about introductory offers and special membership deals. Make sure that you read the fine print and understand the terms of the contract. Watch out for long-term membership deals, low initiation fees without mention of monthly or annual charges, and other hidden costs. A reputable health club should be forthright about all its fees. Review the cancellation policy and know in advance what fees will be incurred should you need to terminate your membership. Beware of deals that sound too good to be true.
- **Special needs.** Before you sign up, make sure that the health club offers what you want, whether it is aerobic classes, nutrition counseling, cardiac rehab programs, or massages. Don't be afraid to talk to other members for advice.

A Few Words on Etiquette.   Even in a gym filled with casually attired fitness buffs, good manners still need to prevail. Here are a few pointers:

- It is courteous to wipe off the machines and equipment with a towel after using them—whether it be a bike seat or a dumbbell in the rack.
- Familiarize yourself with the rules of your club. Ignorance is not an acceptable excuse.
- Abide by posted time limits on equipment during periods of heavy usage. (Think about all the benefits of cross-training on another machine.)
- Return all equipment to its proper place—dumbbells to the rack, kickboards to the shelves, and magazines to the racks.
- Keep in mind that it is OK to socialize at the gym, but do not prevent another exerciser from using the equipment.
- Popular machines may have waiting lists. Be patient and wait your turn. No one likes to feel rushed through a routine, and shouldn't be unless posted time limits have been exceeded.
- Clean up after yourself in the locker room and avoid long showers if others are waiting.

If you are a new enrollee in a club or are in doubt about proper etiquette, just ask the management. If you find some folks violating the rules of game, you should feel free to inform the staff. You should feel comfortable and have fun as you work out.

What We Know

Sizing Up a Health Club

- *Is the club near your home or workplace?*
- *Would you feel comfortable working out there?*
- *What type of equipment is available?*
- *What are the club's hours of operation?*
- *What other amenities does the club offer?*
- *Is a certified trainer available?*
- *What does membership cost? Annual dues?*

Finding a health or fitness club that suits you is not an easy task. But if you do your homework, there should be no surprises in store for you. Enjoy your membership!

Fitness Spas

In the past, January was a golden time for health spas (and health clubs as well) as thousands of Americans made resolutions to lose weight. Nowadays, customers are looking for more than just weight loss. Fitness training and stress management are now included in spa packages. Is a fitness spa for you? Possibly, if you need an intensive exercise regime while being pampered. The drawback? Cost. The fees can range up to thousands of dollars per week.

Other Options

If you want to use a health club, but don't like the available commercial options or are short of funds, you might consider nonprofit organizations like YM-YWCAs or Jewish Community Centers. Colleges and universities often have facilities that may be available to the public. Some apartment complexes or hotels have workout rooms, which may be made available for a fee to non-residents or guests.

Lastly, a recent trend in corporate America is Wellness Centers. Many large companies have exercise equipment that employees may use during off hours or during lunch. For thousands of workers, on-the-job fitness centers, with low or no fees, are becoming an important employment perk.

Home Videos

In spite of the vast assortment of exercise videos on the market, they are not for everyone. Exercise videos can be categorized as follows: aerobic, strength training, stretch, and combinations of the above. The aerobic videos include high- and low-impact and step routines. The strength-training videos are also marketed as muscle conditioning and may require you to use equipment such as dumbbells or other weights. If you want instruction in stretching and yoga, there are videos sold specifically for these purposes.

You cannot judge an exercise video by the celebrity or the instructor promoting it. While you may normally skim the back cover of a movie video before renting, you should be sure to do more when choosing an exercise video. Look for details. See who the video is geared for: beginners or experts. If you are able to rent a video before purchasing, go home and test it out. Make sure that the aerobic and strength training tapes provide tips on proper form and technique without being too boring. Ask yourself whether you will be motivated to use this tape after the first couple of sessions. If you lack motivation, will the tape give you the incentive you need to start exercising? If it is a fast-moving aerobic tape, do you get lost in a move or does the instructor cue you appropriately? Is the routine filled with high kicks, twists, and overextended lunges? Does the video incorporate safeguards such as effective warm-up and cooldown times?

Safety First. When your home exercise companion is a videotape, make sure that you pay proper attention to safety factors. Arrange your furniture to allow enough space so that you do not bump into the TV screen. Make sure that the flooring is not too hard and slippery for the exercises you will be performing. If you have any precious *objets d'art* on the shelf, make sure they are out of harm's way. Don't overdo the workout. It takes time to build up to certain routines. Pressing the pause button is not cheating—it's being sensible.

The Software Option

Computerized exercise software can be programmed to the user's age, height, weight, and gender. As exercising at home continues to become more popular, the video and software market gets more crowded with choices for buyers like you. You can now tailor workouts to best meet your needs and goals. If you find these home fitness guides informative and motivational, great!

Tips for Safety

- Clear the area around the TV to avoid tripping over furniture.
- Avoid exercising on a slippery floor.
- Work at a comfortable pace.
- Warm up and cool down during each workout
- Vary the workout with different videotapes.

MUSIC TO YOUR EARS

I jog outdoors daily. Last year, office colleagues gave me a portable tape machine so I could enjoy some sound while exercising. I tried it a few times, but it never became a part of my running outfit. I guess I just fancy being outdoors and listening to natural sounds such as birds chirping. —Lilly, age 39

What We Know

Music has been found to increase exercise endurance. This may be particularly true for easy listening "elevator" music.

In the June 1992 edition of *Prevention* magazine, it was reported that "easy listening" music allowed joggers to exercise for longer periods of time. Endurance was improved because of the relaxing effect of the slower music. In contrast, loud, fast rock music raised heart rates and caused earlier fatigue.

In a more recent study, researchers asked young adults to vigorously ride a stationary bike with and without music. Both women and men rode an average of 25 percent longer with music than without.[26] While the type of music was not specified, athletes who listened to music certainly seem to have improved their endurance levels.

The Music Makers

Personal stereos come in several varieties: radios, cassette tape players, combination radio-tape players, and portable CD players. Dozens of different models are available, all with different features and prices. Start by thinking carefully about which format best meets your needs. Although most portable units produce surprisingly good sound, they generally will not be able to match the quality of sound you can achieve with a home stereo unit. Part of the problem lies in the quality of the headsets.

If possible, try out the headset of the portable music system in the store before you purchase it. The headphones should sit comfortably on or in the ear both at rest and during activity. Those covering the ear—"muff" or "ball" types—tend to produce better sound than the "bud" style, which sit in the ear canal. However, the latter type stays in place better and blocks out a lot of outside noise.[27]

Determine if the stereo can withstand being jiggled and bounced around as you exercise. CD players may be able to withstand the bounce of walking, but not jogging. Some tape models warble more with exercise than at rest. Depending on where you attach your unit, your "stress" test results will vary. For example, clipping the walkabout to the small of the back or middle of the abdomen rather than to your hip while jogging may reduce the flutter of some tape players.[27]

Make note of the size and weight of your unit, including batteries. Ask yourself how comfortable it will be to carry or wear while exercising. Some models now come with rechargeable nickel-cadmium batteries, which have a shorter life than disposable ones.

An Ear to Safety.   Before you turn the music on during your next workout, think twice. Music can be hazardous to your health if you exercise outdoors. Walkers and runners who tune out the world while exercising may not hear warning sounds of approaching cars or other vehicular traffic. If you exercise alone outdoors with headphones on, you might not hear another person approaching. Listening to very loud music has also been associated with hearing loss. While you might not want to sweat in silence, you should weigh the personal safety issues as well.

OTHER GADGETS

Many of the exercise machines built for home and gym use come adorned with fancy monitors. Displays that tell you the number of miles you have run or pedaled, the number of calories burned, and the amount of time you have exercised are commonly found on some of the mid-price models. More sophisticated treadmills and bikes come with optional heart rate monitors.

If you like gadgets and gizmos, plenty of accessories and monitors are around to make you happy. Sport watches may do more than tell time. Aside from stopwatch functions, lap times, and split times, some devices can help you determine your heart rate and blood pressure. Some basic models have beeping tones that help to motivate you and act as substitute coach to help you keep a certain pace. Important features to look for in sports watches include water resistance or waterproofness and easy-to-read digital displays.

While most athletes keep a close eye on their heart rates by checking their pulse or paying attention to their exertion level, many like the novelty of having it done electronically. Before taking out your credit card and purchasing a heart rate monitor, think about your needs. Do you need a device to monitor your pulse? While the immediate feedback telling you when you go above or below your target heart rate zone can be a helpful training tool, some athletes prefer to adjust their training session according to the way they feel. Heart rate monitors that have a sensor in a chest band work the best under a variety of conditions. Similar to an EKG, the device worn on your chest senses your heart beat and transmits a signal to a receiver worn on your wrist. Women interested in heart rate monitors may want to purchase a special bra into which the sensor is inserted to avoid having to wear a chest band. Look for a monitor that is wireless, simple to operate, and equipped with an easy-to-read display. Only you can tell if you will use these gadgets on a regular basis to help you gain and maintain fitness.

WETSUITS

I celebrate the arrival of each springtime with a weekend of white-water rafting. I also seem to always end up with a urinary tract infection after spending two days outfitted in a one-piece wetsuit. —Marcia, age 23

Whether you are a triathlete, snorkeler, open water diver, or kayaker, you may want to purchase a wetsuit. Wetsuits are designed to keep you warm, but, unlike drysuits, they also allow you to get wet. Wetsuits come in a variety of designs: sleeveless, full length, shorty (one piece with short legs and sleeves), and Farmer John or Jane (a sleeveless one piece with a vest-like neckline). Your sporting activity and desired degree of protection will determine which type of wetsuit is best for you.

Sleeveless models allow more upper body movement, so they are preferred by kayakers. The versions with short legs and sleeves may be selected when water and air temperature are not such crucial factors.

Most wetsuits are made of either spandex, thermoplastic, or neoprene. Spandex suits are lightweight and often used as undergarments for other wetsuits. Wetsuits made of thermoplastic are suitable for tropical temperatures, although they tend to be warmer than spandex. Neoprene wetsuits come in various thicknesses, which help to determine the insulating properties. Neoprene suits tend to be buoyant, which may be beneficial or treacherous depending on your sport. One drawback to neoprene compared to the other materials is the longer drying time required.

One wetsuit feature to evaluate carefully is the zipper arrangement. More and longer zippers result in more water entering the suit and a greater loss of heat. This needs to be counterbalanced with the convenience that zippers afford when it comes to donning and removing the suit. You don't want to be like Marcia (quoted above), trapped in a wetsuit for hours at a time with a full bladder. Not very comfortable!

Wetsuits should fit snugly to limit the amount of water that travels between the suit and your skin. However, the suit should not be so tight as to restrict movement and make you feel uncomfortable. Women need to pay particular attention to the fit, especially with unisex sizing. If you are unable to find a comfortable suit, you may want to go to the expense of having a wetsuit custom made.

When the water temperature is less than about 60°F (15.6°C), you should consider a drysuit. Drysuits are warmer than wetsuits because there is air in contact with the skin rather than water. Drysuits are also more expensive.

Wetsuits vs. Drysuits

Wetsuits

- good for water temperatures between 60° and 80°F
- body gets wet
- generally less expensive
- available in different styles

Drysuits

- useful when the water temperature drops below 60°F
- body stays dry
- more expensive
- may last longer with proper care
- controlling buoyancy may be difficult
- often bulkier than wetsuits

THE BOTTOM LINE IN GEAR

Here are the facts: Women are built differently than men. Most sporting gear is designed for men, even though an equal number of women may participate in that activity. Sporting gear labeled "ladies'" does not always signify an appropriate fit for women. For safety's sake, women should be informed consumers and customers. We need to continue to critically assess sporting gear and advocate for appropriate women's equipment in order to continue to enhance our performance and comfort.

ENDNOTES

1. Martin, S. Cycling sisters. *Women's Sports and Fitness*, April 1996, 18 (3), 58–64.

2. Weaver, S. The best of '96. *Women's Sports and Fitness*, April 1996, 18 (3), 46–51.

3. Weiss, B. D. Nontraumatic injuries in amateur long distance cyclists. *American Journal of Sports Medicine*, 1985, 13, 187–192.

4. Kurland, D. N., & Brubaker, C. E. Injuries on the bicentennial tour. *Physician and Sportsmedicine,* 1978, 6, 74–78.

5. Yesko, J. Is your bike right? *Women's Sports and Fitness*, April 1996, 18 (3), 52–53.

6. Ellis, T. H., Streight, D., & Mellion, M. B. Bicycle safety equipment. *Clinics in Sports Medicine*, January 1994, 13 (1), 75–98.

7. Neporent, L. Fit for a woman: the top innovations in sports equipment made just for us. *Women's Sports and Fitness*, Jan–Feb 1994, 16 (1), 76–84.

8. Carbone, C. Skiing sweet. *Women's Sports and Fitness*, October 1995, 17 (7), 42–44.

9. Getchell, A. Tour allure. *Women's Sports and Fitness*, October 1995, 17 (7), 47–48.

10. Burns, H. Get a grip: from telescoping tubes to grips that grab, ski poles are more fun than they used to be. *Skiing*, December 1995, 48 (4), 66–68.

11. Kurylko, N. Skates that rate. *Women's Sports and Fitness*, March 1996, 18 (2), 42–44.

12. Miller, R .K., & Stanton, B. How to pick a stick: Start by knowing your game. *Tennis*, March 1994, 29 (11), 69–70.

13. Stone, A. Getting a grip on high-tech tennis. *Business Week*, June 7, 1993, 118.

14. Der, B. Choosing a racket. *Sports Illustrated for Kids*, June 1995, 7 (6), 48.

15. Gray, B. Long time coming. *Tennis*, September 1995, 31 (5), 32–36.

16. Gray, B. Is the extra-long for you? *Tennis*, December, 1995, 31 (8), 28–32.

17. Workman, J. String gauge. *Tennis*, July 1993, 29 (3), 117.

18. Der, B. Choosing a racket. *Sports Illustrated for Kids*, June 1995, 7 (6), 48.

19. Gothard, S. A. Get a handle on your grip size. *Tennis*, October 1990, 76.

20. Chirls, S. Getting a grip on your racquet. *Tennis*, April 1994, 29 (12), 83–84.

21. Stone, A. Getting a grip on high-tech tennis. *Business Week*, June 7, 1993, 118.

22. Bryan, M. Getting a grip on golf. *Esquire*, April 1994, 121 (4), 127–130.

23. Pelz, D. How to pick a putter. *Golf Magazine*, May 1995, 37 (5), 100–101.

24. Neporent, L. Fit for a woman: the top innovations in sports equipment made just for us. *Women's Sports and Fitness*, Jan–Feb 1994, 16 (1), 76–84.

25. Getting in shape: It's more important than ever. *Consumer Reports*, January 1996, 61 (1), 14–30.

26. Music to our rears. *Tufts University Diet & Nutrition Letter*, April 1996, 14 (2), 3.

27. Music to go: How to buy a personal stereo. *Consumer Reports*, December 1995, 60 (12), 776–783.

10 *Food for Fitness*

SUSAN L. PURETZ, ED.D.

It's been said that you can eat to live or live to eat. I love to eat and in order to do that and still look good, I have to exercise. —Susan, age 54

NUTRITION: FACT AND FICTION

Why We Eat

Like Susan, many of us eat because we enjoy it. But apart from the pleasure, eating is essential to life. Our bodies require food to grow, to repair damaged cells, to regulate our temperature, and to give us energy. No one food provides everything that our bodies need. For that reason, we are advised to consume a variety of nutrients, including water, proteins, carbohydrates, fats, vitamins, and minerals.

This chapter on nutrition is divided into two major sections. The first describes the basics of everyday nutritional requirements; the second (beginning on page 235) discusses food for fueling fitness and the special nutritional needs of the exercising woman.

FOOD FACTS

Water: The Essential Fluid.   Water is so prevalent throughout our bodies that an anonymous humorist once declared that water must have invented human beings so that it would have a method for transporting itself from one place to another. Water makes up approximately 55 to 70 percent of the human body's weight. For example, bone is more than 20 percent water, and muscle as much as 75 percent water. From food and liquid together, we consume almost three quarts of water per day, and excrete a similar amount.

Water is essential. It moves nutrients and other substances to all parts of the body; it is necessary for the chemical reactions that permit us to use the food we ingest; and it regulates our body temperature. Although we can survive without food for a long time, we cannot live without water for more than a few days. And, if we are active, we may feel the effects of insufficient water in less than one hour.

Protein's a Builder.   Whether the protein comes from meat, dairy products, or vegetables, the body will use it. Besides being an important part of muscles, bones, blood, enzymes, some hormones, and cell membranes, protein is necessary for repair, maintenance, and growth.

Protein is made up of approximately 23 building blocks known as **amino acids**. Of the 23, 8 to 10 are called **essential** because they cannot be manufactured by the body and must be obtained from the food we eat. If that food lacks or has inadequate amounts of any of the essential amino acids, it will be impossible for our bodies to use the other amino acids properly. For that reason, proteins that supply all of the essential amino acids are known as **complete proteins**. They come only from animal sources because the animals have done the manufacturing for us. While the proteins in vegetables are incomplete, they can be combined to give us complete proteins. Table 10.1 provides examples of protein choices.

The National Academy of Sciences expresses our body's need for nutrients as **RDA**, that is, **Recommended Dietary Allowance**. You will see the RDA for protein expressed as .8 grams per kilogram of body weight (since a kilogram equals approximately 2.2 pounds, the protein RDA is less than .4 grams for each pound that you weigh). A 120-pound woman needs about 43 grams a day, while a woman who weighs 150 pounds needs about 55 grams. Most major nutritional agencies and organizations recommend that protein make up 12 percent of the diet; however, the American Heart Association recommends 15 percent. So somewhere in between may be a good target. This amount satisfies the needs of 99 percent of people living a "normal" life. Individuals who engage in very strenuous endurance or weight training have increased protein requirements. However, the typical American diet provides these amounts, as we will see later in this chapter. If we eat more protein than we can use, it is converted to fat and stored, used as a source of energy (an expensive one!), or excreted. And that, pardon the pun, is a waste.

What We Know

All carbohydrates eventually end up as glucose before they can circulate through the body.

Carbohydrates for Calories.   Carbohydrates supply **glucose**, the fuel burned by our cells to generate energy. While 66 percent of our total circulating glucose goes to fuel the brain, the rest is needed to provide energy for all other cells throughout the body. Nutritionists

TABLE 10.1

Protein Sources

To get adequate amounts of the essential amino acids on a daily basis, you should:

▶ *Choose from animal proteins (preferably low-fat)*　**or**

▶ *Mix foods from two or more of the vegetable protein groups*　**or**

▶ *Mix one vegetable protein group with a small amount of animal protein (preferably low-fat)*

Low-Fat Animal (Complete) Proteins

	Protein (*grams*)
Nonfat dry milk　1 cup	24
Nonfat milk　1 cup	8
Low-fat cottage cheese　1 cup	6
Egg white　1 large	4
Beef roast (lean)　3 oz.	21
Poultry (without skin)　3 oz.	21
Fish　3 oz.	21

Vegetable (Incomplete) Proteins

	Protein (*grams*)		Protein (*grams*)
Legumes		**Vegetables**	
Baked beans　1 cup	14	Corn　½ cup	3
Lentil Soup　10.5 oz.	11	Peas, fresh　1 cup	9
Hummus　1 cup	6	Potatoes, baked　1 large	4
Tofu　4 oz.	9		
		Nuts and Seeds	
Grains		Almonds*　1 oz.	6
Brown Rice　1 cup	5	Seeds*　2 tbs.	3–5
Pasta　1 cup	7	Peanut Butter*　1 tbs.	4
Breads　1 slice	2–3		
Oatmeal, cooked　1 cup	5		
Bran Cereal　½ cup	5		

* High in fat

Note: To get adequate amounts of the amino acids lysine and methionine from a vegetarian diet, you would need to eat both legumes and grains since the other two groups are not very good sources.

Source: Adapted from Society for Nutrition Education Information

Calorie, the word we use to describe how "fattening" foods are, is the term used to measure the potential energy contained in foods. Carbohydrates, fat, and proteins provide energy, but an equal amount of each does not provide an equal number of calories. Carbohydrates and proteins have the potential to produce four calories per gram, whereas fat produces nine. When we use the popular term calorie to describe the amount our bodies need, how many we are eating, or the number in a particular food, we are actually referring to kilocalories (k-calorie). A kilocalorie is the amount of heat required to raise the temperature of one kilogram of water one degree Celsius. The term kilocalorie is usually reserved for scientific work and technical journals. One kilocalorie is equivalent to 1,000 calories. However, in common usage and in this book the term calorie is used to refer to kilocalorie. Most adults use between 1,500 and 3,000 calories (or k-calories to be precise) in a day.

say that carbohydrates should provide 50 to 60 percent of our daily calories.[1] The recommendation for serious endurance athletes (for example, triathletes, cyclists, and marathon runners) is to consume 60 to 70 percent of calories from carbohydrates.[2] See the sidebar for more information about calories.

Carbohydrates can be categorized as either simple or complex. Complex carbohydrates include starches and fiber; simple carbohydrates are the sugars. Regardless of whether they are complex or simple, all carbohydrates are ultimately broken down during digestion into monosaccharides, the most important of which is glucose. Glucose, known as "blood sugar," reaches its destination in two ways: either it's absorbed from our intestines after a meal, or it's released from the liver or muscles where it has been stored in the form of **glycogen.**

Fats Are Functional.   Fat serves as the most concentrated source of energy in the diet, supplying twice the energy of carbohydrates and proteins. Fat is also a source of body insulation, support and cushioning for organs, a medium for absorption of fat-soluble vitamins (to be discussed shortly), and a structural component of cell membranes. Fat currently represents almost 40 percent of all calories in the typical American diet—a number that nutritionists say is far too high.

The fats in our diets and in our bodies are technically known as **lipids,** a general term for a number of different water-insoluble substances. In ordinary usage and in this book, we often say "fats" when we actually intend the broader meaning of lipids; for example, we refer to a "high-fat diet" when it would be more accurate to say a "high-lipid diet." Technically, fats are lipids that are solid at room temperature, while oils are lipids that are liquid and pourable at room temperature.

Lipids are categorized as triglycerides, phospholipids (including lecithin), and sterols (of which cholesterol is the best known).

• **Triglycerides.**   **Triglycerides** make up about 95 percent of the lipids in foods and in our bodies. They consist of a molecule of glycerol to which three **fatty acids** are attached. While many fatty acids can be manufactured by the body, some cannot and must be ingested—those are known as **essential fatty acids.** Fatty acids are found in both plant and animal foods.

You often hear the lipids in foods referred to as saturated fat (or unsaturated fat). **Unsaturated** fats, generally liquid at room temperature, are derived primarily from plant sources such as corn, soybean, and peanut. Unsaturated fats are further divided into monounsaturated and polyunsaturated, depending on their chemical structure. **Saturated** fats are derived mainly from animal sources such as meats, egg yolks, and dairy products.

As with any rule, there are exceptions. For example, coconut and palm oils, derived from plants, are highly saturated. That's why they're listed separately on food packages. Vegetable oils are initially polyunsaturated, but when made into margarine through a process called hydrogenation, they become partially saturated. Although margarine might be considered a healthier fat, it is more saturated than the oil from which it is made. Additionally, because questions have been raised recently about possible harmful health effects that might occur from the process of hydrogenation (in which trans fatty acids are produced), the Dietary Guidelines for Americans suggests limiting the intake of margarine (and not switching to butter).

· **Fat Is Not Cholesterol.** The difference between fat and **cholesterol**, although simple, causes much confusion. Cholesterol is a substance that is manufactured by the body and is also found in the animal foods we eat. Cholesterol is *not* found in fruits, vegetables, nuts, grains, or other plant sources. So, margarines are automatically cholesterol-free if they are made from a vegetable oil, even though they may contain saturated fats. Fat, as we discussed earlier, is a substance found in food from *both* plants and animals. Lipids from animals (and dairy products) contribute most heavily to our total dietary cholesterol because they contain cholesterol as well as saturated fat.

Cholesterol is an essential component in the formation of cell membranes and in several hormones, such as testosterone. In elevated quantities, however, cholesterol has harmful effects and may build up in the arteries and contribute to coronary artery disease. Diets that are high in saturated fats from meat and dairy products usually are high in cholesterol. In addition, saturated fats, independent of dietary cholesterol, promote cholesterol synthesis. Thus, people with elevated cholesterol levels are often advised to reduce their intake of saturated fats. Although both fat and cholesterol are necessary to maintain bodily functions, a diet with fat intake as low as 10 percent is sufficient to provide the necessary substances for the body to manufacture cholesterol.[3]

Vitamins. Vitamins promote specific chemical reactions within our cells. There are 13 known vitamins. Nine are water-soluble (the eight B vitamins and vitamin C) and are found in the watery parts of food. If we take more of these **water-soluble vitamins** than the body needs, the excess will usually be excreted; however, high doses may sometimes cause adverse side effects and interfere with medications.

Caution! The four **fat-soluble vitamins** (A, D, E, and K) should not be taken in excess of the amounts required. The extra is stored in our bodies, sometimes causing toxicity.

Normal vitamin dosage recommendations have been established by the National Academy of Sciences/National Research Council and include a substantial margin of safety, taking into account differences among individuals and establishing a range within which most people's nutritional needs will be covered.

TABLE 10.2

....

Good Sources of Vitamins and Minerals

Vitamin A:
Fortified dairy products, eggs, liver, yellow and green leafy vegetables, apricots

Vitamin B₁ (Thiamine):
Meats, legumes, whole grains, some vegetables

Vitamin B₂ (Riboflavin):
Milk and dairy foods, meats, eggs, whole grains, dark green vegetables

Vitamin B₃ (Niacin):
Whole grains, meats, fish, nuts, legumes

Vitamin B₆:
Meats, whole grains, green leafy vegetables, bananas

Vitamin B₁₂:
Meats, eggs, milk and dairy products; not found in vegetables

Folic Acid:
Green leafy vegetables, orange juice, legumes

Pantothenic Acid:
Widespread in foods

Biotin:
Widespread in foods

Vitamin C:
Citrus fruits, tomato, bell pepper, cabbage, potato, melons

Vitamin D:
Sunlight, fortified milk and other dairy products

Vitamin E:
Wheat germ, vegetable oils, egg yolk, nuts, green leafy vegetables

Vitamin K:
Liver, vegetable oils, green leafy vegetables, tomato

Calcium:
Milk, cheese, dark green vegetables, dried legumes, yogurt

Copper:
Meats, seafood, drinking water, nuts

Iodine:
Iodized salt, seafood

Iron:
Eggs, meats, legumes, whole grains, green leafy vegetables

Magnesium:
Whole grains, green leafy vegetables, nuts, legumes

Phosphorus:
Milk, cheese, meats, whole grains

Potassium:
Meats, milk, whole grains, many fruits and vegetables

Sodium:
Salt, soy sauce, pickles, processed foods

Zinc:
Red meat, poultry, shellfish, beans

Minerals.   Minerals, of which there are about 20 commonly found in our bodies, constitute only about 4 percent of our body's weight, yet are essential to our functioning.[4] Minerals help to regulate body functions, aid in growth and maintenance of body tissues, and serve as catalysts for the release of energy. They are sometimes referred to as either **macro minerals**, such as calcium, magnesium, potassium, phosphorus, and sodium, because they are needed in relatively large amounts; or **trace minerals**, such as iron, zinc, and copper, because—as the name implies—they are needed in minute amounts. Table 10.2 provides examples of some foods in which essential vitamins and minerals are found.

Good Nutrition

Generations of Americans were reared to worry about eating enough to obtain the nutrients vital to health. Today eating enough is not the problem for most of us—eating wisely is. We are faced with a superabundance and wide variety of food, including many products that are highly attractive but of dubious health value. In some cases, the foods we were taught to cherish are now accused of undermining health and contributing to early death.

Should there be a national policy on nutrition to keep Americans from killing themselves? This seemingly simple question has produced a great deal of angry debate. What should the government suggest that the public eat? How much proof is necessary? Should broad recommendations be avoided until there is proof that the average American will benefit, or is it important to wage an aggressive public health campaign now, while the data are still preliminary? The battle is not over.

The Government has issued various versions of *Dietary Guidelines for Americans* since 1980. The 1995 *Guidelines* generally concurred with the message presented in the 1990 version; however, there were a few changes that appeared in the text accompanying the 1995 report.

The new *Guidelines* continue to stress eating a variety of foods. The health benefits of a vegetarian regimen are acknowledged for the first time. However, vegetarians are cautioned to pay special attention to ingesting adequate amounts of iron, zinc, calcium, vitamin B (especially B_{12}), and vitamin D. *Note:* B_{12} comes only from animal foods. Vegetarians who do not eat meat, eggs, and dairy products can substitute Vitamin B_{12}-fortified soy beverages or B_{12} supplements. The 1995 *Guidelines* also stress the necessity of both weight control and physical activity in maintaining a healthy body.

The Food Pyramid: A Smorgasbord of Choices

In 1992, the *Food Guide Pyramid*, a schematic representation of the *Dietary Guidelines*, was introduced (see next page). The Food Pyramid is a pictorial guide for daily food choices. It recommends getting most of our calories from foods in the groups closest to

Food Guide Pyramid
A Guide to Daily Food Choices

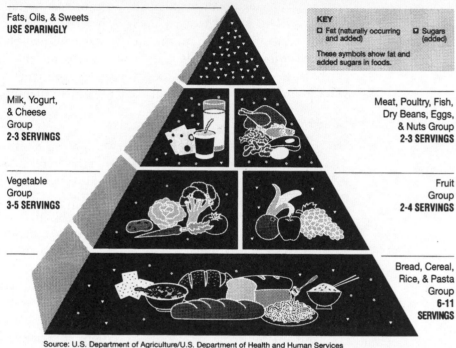

Fats, Oils, & Sweets
USE SPARINGLY

KEY
☐ Fat (naturally occurring and added)   ☑ Sugars (added)
These symbols show fat and added sugars in foods.

Milk, Yogurt, & Cheese Group
2-3 SERVINGS

Meat, Poultry, Fish, Dry Beans, Eggs, & Nuts Group
2-3 SERVINGS

Vegetable Group
3-5 SERVINGS

Fruit Group
2-4 SERVINGS

Bread, Cereal, Rice, & Pasta Group
6-11 SERVINGS

Source: U.S. Department of Agriculture/U.S. Department of Health and Human Services

the pyramid's base: grains (6 to 11 servings per day), vegetables (3 to 5 servings per day), and fruits (2 to 4 servings per day). It recommends eating moderate amounts of food from the dairy group (2 to 3 servings per day) and the meat and beans group (2 to 3 servings per day); and urges fewer choices from foods high in fats, oils, and sweets ("use sparingly" is their advice concerning foods in the small top segment of the pyramid).

The recommended servings sound like you can't possibly eat that much, yet if you thought about what you usually eat, you'd be surprised. Let's look at the grains and what seems to be a whopping 6 to 11 servings per day. Start with breakfast—a small bowl of cereal and a slice of toast are two servings. If you have a few crackers for a snack, that's a third serving. A sandwich for lunch counts as two more servings, while rice and a roll eaten as part of dinner bring your total to seven servings. There, you've made it. That's all it takes. Table 10.3 gives examples of nutritional choices from each group.

TABLE 10.3

....

The Pyramid Guide to Daily Food Choices

Food Group
Suggested Daily Servings

Breads, Cereals, Rice and Pasta
6 to 11 servings
   What counts as a serving:
   1 slice bread
   ½ hamburger bun
   ½ English muffin
   1 small roll, biscuit, or muffin
   3 to 4 small or 2 large crackers
   ½ cup of cooked cereal, rice,
     or pasta
   1 ounce of ready-to-eat cereal

Fruits
2 to 4 servings
   What counts as a serving:
   a whole fruit such as a medium
     orange, banana, or apple
   a grapefruit half
   a melon wedge
   ¾ cup fruit juice
   ½ cup berries
   ½ cup chopped, cooked, or
     canned fruit
   ¼ cup dried fruit

Vegetables
3 to 5 servings
   What counts as a serving:
   ½ cup cooked vegetables
   ½ cup chopped raw vegetables
   1 cup leafy raw vegetables, such
     as lettuce or spinach
   ¾ cup vegetable juice

Meats, Poultry, Fish,
Dry Beans and Peas,
Eggs, and Nuts
2 to 3 servings
   What counts as a serving:
   Amounts should total 5 to 7 ounces
     of cooked lean meat, poultry
     without skin, or fish each day.
   Count 1 egg, ½ cup cooked beans, or
     2 tablespoons peanut butter as
     1 ounce of lean meat.

Milk, Yogurt, and Cheese
2 servings from entire group
   What counts as a serving:
   1 cup milk
   8 ounces yogurt
   1½ oz. natural cheese
   2 oz. processed cheese

Fats, Oils, and Sweets
   What counts as a serving:
   Use fats and sweets sparingly.
   If you drink alcoholic beverages,
   do so in moderation.

Source: U.S. Department of Agriculture, 1995

Good nutrition means eating for variety, balance, and moderation. Seven basic elements suggested by the Dietary Guidelines for Americans *should be kept in mind.*

1. Eat a variety of foods.

2. Maintain weight by balancing the food you eat with physical activity—calories ingested should equal calories burned.

3. Avoid too much fat, saturated fat, and cholesterol.

4. Choose a diet with plenty of grain products, vegetables, and fruits.

5. Avoid too much sugar.

6. Avoid too much salt.

7. If you drink alcohol, do so in moderation.

What to Do

When you increase fiber intake to recommended amounts:

1. Increase it gradually over the course of several weeks to avoid excessive gas.

2. Drink plenty of water and other liquids.

3. Spread your intake throughout the day.

The Ideal Diet

While we may think our eating patterns have changed in recent years, nutritionists would disagree. For most Americans, the current diet consists of approximately 45 percent carbohydrates, 12 to 15 percent proteins, and 38 percent fats. In a 1991 nationwide survey of food consumption, it was reported that only 9 percent of American adults had eaten five fruit and vegetable servings (the minimum number recommended in the pyramid) on the day of the survey and 11 percent had not eaten any on that day.[5] Nutritionists now stress that the healthiest diet should include about 58 percent carbohydrates, 12 percent proteins, and no more (and hopefully less) than 30 percent fat.[6] Saturated fats should constitute 10 percent or less of total caloric intake.

Vitamins and Minerals. If you follow the guidelines provided in the food pyramid, you should be receiving all the vitamins and minerals your body needs. The discussion later in this chapter on vitamin myths explodes many common misconceptions.

Don't Forget Fiber

Dietary fiber is a term used for the indigestible components of plants. Dietary fiber can be divided into two main categories: that which is soluble in water and that which is not. During digestion, **water-soluble fiber** becomes gel-like and is fermented by bacteria in the colon; **water-insoluble fiber** remains essentially unchanged.

Fiber in the diet exerts a variety of effects. Some benefits that have been attributed to both soluble and insoluble fiber include: increased satisfaction after eating (i.e., your belly feels full!); rapid passage of food through the intestines and out of the body; and greater bulk and frequency of bowel movements. While both types of fiber provide those benefits, soluble fiber has been shown to have additional beneficial effects, including lowering insulin requirements and decreasing levels of serum cholesterol and triglycerides.

Because it is important to get both soluble and insoluble fiber, and because the type and amount vary in different foods, we must eat as many sources of fiber as possible in order to ensure that we get enough of both kinds. Table 10.4 gives some examples.

In general, grains are high in overall fiber, and fruits and vegetables are among the best sources of soluble fiber. While both carrots and celery are much higher in total fiber than tomatoes, carrots provide 50 percent more soluble fiber than celery. On the other hand, bran is one of the best sources of total fiber, but it has a low percentage of soluble fiber. When you select a wide variety of fiber-rich foods daily, it ensures that you get a mix of the types your body needs.

The majority of Americans eat only about 10 to 15 grams of fiber each day. Various

TABLE 10.4

....

Good Sources of Dietary Fiber

Insoluble Fiber	Soluble Fiber
More than 5 grams	
1 oz. high-fiber wheat-bran cereal	½ cup cooked beans
1 cup cooked lentils	
2 to 5 grams	
6 whole-wheat crackers	1 cup cooked oatmeal
Medium banana	¾ cup cooked bulgur
Medium potato (with skin)	Medium apple, pear
⅔ cup cooked brown rice	Medium orange, grapefruit
½ cup cooked spinach, broccoli	½ cup cooked peas, cabbage
1 to 2 grams	
1 slice whole wheat bread	½ cup cooked carrots
1 cup cooked pasta	Medium peach, nectarine
½ cup corn	Two apricots
½ cup cooked cauliflower	

....

Note: Only a few representative examples are listed. There are many other sources.

Adapted from: *Therapeutic Fiber in the Treatment and Prevention of Disease*, 1987, Proctor and Gamble.

health organizations recommend that we get 20 to 35 grams per day. To get that amount, we should eat approximately six servings of whole grain breads and cereals and four servings of fruits and vegetables. Cooking, canning, freezing, and freeze-drying do not appear to significantly decrease the fiber content of most foods, but peeling fruits and vegetables does. Making juices of fruits and vegetables also causes much of the fiber content to be lost, especially if the juice is filtered or the skins have been removed.

Vitamin Myths

Sixty-nine percent of the women in our sample said they took vitamins. Of that number, most of them popped multivitamins daily. That flies in the face of the prevailing wisdom, which states that a daily diet chosen from the Food Guide Pyramid will satisfy all our vitamin and mineral needs.

Supplemental vitamins are taken by both recreational and competitive exercisers because they believe that extra vitamins will enhance their performance and perhaps give them a competitive edge. If these beliefs were based on fact, then all of us should be gobbling up vitamin pills. However, five organizations (including the American Dietetic Association and the American Society for Clinical Nutrition) have issued statements in support of research concluding that there is no demonstrated benefit of vitamin supplements in excess of the RDA's. Yet, claims that vitamin supplements enhance performance continue unabated. A look at those claims reveals the distance between fact and fiction.

The Water-Soluble Vitamins

• **Vitamin C.** Many athletes take vitamin C supplements.[7] While research clearly shows that inadequate amounts of vitamin C can impact athletic performance,[8] no well-conducted scientific study has reported any benefit in taking quantities in excess of the RDA found in a well-balanced diet.[9]

• **Thiamine (B_1).** Although few studies have evaluated the effects of B_1 supplements, two that did showed no improvement in endurance or other performance parameters.[10]

• **Riboflavin (B_2).** The National Research Council stated that the requirement for riboflavin does not appear to be related to energy utilization or muscular activity.[11]

• **Niacin.** Three well-designed studies showed no beneficial effect of niacin supplements on endurance capacity, efficiency of work, or anaerobic and aerobic capacity.[12]

• **Vitamin B_6.** Supplementation has not been shown to enhance performance.[13]

• **Vitamin B_{12}.** Supplementation has not been shown to enhance maximum oxygen consumption or other tests of strength, power, and muscular endurance.[14]

• **Pantothenic Acid, Folate, and Biotin.** Not enough data is available to make any conclusive statement.[15]

The Fat-Soluble Vitamins

Since excess amounts of these vitamins are stored in the body (unlike the water-soluble ones whose excess is excreted), there does not seem to be any purpose in taking supplements. Athletes generally don't take extra vitamin A, D, or K.[15] But a mystique has arisen concerning vitamin E. Because it may act as an antioxidant, vitamin E has been viewed as helping red blood cells stay intact during exercise by preventing oxidation in the cell wall. But to date, no studies have shown any association between these fat-soluble vitamins and enhanced athletic performance.[16]

Mineral Misconceptions

Information on minerals and their association with physical performance is even clearer than the information available about vitamins.

• **Calcium**. We discuss the importance of calcium for women in Chapter 14, Keeping It Going. Although calcium is needed to maintain skeletal strength, it has not been shown to enhance performance. Thus calcium supplementation for the sole purpose of performance improvement is not widely practiced.[17]

• **Potassium**. Media hype to the contrary, potassium losses in sweat are negligible, except in a few instances, such as during hard and long exertion in extreme humidity.[17] Potassium supplements are unnecessary because we are adequately resupplied with potassium by the foods we eat, such as meats, milk, and many fruits—including the especially popular banana.

• **Sodium**. Under normal conditions, sweating causes sodium loss—but not depletion. The use of salt tablets is usually unnecessary because research indicates that the body very efficiently regulates its supply of salt.[18] Normal dietary intake after exercise will restore any loss. Under extreme conditions, however, such as triathlons, marathons, and other super-endurance events, electrolyte replacement may be advised. *Note:* Salt tablets may have side effects like nausea, vomiting, and dehydration.

• **Iron**. There are several issues to consider regarding iron supplements. The first is whether exercisers need to take them. Thus far there seems to be no evidence for the necessity of increased iron intake as a result of exercise unless you are iron deficient. The second issue is whether extra iron enhances performance. Research does not indicate any performance benefit of additional iron to individuals who are not iron deficient. *Note:* While iron-deficiency anemia clearly can reduce physical and intellectual performance, excess amounts of iron can also endanger your health. Iron is stored by the body and large amounts can be toxic to the heart, liver, and pancreas.

While pregnant women and some year-old babies may have iron-deficiency anemia, most Americans do not.[19] According to a recent report, people who eat a well-balanced diet—even if it is a fast-food diet—generally have all the iron they need. That being said, there is still a concern in the athletic community that iron-deficiency anemia may be a problem in female exercisers who are involved in endurance training, are of low body weight, or do not eat red meat.[20]

Clearly, if you have any of those risk factors, or if you tire easily despite your high level of fitness, then medical assessment, including a dietary and laboratory evaluation, may be advisable. For more information on iron deficiency, see page 264–265 in this chapter.

• **Zinc, Selenium, Copper, Chromium.** There is no documentation that supplementation with these minerals will benefit performance in healthy people who have adequate amounts of these trace elements. Remember, a well-balanced diet assures that you will get plenty of these minerals. (See page 233 for more on chromium.)

If Some Is Good, More Will Be Better. It has been estimated that anywhere from 30 to 80 percent of athletes use supplements.[21] To use vitamin and mineral supplements with the expectation that they will improve performance puts us in a no-win situation. This is especially true if we neglect things that could enhance performance, such as a balanced diet, adequate sleep, and proper training.

Most athletes are unaware of the possible dangers of megadosing. When you megadose, that is, take the vitamin or mineral in doses that are many times the RDA requirements, once-friendly vitamins begin to function more like designer drugs and can produce toxicities and serious side effects. For example, long-term megadoses of niacin have been associated with liver damage, skin rashes, and elevated uric acid levels[22]; high levels of potassium can cause cardiac rhythm problems.[23]

Athletes often hear through the grapevine that large quantities of vitamins provide energy, thereby supercharging the body.[23] That is patently false. No research supports that assertion. Moreover, if vitamins are taken to achieve that aim while caloric intake is shortchanged, the end result will be less energy.

You should be aware that a typical ploy of supplement manufacturers is to use scare tactics such as describing extreme cases of vitamin and mineral deficiencies, and claiming that we are all in danger of having the same happen to us if we don't buy their products.

Hedging a Bet. Despite sound information to the contrary, athletes continue to take supplements. If you've ever watched professional sports on television, you are probably familiar with the idiosyncratic behavior of athletes. For example, before taking a foul shot, some basketball players bounce the ball several times, bring the ball up, spin it or make some other kind of motion, bounce the ball again, and then finally shoot for the basket. Sport psychologists call those actions superstitious behavior; through reinforcement (the ball going in the basket), the behavior becomes a ritual.

Taking nutritional supplements is another example of superstitious behavior. The athlete has become convinced that it is the supplement (above and beyond the training) that gives the competitive edge. Dispelling the association between excelling and nutritional

While vitamin and mineral supplements will generally not impair performance, there is no scientific evidence that taking amounts in excess of the RDA is either necessary or enhances performance in well-nourished athletes.

We must not make the mistake of skimping on our diets and relying on supplements. It's a waste of money, it doesn't work, and it may harm us.

supplements becomes very difficult because there is a tendency to disregard scientific information. Athletes say "it works for me" without ever putting themselves to a proper scientific test. In almost every case, taking extra vitamins does not work for you, or anybody else. We all look for that something extra beyond our training. Supplements will not provide it.

The placebo effect can be very strong and we wonder how important it is to argue against supplements in this instance. Perhaps the battle should be reserved for issues where the stakes are higher and athletes can do themselves serious injury—as when they take steroids. We discuss this in Chapter 18, Beware of the Danger Zones.

Beware of Other Supplements. Vitamins and minerals are not alone in being credited with special powers. Some other substances that are used in the misguided hope that they will enhance our abilities are described below.

• **Amino Acid Supplements**. Certain amino acids, such as arginine and ornithine, are purported to enhance muscular development and to decrease body fat. Studies do not support these claims.[24]

Promoters point to the fact that the protein in amino acid supplements is pre-digested, hoping that you will think that it is easier and faster for your body to use these supplements. Not so! It's been shown that they absorb water into your stomach, which can cause cramping and/or diarrhea. Whether you are looking at arginine and ornithine; leucine, isoleucine, and valine; or l-tryptophan, the bottom line is that your body (remember from section one of this chapter) converts and then stores extra protein as fat. Your normal exercising diet will supply you with enough protein. Any extra protein (supplement, powder, or from your food) is wasted as protein and can contribute to weight gain. Protein supplements are an expensive way to become fat. If you want to build larger muscles, you need to exercise, not take pills.

• **Aspartates.** Some research on these salts of aspartic acid, a non-essential amino acid, reported that aspartate supplementation increased endurance capacity; other studies found no such effect.[25] Because of the conflicting results, it has been suggested that additional double-blind placebo studies are needed to confirm possible performance benefits.

• **Bee Pollen.** Bee pollen, touted as providing extra energy, has been found to have no training or performance benefit.[26]

• **Carnitine.** This vitamin-like molecule is found in meat and dairy products and in small amounts in grains, fruits, and vegetables. At this time, no research has substantiated its use,[27] and one study indicated that d-carnitine and D,L-carnitine may be toxic.[28]

• **Chromium Picolinate.** This product, a new darling of health food aficionados, is advertised to increase lean body mass and delay fatigue but has not been shown to do so. Recent attention has focused on its use for diabetics, but its effectiveness in controlling glucose levels has not yet been documented. It is necessary only if you are one of those rare individuals who is chromium deficient. In the U.S., this condition is almost non-existent, so taking chromium picolinate is unnecessary. Further, a recent study found that it may be carcinogenic.[29]

• **Gelatin.** Gelatin is derived from collagen and contains approximately 25 percent of the nonessential amino acid glycine. Research has not shown that it benefits physical performance. *Note:* Since dessert gelatin contains about 4 grams of protein and 34 grams of carbohydrate per cup, you might find it appetizing enough to use after workouts to replace carbohydrates, for example, instead of fig bars.

• **Honey.** Basically, a sugar is a sugar is a sugar. No scientific evidence has supported any claims made for honey, outside its benefits as a carbohydrate. Once again, if you use it as a source of carbohydrate to replenish muscle glycogen stores during recovery from exercise, it is no better or worse than other carbohydrate sources—regular sugar, for example.

• **Phosphate Salts.** The verdict is still not in as to whether there are any performance benefits from taking phosphate salt supplements. *Note:* Some athletes have experienced gastrointestinal problems when the salts were consumed on an empty stomach.[30]

• **Wheat Germ Oil.** Researchers have not supported any peak performance effect for wheat germ oil.[30] This is despite the book, *The Physiological Effects of Wheat Germ Oil on Humans*, which documents studies by Thomas Cureton and his associates over a 20-year period claiming benefits for this oil.

What We Know

An inadequate diet is not redeemed by supplementation. Pills and potions are not an alternative to eating a healthy diet. While increasing our activity may expand the need for vitamins and minerals, it also raises our need for other nutrients as well. This can, and should, be met by increasing calories in a well-balanced diet. Go with food, not pills.

The Supplement Dilemma. A wise physician once said, "If you don't have a problem, don't treat it." That seems like good advice regarding vitamin and mineral supplements. Obviously, if there is a proven dietary deficiency of a vitamin or mineral, it makes sense to take supplements. But a doctor, not you or I, should determine whether they are needed. When nothing is wrong, why waste money?

• **A Partial Solution.** There is one big caveat. If your work or lifestyle precludes a nutritious daily diet, then vitamin supplements should be considered. Ordinary multiple vitamin pills, not therapeutic or megavitamin doses, are all that are necessary as supplements. They should not contain more than 100 to 150 percent of the RDAs for each vitamin or mineral, and they should be taken no more than once daily. Since the important components of any particular vitamin are chemically the same, in general, we recommend buying generic vitamin pills and not spending extra money on name brands. Check expiration dates on the labels to ensure freshness and note what vitamins and minerals are included. The label should indicate that the ingredients meet USPS standards, one of which is that the pills have to disintegrate and dissolve thoroughly in your stomach within a certain amount of time.

Energy Requirements.   As exercising women, our metabolic needs are quite different from those of our sedentary sisters. While they might survive on an estimated 1,600-calorie diet, we might not. Depending upon training regimens, some of us might lose weight and lack energy if we consumed only 1,600 calories while leading physically active lives.

Protein, fat, and carbohydrate requirements are increased as a result of exercising. The amount of food we need to maintain weight and energy is dependent on many factors, including the type of sport/exercise we do; duration, frequency, and intensity of the activity; our fitness level; and our proper body weight. In general, as our level of physical activity increases, so do our energy needs and caloric intake. Bowling is less physically demanding than recreational badminton, which is less demanding than cross-country skiing, etc. A small woman may require 1,800 calories on a bowling day, but may need twice as many calories when she engages in cross-country skiing. On average, elite endurance athletes (cyclists, rowers, runners, swimmers, and triathletes) consume about 55 calories per kilogram of body weight per day.[31] For a woman who weighs 130 pounds (59 kg), this would be equal to 59 times 55, or 3,245 calories.

Protein for Growth

Athletes once consumed large steaks before a major competition. Today, the emphasis has shifted to carbohydrates. Nevertheless, research has shown that protein requirements do increase with exercise. While we exercise, our muscle's proteins are being broken down; afterwards, they are repaired and rebuilt. For moderate daily exercise, some researchers have recommended an increase in our protein intake from .8 grams per kilogram (2.2 pounds) of desirable body weight per day (abbreviated as g/kg per day) to as much as 1.2 g to 1.7 g/kg per day.[32] For athletes involved in high-intensity endurance training, an increase to more than 1.7 g/kg per day is recommended.[33] Table 10.5 illustrates the recommended increase in protein and carbohydrates (based on body weight) necessary for exercising women.

In practical terms, if a sedentary woman weighs 125 pounds, her normal protein requirement would be approximately 45g of protein per day. We get that number by multiplying the protein RDA of .8 g/kg per day by 125/2.2 (the conversion of her weight from pounds to kilograms). Since protein needs are also expressed as a percentage of total calories, that woman's normal daily diet would be 180 calories from protein, representing approximately 12 percent of her estimated 1,600 total daily calories. To get that we multiplied 45 grams of protein by 4 calories per gram—the caloric value of each gram of protein ($45 \times 4 = 180$).

If our 125-pound woman were to start exercising, she would need to increase her

TABLE 10.5

Recommended Nutrition for the Exercising Woman

If you weigh		You will need	
		Protein[1]	Carbohydrate[2]
Pounds	Kg	(grams)	(grams)
90	41	49–70	205–410
100	45	54–76	225–450
110	50	60–85	250–500
120	54	65–92	270–540
130	59	71–100	295–590
140	63	75–107	315–630
150	68	81–115	340–680
160	73	87–124	365–730
170	77	92–131	385–770

1. Based on 1.2 to 1.7 g/kg body weight
2. Based on 5 to 10 g/kg body weight

Note: To get the equivalent in calories, multiply the grams of protein or carbohydrates by 4. For example, the recommended calories from carbohydrates for a 100-pound woman would be 900 to 1800 calories, depending upon the intensity and duration of her exercise.

What We Know

The additional protein required by most exercising women can be met by a varied diet that has enough protein calories to adequately meet overall increased energy expenditure.

protein intake to anywhere from 68 to 97 grams (272 to 388 calories), based on the recommendation of 1.2 to 1.7 g/kg per day. This is normally accomplished by simply eating more of the recommended balanced diet. *Note:* With the exception of those athletes who are in highly intensive endurance training, most female athletes and exercisers consume adequate amounts of protein in their daily diets. Despite this, many athletes still needlessly consume larger quantities of protein foods and expensive protein supplements.

Fuel for Energy: Carbohydrates and Fat

Our bodies can use fat, carbohydrates, or protein as a source of fuel. But the type, intensity, and duration of our activities determine which fuels our bodies use. This is a highly complex subject, and in the discussion that follows, we try to simplify the topic so it can be readily understood. Our goal is not to make athletes into nutritionists but rather to help athletes become better informed about their nutritional needs.

Fuel that is available for a muscle's use can be found in four places: the muscles, bloodstream, liver, and fat tissue.

The carbohydrates we eat circulate in the bloodstream as glucose. Excess glucose is stored as glycogen in our muscles and liver and then converted back to glucose as needed. Any extra fat, whether we like it or not, gets stored as body fat in fat tissues (known as adipose tissue) or in, believe it or not, our muscles. When you eat a piece of meat that is labeled "prime cut" and you savor its tenderness, it is because that animal's muscle is laced with fat. The same thing happens to our muscles. Fat stored in our muscles is immediately available for use. The fat in our adipose tissues has to be broken down by enzymes into fatty acids, which are then transported by the blood to our muscles. It's been estimated that the average body contains enough stored fat for about 119 hours of exercise, enough stored muscle glycogen for 1.5 hours of exercise, and enough stored liver glycogen for 6 minutes of exercise.[34]

What We Know

Fuel for Exercise

Type Fuel	Where Found	What Form
Carbohydrates	Bloodstream	Glucose
	Muscles and Liver	Glycogen
Fats	Fat Tissue	Fat
	Muscle Tissue	Fat

Decisions

Our muscles sense when different amounts of energy are required. By thinking of our physical movements as falling into three categories of intensity, it will be easier to understand our fuel choices. The categories are: 1. low-intensity activities, characterized by normal breathing and including our daily chores such as light housework, shopping, or walking about; 2. moderate-intensity activities, characterized by an elevated breathing rate and more vigorous activity such as gardening, housecleaning, or jogging at a pace of ten-minute miles; 3. high-intensity activities, characterized by very vigorous movement coupled with gasping breaths, such as occurs during sprinting on a track or for a bus. See Table 10.6 for further examples of different activities categorized by intensity.

TABLE 10.6

··

Activities Classified by Intensity

Type of Activity

Low Intensity of Short or Long Duration

Walking	Bowling
Badminton	Golf
Archery	Light Housework

Moderate Intensity and Prolonged Duration

Distance Running	Swimming
Hiking / Backpacking	Cross-Country Skiing
Calisthenics / Aerobics	Housecleaning
Bicycling	

High Intensity and Short Duration

Weight Lifting
Sprint Training

Alternating High Intensity with Moderate Intensity

Interval Training for Swimming / Running
Soccer
Basketball

• **Oxygen.** Oxygen is an important component in the decision about which food is used as fuel. Unlike our brain's need for almost constant oxygen, our muscles can function without oxygen for short periods of time. When muscle cells utilize oxygen to contract, they are working **aerobically**; when oxygen is not used, they are performing **anaerobically**.

In Chapter 3, Body Works, we described some of the chemical reactions that are involved when muscles use food to get energy. When we are working aerobically, for example, doing everyday minimal physical movements, our skeletal muscles utilize very little glucose, deriving 85 to 90 percent of their energy from fat.[35]

• **Intensity.** As we increase the intensity of our movement, this all changes. To meet the abrupt increase in energy requirements, for example, when we are sprinting on the track or for a bus, our muscles immediately draw on the glucose stored within the muscle tissue itself, and "burn" it anaerobically. Thus, as the exercise intensity increases, the relative utilization of carbohydrate increases.

Tip: You can use your breathing rate as a rough gauge of which fuel you are using. If you can't talk normally during your exercise, you are probably burning more glucose than fat.

• **Duration.** Lastly, the duration as well as the intensity of our activity also is involved in the muscle's choice of fuels. As the duration of our exercise increases, the intensity usually must decrease. Therefore, our bodies can provide necessary energy for longer periods of time.

• **The Interaction.** The contribution of fat as a fuel choice increases during prolonged moderate exercise. If we exercise at moderate intensity—up to 60 percent of our aerobic capacity, for four to six hours—fat can supply as much as 70 percent of our energy needs.[36] For example, a group of novice bicyclers, working at 30 percent of their aerobic capacity, were found to increase burning of fat from 37 percent after 40 minutes of exercise to 62 percent after four hours.[37]

What We Know

*The longer the **duration** of an activity, the greater the likelihood of fat being the primary fuel source (see Chart 2).*

*On the other hand, as the **intensity** of exercise increases, glucose becomes the major contributor to the fuel mixture (remember, carbohydrates are the only fuel that can be burnt with or without oxygen).*

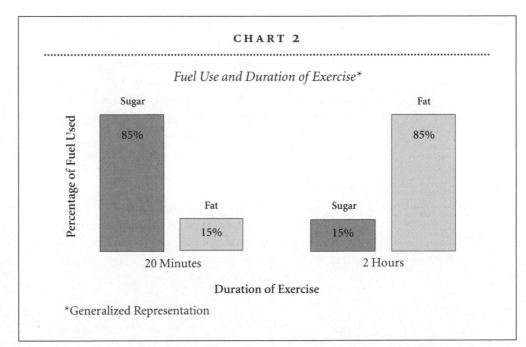

CHART 2

Fuel Use and Duration of Exercise*

Percentage of Fuel Used

Sugar 85%

Fat 15%

Sugar 15%

Fat 85%

20 Minutes

2 Hours

Duration of Exercise

*Generalized Representation

Advantages

Carbohydrates
Easier to burn
Can be used initially
without oxygen

Fats
Lots of it available

Disadvantages

Carbohydrates
Short supply
Oxygen must eventually
be present to get rid
of lactic acid

Fats
Must have oxygen to use

• **Fat vs. Carbohydrates.** Our bodies have 30 times more fat than either stored glycogen or free floating glucose. Why, then, don't our muscles burn *only* our fat? The reason is simple: Glucose is much easier to burn, and has the advantage of being able to be used for a short period without oxygen. But that's the catch: In order for the muscles to continue to use glucose, oxygen must soon be present. Two important metabolic factors influence the body's choice of fuels: 1. glucose is in short supply, a condition which limits the length of time we can sustain short, intense bursts of activity; and 2. lactic acid (remember from Chapter 3—it's the end product of muscle work) builds up when glucose is used without oxygen. This further puts a crimp on intense bursts of action, and may, figuratively speaking, cramp us up. Thus we have a working relationship with fats and carbohydrates that dictates when, where, and how each of them will be used as a fuel source.

Practical Terms: 100-Yard Sprint vs. Three-Mile Jog. Putting it together, here's what happens when we exercise. When sprinting, our bodies perform with what oxygen we have, and the main energy source powering our muscles is glucose. When oxygen and glucose are depleted and lactic acid builds up, we can go no further until we get more fuel and get rid of the lactates. But for those things to occur, we need oxygen. Because we don't have enough, we must either stop or walk to catch our breath. Our oxygen regained, we can sprint once more. This use and recovery is the mechanism that allows us to do fartlek or interval training (which we described in Chapter 5, Routines: The Stars Are the Limit).

When jogging or running distances—where we are not out of breath—oxygen is constantly used by the muscles. Waste products don't accumulate and our activity can continue until we choose to stop. When we first start an activity, our muscles use primarily glucose and a small amount of fat that is circulating in the blood. Gradually, as our activity continues for more than 20 minutes, we rely more on fat as a fuel. Table 10.7 summarizes our use of fat and sugar for fuel.

Training Effects

Why Do We Train?

> When I turned 40 I weighed 225 pounds. I knew I had to do something about it. I gave myself a year to lose the excess. After losing 35 pounds, I started running and another 65 pounds came off in about four months. I now weigh 125 to 128 pounds. I'll turn 50 by the time you get this survey, and I'm still running and I also lift free weights. —Rita, age 50

Losing weight and improving performance are, of course, common reasons to train. Of equal importance is to increase our capacity to expend energy. One factor that limits per-

TABLE 10.7

....

Fuel Use and Intensity of Exercise

Low intensity: Normal breathing
e.g. Walking 1 mile in 20 to 30 minutes
Fuel: Body and muscle fat (approximately 90%)
    Blood glucose (10%)

Moderate intensity: Moderately labored breathing
e.g. Jog 3 miles in 30 minutes
Fuel: Begin with glucose
Increasingly rely on fat and glucose
    Note: Fat will be the primary fuel after approximately 2 hours.

High intensity: Labored breathing
e.g. Sprinting
    Fuel: Glucose plus a small amount of fat

....

Note: Glucose is used here generically to refer to both muscle glycogen and blood glucose.

formance and causes fatigue is the depletion of fuel; another is the failure of our bodies to maintain their internal chemical balance (homeostasis).

In the previous section, we discussed "fuel for energy," so let's look now at how our training programs enable us to produce more energy, more efficiently, and for longer periods of time.

Training and Fats. An endurance-trained muscle is well equipped to use fat for fuel. When it uses fat, glucose, in effect, is spared.

Good aerobic conditioning has a marked effect on all aspects of fat metabolism. Training improves our capacity to both mobilize and utilize fat.[38] A variety of biochemical adaptations in a well-conditioned body shunt fat into the muscle fibers faster and make energy from fat available at a faster rate than in an unconditioned body.[39] Training also results in increased release of fatty acids for fuel; a larger cardiac output, which allows a more rapid delivery of fuel and oxygen to the muscles; and decreased levels of cholesterol and triglycerides.[40]

As a result of training, more fat will be used for energy at a given workload. This helps save our stored carbohydrates, important because it has been estimated that we have only enough glycogen to fuel 1.5 hours of intense aerobic activity.

Training and Carbohydrate Usage. Our level of fitness and our aerobic capacity will influence what fuel our muscles use. Enhancing aerobic capacity through endurance training enables us to not only burn more fat and less glucose, but also to increase the capacity of our muscles to store glycogen. Muscle glycogen stores will thereby be higher at the outset of exercise, and fit women will deplete them at a slower rate than will those who are untrained. Additionally, when we are fit, our bodies can quickly replace spent glycogen when carbohydrates are ingested after exercise.[41]

Performance Food

Because of the great variety of activities in which we engage, and the multitude of ways we participate in them, it is difficult to prescribe nutritional advice to fit every individual's needs.

Note: In presenting the information in this section, we have directed our advice to a wide audience. By looking at Table 10.8, you can determine which information is

---

TABLE 10.8

....

Exerciser Definitions

Type of Exerciser

Recreational Exerciser—You don't train. You just participate intermittently in exercise or activity for fun.

Fitness Enthusiast—You participate in regular exercise or activity for a multitude of reasons, including health, self-image, and feeling good. You are not competition-oriented, although you consider your exercise as training.

Competitor—You exercise/train in order to compete in local, state, or national events.

---

most appropriate for you. When there are changes in your exercise status, you can use this information to help reevaluate your nutritional requirements. Please recognize that these are general categories for women who exercise; you may not necessarily match any definition.

When we work out, whether as fitness enthusiasts or competitors, we eat in order to maintain our energy levels and maximize our daily performance. The facts about food that we discussed in this chapter's first section should be our nutritional focus—the nuts and bolts approach to our daily diet. Our goal should be a healthy balanced menu, which can be achieved by following the Food Pyramid discussed earlier.

Fitness enthusiasts and competitors need additional calories to meet increased energy expenditures. Adequate fuel, particularly sufficient muscle glycogen, is a key factor for good performance. For activities of less than 60 to 90 minutes of continuous exercise, a normal well-balanced diet should provide adequate carbohydrates to meet your energy requirements.

Figuring Your Caloric Needs

I once attended an exercise workshop that suggested we keep a food diary over a two-week period to find out exactly what we consume. Until then, I had no idea of how much food I ate. Well, I guess I'm a bit compulsive, because I'm still maintaining the diary five years later—it helps me count my calories. —Betty, age 39

Energy requirements vary, but are dependent upon your basal metabolic rate, your lifestyle, and your exercise expenditure. For a fast and rough calculation of your energy requirements, see Table 10.9.

BMR + Lifestyle Component + Exercise Rate = Energy Requirements

- **Basal Metabolic Rate (BMR).** This is the basic number of calories we need to keep our bodies going when we are doing absolutely nothing. Among other things, the base rate is dependent upon body size, age, and gender. Basal metabolism is higher in larger people compared to smaller, in younger people compared to older, and in males in contrast to females.

You can calculate your BMR in several different ways. All methods use variations of body weight assessment. Whichever method is used, keep in mind that the value is an estimate. In order to get a truly accurate value, a standard BMR test is needed; however, to roughly estimate your BMR, multiply ten calories per pound of body weight. Using that formula, a 125-pound woman would have a BMR of 1,250 calories, which is the

What to Do

Make sure you have adequate calories in your diet to balance your increased exercise energy expenditure. Later in this chapter we will offer special advice for those who frequently exercise intensely or for prolonged periods of time (longer than 1.5 hours).

TABLE 10.9

....

Calculating Daily Caloric Expenditure—A Fast and Rough Method

I.   **Basal Metabolic Rate (BMR)**
For adult females: multiply 10 × your weight in pounds
        I._____calories

II. **Lifestyle Component (choose the one which best describes what you do
     and then do the calculation)**
    a. Sedentary: limited standing and walking—you sit, drive, or ride whenever possible rather than walk.
        Calculate 25 percent of your BMR calculation from above

    b. Lightly active: you sit most of the day, but move around two to four hours a day.
        Calculate 40 percent of your BMR calculation from above

    c. Moderately active: walking, housework, garden, recreational activities, little sitting.
        Calculate 50 percent of your BMR calculation from above

    d. Physically active: little sitting, lots of physical—often heart-thumping—activity.
        Multiply 60 percent of your BMR calculation from above

        II._____ calories
        SUBTOTAL I. + II. _____ calories

III. **Exercise Component (assumes the equivalent of 30 minutes of activity. If you don't meet this
     assumption, write 0.)**
Multiply 0.12 × the subtotal from above steps I and II.
        III._____ calories

IV. **Total Daily Caloric Expenditure:**

Add your BMR, your Lifestyle Component, and your Exercise Component to get your approximate daily caloric expenditure.

Total Daily Caloric Expenditure = I. + II. + III.
        IV._____ calories

....

Adapted from: Boyle, A.M., & Zyla, G., (eds.). *Personal Nutrition*, 3rd ed., 1996 and Reid, J.G., & Thomson, J.M., (eds.). *Exercise Prescriptions for Fitness.* 1985.

TABLE 10.10

....

Calories Expended in Various Activities

Activity	Approximate Calories Expended per Hour* (* For a 125-pound woman)
Aerobic Dancing (vigorous)	456
Cross-country skiing (moderate—4 mph)	492
Cycling	
outdoor, 5 mph (level)	144
outdoor, 10 mph	318
Dancing (waltz, fox-trot)	300
Handball/Squash/Racquetball	492
Hiking with pack (3 mph)	336
Horseback riding	144
Roller skating (9 mph)	330
Running	
12:00 min./mile	425
10:00 min./mile	605
8:00 min./mile	710
6:00 min./mile	860
Swimming: crawl (45 min./mile)	435
Tennis	
Doubles	255
Singles	370
Volleyball (recreational)	216
Walking	
2 mph (30 min./mile)	156
4 mph (15 min./mile)	318
5 mph (12 min./mile)	408
Weight Training	390

....

Adapted from: Williams, M. H. *Nutrition for Fitness and Sport*, 2nd ed., 1988, and Kostas, G. *The Balancing Act: Nutrition and Weight Guide*, 1993.

Note: There is a wide variation in values for the same activity from one source to another, so these numbers are all ballpark figures.

TABLE 10.11

....

Sample Diets for a Day of High-Carbohydrate Eating at Six Calorie Levels Based on Servings from the Food Pyramid

Group	Calorie Level					
	1,500	2,000	2,500	3,000	3,500	4,000
Bread servings	7	11	16	18	20	24
Fruit servings	5	6	7	9	10	12
Vegetable servings	3	3	3	5	6	7
Milk servings	3	3	4	4	4	4
Meat	5 oz.	5 oz.	5 oz.	5 oz.	6 oz.	6 oz.
Fat servings*	2	3	5	6	8	10

....

*A serving of fat is equal to 1 teaspoon of butter or oil.

minimum number of calories per day needed to sustain that weight if she were to do nothing.

• **Lifestyle Component.** Our normal daily physical movements can be thought of as the lifestyle component of our energy requirements. The number of calories expended during daily activities is not as great as the calories we expend for basal metabolism. Using Table 10.9, decide which definition (and accompanying number) describes your lifestyle component. Remember, this is a rough approximation. If our 125-pound woman lives a relatively sedentary existence—grocery shopping, driving to work, sitting at work, she will need an extra 312 calories (.25 multiplied by 1,250, her BMR) to get her through the day. Because our hypothetical woman does not do the equivalent of 30 minutes of activity, Step 3 is not computed. Thus her total daily energy requirement to fuel her sedentary existence is 1,562 (1,250 plus 312)—close to the 1,600 we suggested some pages back!

• **Exercise Metabolic Rate.** Anyone who exercises, works out, trains, or competes now has to factor that additional energy demand into the equation. Look at Table 10.10 and you will see the caloric expenditure of various physical activities. You will note very quickly that one session of exercise or physical activity, no matter how strenuous it may seem, actually expends relatively few calories—rarely more than 10 to 15 percent of total

TABLE 10.11 *(continued)*

Figuring Out Carbohydrate Intake

A rough way to figure out what percentage of carbohydrates you are eating per day is as follows:

1. Choose your calorie level.

2a. Multiply the number of servings in each group by these numbers:

Bread	15	Vegetables	5
Fruit	15	Milk	12

2b. Total the numbers you get for the 4 groups. That will give you the number of grams of carbohydrates.

   Example: Using a 2500-calorie training diet, we get

Bread	16 servings × 15 =	240
Fruit	7 servings × 15 =	105
Vegetables	3 servings × 5 =	15
Milk	4 servings × 12 =	48
		408g carbohydrates

3. Multiply the number from step 2b by 4, because every gram of carbohydrate is equivalent to 4 calories.

   Using our example from above, we get:

   408g carb × 4 cal/g = 1632 calories from carbohydrates

4. Divide the number from step 3 by the calorie level to get your carbohydrate percentage.

   Using our example from above, we get

   1632 / 2500 = 65% Carbohydrates

Source: Based on Exchange List material from the American Diabetic Association

energy expenditure for the day. That is because active energy output usually can't be kept up for very long over the course of a day. If you've walked for a half-hour (15 minutes per mile), you've only used 172 calories. That's the approximate number of calories in one soft granola bar.

Eating for Exercisers.   In order to be successful in our physical pursuits, we must consume enough calories to meet the energy needs that we've just calculated. Our goal is to eat enough calories (primarily from carbohydrates) to replace our muscle glycogen and thereby maintain a quality training program. We also don't want to take in excess calories, which will end up stored as fat. See Table 10.11 for some sample diets based on servings from the Food Pyramid, as well as a formula for figuring out your carbohydrate intake.

Eating Loads of Carbohydrates Is Not "Carbohydrate Loading." We must eat a lot of carbohydrates because our muscles rely on them. The amount of glycogen stored in our muscles and liver is directly related to the amount of carbohydrates in our diet and to our physical conditioning.

Carbohydrate intake for exercising women should provide at least 60 percent of total calories (or two grams per pound of body weight). Carbohydrate calories should come mostly from complex carbohydrates (starches); refined sugars should contribute very little (15 percent). Diets that contain 60 percent or more calories from carbohydrates allow for the greatest storage of glycogen in the muscles. But this is *not* what athletes call **carbohydrate loading**, which is a combination of diet and training prior to a long endurance competition. Rather, eating a 60 percent carbohydrate diet is just a way to provide the body with energy to strenuously exercise day after day. We discuss carbohydrate loading on pages 252–253 and in Tables 10.14 and 10.15.

• **Special Advice.** If you are in heavy aerobic training (more than 1.5 hours daily), it is advisable to increase carbohydrates to 65 to 70 percent of your total diet's calories. These should be mostly complex carbohydrates and, at the same time, you should reduce your total fat intake to 20 percent.[42] *Note:* While the recommendation is to eat substantially more complex than simple carbohydrates, the research supporting each type's effect on muscle glycogen is not clear-cut.[42] One advantage of complex carbohydrates, however, is that they provide more B vitamins (for energy metabolism) and more fiber and iron.

• **Fat Loading.** While eating lots of rich ice cream to increase your fat intake for food energy may be appealing, fat loading for extra energy has not yet been supported by research, and it may even decrease endurance.[43] The major disadvantage of fat loading is the potential effect on health: increased risks of cardiovascular disease, obesity, and certain kinds of cancer. Besides, with the exception of the elite endurance athlete, most of us have adequate amounts of body fat.

> *If you don't look like a racehorse,*
> *don't run like a racehorse,*
> *are not a racehorse,*
> *why eat like one?*

Food for One-Hour Exercisers. If you engage in household physical activity, work out, exercise, or compete for less than 90 minutes at a time, you don't need to carbohydrate load; your muscles have enough sugar reserves (glycogen) to fuel 1.5 hours of activity.[44] Glycogen isn't likely to run out during 1.5-hour sessions, no matter how intense they are. You should eat a lot of carbohydrates, but there's no need to practice the strategy of carbohydrate loading.

Preventing Staleness. We also need to allow our muscles recovery time before working them again. During each moderate-to-strenuous training session, depletion of the glycogen stores in both the muscles and the liver takes place. If this reserve is not replenished before the next training session, we will not be able to maintain the intensity of a workout and we will experience no improvement even though we are "in training." We may feel "burnt out" or "stale." (*Note:* This feeling may be caused by dehydration as well as overtraining.) Full recovery of glycogen stores in working muscles takes approximately 24 to 48 hours.[45] Planning a workout or training program to allow for muscle recovery is important and is covered in Chapter 5, Routines: The Stars Are the Limit, and Chapter 6, A Sampler of Activities.

Eating Beforehand. If you exercise before breakfast, your fuel tank will hold out, providing the workout or competition is less than one hour. The reason is simple: Your overnight fast has lowered, but not depleted, your glycogen reserves (your body's main source of glucose until you eat and are refueled). If your activity is less than one hour, your body can handle it, and you don't have to eat if you don't feel like it.

If you decide to breakfast before you exercise, don't be overly concerned about what you may have heard: that carbohydrates raise blood insulin and consequently lower your blood sugar (causing hypoglycemia), which may possibly cause fatigue. New information indicates these effects are transient and probably of no great effect on performance. If you find that you are sensitive to a drop in blood sugar, don't eat, or eat very lightly before you exercise.

If, however, you exercise heavily for more than one hour, your performance will be

TABLE 10.12

*Examples of Pre-exercise Breakfast Menus
at Three Different Calorie Levels*

	Calories	Carbohydrate (grams)
Menu 1		
1 cup coffee	5	1
½ cup strawberries	23	5
8 oz. low-fat milk	102	12
1 cup cereal (e.g. bran flakes)	127	31
Total	**257**	**49**
Menu 2		
1 cup coffee	5	1
8 oz. low-fat milk	102	12
2 pieces whole-wheat toast	69	13
1 tablespoon jelly	49	13
½ cup orange juice	66	13
1 cup oatmeal	234	25
Total	**525**	**77**
Menu 3		
1 cup coffee	5	1
2 Pancakes	120	18
with syrup	227	60
8 oz. low-fat milk	102	12
Small piece of fruit (banana)	104	27
1 cup breakfast cereal (bran flakes)	127	31
Total	**685**	**149**

Note: Stay away from foods high in fats and proteins such as meats, cheeses, nuts, cream, muffins, croissants, butter, pies.

TABLE 10.13

Liquid Supplements

	Quantity	Calories	Carbohydrates (grams)	Protein (grams)	Fat (grams)
Nutrament	12 oz.	360	52	16	10
GatorPro	11.6 oz.	360	59	17	6

Source: Food labels

impaired if you don't eat breakfast, regardless of whether or not you are sensitive to lowered blood sugar.

Eating carbohydrates before exercise will provide readily available glucose to fuel your exercise and thus will spare your liver and muscle glycogen stores. If you are worried about food in your stomach when you start exercising, you can drink a liquid meal, or eat two or so hours beforehand to allow adequate time for your meal to exit your stomach. *Note:* Because of individual variations, you should experiment so that you know what your body will tolerate and what makes you comfortable.

• **How Much Carbohydrate in Your Pre-exercise Meal?** The general recommendation is 1 to 4 grams per 2.2 pounds of body weight, 1 to 4 hours before prolonged exercise (more than 1.5 hours).[46] As you get closer to your exercise time, you would eat less—perhaps 1 gram per 2.2 pounds of body weight, 1 hour before; the further away, the more you can consume without worrying about stomach distress. For our 125-pound woman, she would eat 57 g (or 228 calories) of carbohydrates if she were going to begin exercising in 1 hour and 227 g (or 908 calories) of carbohydrates 3 to 4 hours before her scheduled exercise. (We got those numbers by dividing her weight, 125, by 2.2 pounds and multiplying that by 4 to get the number of grams. Next we multiply the number of grams by 4, which is the number of calories per gram of carbohydate.) Obviously the intensity and duration of the exercise would also influence the amount of carbohydrate.

• **What's Recommended?** Solid, high-carbohydrate food choices include fruit, bread (add jam for additional carbohydrates), and low-fat or nonfat yogurt. For liquids, fruit juices and nonfat milk are good choices. See Table 10.12 for some sample pre-exercise breakfasts.

TABLE 10.14

....

Carbo Loading Techniques
(Exercise and Food)

Countdown: Days before competition

Training	Diet
Six Days	
Intense to moderate (1 to 2 hours)	Usual 60% carbohydrates
Five Days	
Moderate (40 to 60 minutes)	Usual 60% carbohydrates
Four Days	
Moderate (40 to 60 minutes)	Usual 60% carbohydrates
Three Days	
Moderate to light (20 to 40 minutes)	70% carbohydrates
Two Days	
Light (20 minutes)	70% carbohydrates
One Day	
Rest	70% carbohydrates
Competition Day	Your usual pre-event
You're On!	meal (don't experiment)

• **What About Liquid Carbohydrate Supplements?** These commercially prepared formulated liquid meals (see Table 10.13) are tasty and high in carbohydrates. They contribute both calories and fluid and can be consumed closer to exercise time because they exit the stomach faster than solids. But they are costly compared to solid foods or other fluids. Because of the expense, they are probably unnecessary for normal workouts and training. However, they can be useful before competition, especially if you are tense. Tension keeps food in the stomach longer; liquid carbohydrates will counteract that effect.[47]

These products can also be used for supplementation during heavy training, when caloric requirements are extremely elevated and sometimes hard to achieve.

• **Alternatives to Expensive Commercial Products.** You can make your own liquid meals by combining skim milk (use a lactose-free milk if you are lactose intolerant), non-fat milk powder, and fruit in a blender. Add sugar, honey, and flavorings for extra carbohydrates and taste. *Note:* Large amounts of fructose (found in sugar and honey) can cause gastrointestinal distress and diarrhea.[48]

Nutrition for Competition. The focus in this section is on preparation for, maintenance during, and recovery from competitive events. Again, the type of activity and its intensity and duration will make a difference in your food requirements.

Eating for the Competitive Edge: Carbohydrate Loading. A sensible goal in the few days before prolonged and intense endurance competition (exercise of more than 90 minutes' duration that results in exhaustion) is to get high carbohydrate concentrations. To do this, we follow a procedure called carbohydrate loading (aka **carbo loading**). This involves a combination of diet and training for the week before the scheduled event. Athletes who use carbohydrate loading can increase their muscle glycogen reserves by 20 to 40 percent above normal.[49] More fuel may mean better performance. The method described below is the newest modification of the original classic method. It was developed because, in the old method, there were complaints of low blood sugar and increased blood acids with associated nausea, fatigue, dizziness, and irritability.[50] See Table 10.14 for a summary of the technique.

• **Countdown: Days Six, Five, and Four.** Train moderately hard (one to two hours on day six, and about one hour on days five and four) and, believe it or not, eat a moderately low-carbohydrate diet (for the amount of training you're doing). The reasoning behind this recommendation is that you will make your muscles overcompensate later by depriving them now of adequate carbohydrates.

• **Countdown: Days Three and Two.** Do no more than 20 to 40 minutes of moderate- to low-intensity exercise (that is, taper off your exercise from day three to day two) while eating a high-carbohydrate diet of approximately 8 to 10 grams per 2.2 pounds per day, or 70 percent of your total calories. For our hypothetical woman of 125 pounds, that would be 455 to 568 grams (125 pounds divided by 2.2 and multiplied by 8 or 10). This should result in an increase in muscle glycogen stores. See Table 10.15 for a sample daily meal plan for carbo loading.

• **Countdown: Race Day Minus One.** The best advice is to rest, or, if you feel so

TABLE 10.15

....

Menu for Carbo Loading

Breakfast
   8 oz. low-fat milk
   2 pieces whole-wheat toast
   4 tsp. jelly
   1 cup orange juice
   1 cup oatmeal with 1/2 oz. raisins or with 2 tsp. brown sugar

Snack
   1 banana
   3 fig bars
   1 cup low-fat milk

Lunch
   1 orange
   1 cup apple juice
   2 beef and bean burritos
   1 cup lemon sherbet

Dinner
   2 cups macaroni
   ⅔ cup spaghetti sauce
   2 tbsp. Parmesan cheese
   2 slices Italian bread
   ½ cup broccoli
   ½ cup ice cream, with
   ¼ cup strawberries

Snack
   3 cups popcorn, air popped
   1 apple

This menu contains approximately 2,500 cal: 70% carbohydrate, 14% protein, 16% fat.

....

Adapted from: Coleman, E. Carbohydrates: The master fuel. In J. R. Berning, & S. N. Steen, (eds). *Sports Nutrition for the 90s.*

compelled, do a very light workout, and consume the same 8 to 10 g/kg of body weight of carbohydrates.

• **Eating the Night Before**. It's become standard to eat a high-carbohydrate meal the evening before competition. The meal's purpose is to provide a final load to muscle glycogen stores.

• **Countdown: Three to Four Hours Before the Race**. While there may be a slight physiological advantage to fasting before exercise in activities of short duration, researchers do not recommend abstinence prior to endurance competition.[51] Instead, new research suggests eating a large (4 g/kg body weight) carbohydrate meal three to four hours before your competition.[52] Peak performance is thereby sustained until the race's end because our bodies are able to maintain their ability to oxidize carbohydrates. Refer back to Table 10.12 for suggested pre-exercise meals. *Note:* While this is what researchers recommend, many runners indicate that because of prerace nervousness, they have trouble digesting such large amounts. Learn your tolerance beforehand so that you will not suffer during competition.

• **Down to the Wire: One Hour Before Competition**. No one food confers a special benefit before competition; however, some athletes have particular favorites. Although eating carbohydrates one hour before competition may cause a decline in blood glucose at the onset of exercise,[53] most studies have found no adverse effect on performance.[54] The best choices are foods high in carbohydrates and low in fat, protein, and fiber. If you have carbohydrate loaded, you don't have to be concerned about what type of sugar (simple or complex) to consume at this time—either is fine. Let your taste and experience be your guide. Other than plain water, the best pre-event snack is a little fruit juice.

The Race: Eating on the Run. "Hitting the wall": This expression is often used by runners to describe the physiological condition that occurs when muscle glycogen is depleted and blood sugar declines (**hypoglycemia**). At that point, our work rate suddenly drops. Research has shown that after one to three hours of continuous exercise at moderate intensity, we will fatigue. Research has also shown that taking in glucose, sucrose, or maltodextrins during exercise delays fatigue by 30 to 60 minutes—which might be just the amount of time necessary to finish our activity.[55] This extra "spark" comes from providing our muscles with a new supply of blood sugar, which has become almost 50 percent of the fuel source during a prolonged moderate-intensity exercise.

It is generally believed that if we exercise for more than two hours, it is best to ingest carbohydrates during that exercise. Preliminary evidence also suggests that eating during exercise may be beneficial if we exercise for one to two hours.[56]

While what you ingest may ultimately narrow down to what is available and/or your individual preference, we recommend that those carbohydrates be in liquid form,

TABLE 10.16

Eating for Peak Performance
(For Activities of Various Lengths)

	Endurance activity of at least 2 to 3 hours	Activity of 1 to 2 hours	Activity of under 1 hour
Carbohydrate Load	Yes	No	No
Water	Yes	Yes	Yes
Sugared Fluids			
Before	Yes	No	No
During	Yes	May help but water is recommended	Use Water
Minerals	No	No	No
Vitamins	No	No	No
Electrolytes during event	Yes	No	No

What We Know

For maximum performance during prolonged endurance exercise, you should follow a carbohydrate-loading regimen (both eating and training) the week before, and combine that with continued carbohydrate intake during the exercise. Following both the eating and training strategies together may produce better performance than one alone.

because then they serve double duty as a fuel source and as a fluid replacement. You should consume about 15 to 30g (60 to 120 calories) of carbohydrate-rich foods or fluids every half hour.[57] Drinking 8 ounces of any sports drink containing 5 to 8 percent carbohydrate every 15 minutes or so provides this amount and also helps prevent dehydration. Table 10.16 provides a quick summary of what you should do for peak performance in events of various lengths.

Eating After Prolonged Exercise. Sufficient carbohydrates should be eaten as soon after prolonged endurance exercise as is practical to provide the most time for resynthesis of your muscle glycogen. In the first two hours after exercise, resynthesis occurs at a faster rate than normal.[58] However, if you are like most people, you probably will be more thirsty than hungry immediately after exercising vigorously. It would be beneficial to drink beverages containing simple sugars like glucose or sucrose, such as fruit juices, or one of the liquid nutritional products listed in Table 10.13.

When your appetite returns, our advice is to eat meals containing more than 70 percent carbohydrates to the tune of approximately 8 grams per 2.2 pounds of body weight during the next 24 hours. For our hypothetical woman of 125 pounds, that amounts to 455 calories from carbohydrates. During this time, stay away from high fat and protein foods because they will have a tendency to suppress your appetite and limit your carbohydrate intake. *Note:* For typical endurance training, the dietary recommendation is 60 percent carbohydrates.

Fluids for Everyone.   Gabriele Anderson-Schiess, the Olympic marathon runner who collapsed, became delirious, and staggered over the finish line in the 1984 Olympics in Los Angeles, is an example of what dehydration can do to you. We sometimes dwell on nutritional requirements, focusing on carbohydrates, protein, and fat, and forget that water is essential in order for our bodies to work right. Mild dehydration impairs exercise capacity and prevents us from achieving maximum performance; severe dehydration can be fatal. Because exercise blunts our thirst mechanism, it is most important to monitor and meet fluid needs during exercise.[59]

Fluid Problems. Like water in a car radiator, water in our blood (plasma) serves to dissipate heat. Blood collects heat from our muscles and transports it to our skin, to be expelled primarily through evaporation of sweat. The amount of heat from our muscles is enough to raise internal body temperatures by one degree centigrade every five to eight minutes. When we sweat, we lose both water and heat. Our lost water must be replaced. If we don't drink, our bodies pull water from other places. Our muscles become a prime source and end up contributing the greatest amount of water, since approximately 45 percent of total body water is stored in muscle.[60]

As more water is lost from the body, cramps, fatigue, decline in performance, weakness, nausea, and dizziness may occur. Ultimately, heat illness—exhaustion or stroke—may occur. A water loss equal to 4 to 5 percent of body weight can reduce muscular work capacity by 20 to 30 percent.[61]

Depending on our activity and the weather, we can lose from 1 to 2.5 quarts of fluid during every hour of heavy exercise; athletes can dehydrate by 2 to 6 percent of their body weight during exercise in the heat.[62] Thirst is not a reliable indicator of needs, because it often comes too late. One study found that when you are exercising hard, you might not feel thirsty until you have lost 1 to 2 percent of your weight through dehydration.[63] Sometimes the color of your urine is a helpful indicator. A darker color indicates that your kidneys are concentrating your urine because adequate water is not available. *Hint:* To see how much water you need during your usual activity, weigh yourself before and after. The difference is all water. *Recommendation:* To replace that loss, you should drink 16 ounces for every pound of weight lost. You should drink before, during, and after exercise. One suggested schedule can be seen in Table 10.17.

TABLE 10.17

....

Suggested Liquid Consumption

Liquid Amount

Before exercise*

Two hours prior   16 to 20 oz.
15 minutes prior   An additional 16 oz.

During exercise   About 1 qt. per hour—roughly
                               1 cup (8 oz.) every 15 minutes

After exercise   Two cups (16 oz.) for each pound of
(At a comfortable rate)   body weight lost

....

* The final verdict on whether there are performance benefits from hyperhydrating (taking in more fluid than you need) before exercising is not in. Research has produced mixed results.

REMINDER: Thirst is not an adequate indicator of how much fluid you need.

• **Special Considerations.** On some days and in certain geographic locations where high humidity prevails, sweat doesn't evaporate, and body heat isn't lost, but we still lose precious water when we exercise. We must then drink more fluid than usual to replace the quantity lost as our bodies keep trying to dissipate heat.

Fluid Choices: Before, During, and After Exercise. You will never go wrong drinking water before, during, or after exercise. It is cheap, usually readily available, and the most effective fluid. Other choices include fruit juices, sports drinks that contain glucose and electrolytes, and sweet-tasting beverages. If you exercise vigorously for less than one hour, or moderately for less than two hours, the choice between water and the other options is mostly a matter of personal taste and convenience since your body only needs the water from those beverages. If, however, you engage in endurance events, strenuous exercise for more than one hour, or moderate activity lasting longer than two hours, mounting evidence suggests that sweet liquids—juices, sports drinks, etc.—enhance energy and endurance.[64] In choosing between these options you must consider how rapidly it will be absorbed, its taste, and its benefit to your performance. *Note:* You can prepare your own alternative to commercial sports drinks. Just add a pinch of table salt to a quart of water and stir in two to three ounces of fruit juice.

TABLE 10.18

Sports Drinks

	Quantity	Calories	Carbohydrate %
10-K	8 oz.	60	6%
All Sport	8 oz.	70	8%
Exceed	8 oz.	68	7.2%
Gatorade	8 oz.	50	6%
Hydra Fuel	8 oz.	66	7%
Nautilus Plus	8 oz.	60	7%
PowerAde	8 oz.	67	8%

Adapted from *Consumer Reports*, August, 1993

• **Fruit Juices.** If you use fruit juices, they should be diluted—with up to twice as much water—to encourage faster absorption from the stomach. Reminder: Be aware that fructose can be associated with gastrointestinal distress.

• **Carbonated Beverages.** These are usually not advised. The carbohydrate concentration in some of these commercial beverages may exceed 10 percent. In that case, or if they contain caffeine—which has a diuretic effect—they are not recommended.

• **Commercial Sports Drinks: Guidelines for Choosing One.** If you prefer a commercial sports drink, the following guidelines might help you choose the right one.

1. It should contain 6 to 7 percent carbohydrates. Drinks with more than 10 percent carbohydrates may cause cramps, nausea, bloating, and diarrhea; drinks with less than 5 percent carbohydrate do not produce the desired endurance-enhancing effect. See Table 10.18 for comparisons of sports drinks.

2. Too much sodium in the drink may hinder water from reaching the muscles. Since a regular diet provides adequate amounts of salt to replace sodium lost during exercise, large amounts in the fluids we drink during exercise are not necessary. It's recommended that a dilute solution, such as 50 mg per cup (8 oz.)—look at the label—is sufficient to help stimulate fluid absorption and enhance the drink's taste.[65]

3. Each sports drink has its own formulation, but they are usually a mix of sucrose, glucose, and fructose or a glucose polymer like maltodextrin. A glucose polymer tricks the stomach, thereby providing more glucose without affecting how quickly it is absorbed.

Fructose has been found by some researchers to delay fatigue in activities lasting longer than two to three hours.[66] It is absorbed faster in the stomach, but more slowly in the small intestine than glucose.

The downside of fructose is, as previously mentioned, that large amounts may cause gastrointestinal upset. A well-known victim of this problem is Kim Jones, an elite marathoner for more than a decade. In 1996 she was unable to finish the Olympic trials and the Boston Marathon because of severe stomach cramps and diarrhea. Her problems were later traced to a new sports drink loaded with fructose. She has since returned to her previous sports drink of choice and reports no problems.[67]

Caffeine. We do not recommend caffeine. While it may be energizing, researchers are divided about its performance effect. Some suggest that it enhances endurance, but others disagree. Regardless of that debate, caffeine is a diuretic: any potential performance benefit may be offset by increased urinary fluid loss. Furthermore, coffee may also stimulate a bowel movement, which would be inconvenient during a competition. *Caution:* Caffeine is a stimulant banned by the United States Olympic Committee. You can reach banned levels if you are tested within two to three hours after drinking about six to eight cups of coffee.[68]

Cold vs. Warm. Cold fluids—40 to 50 degrees F, i.e., refrigerator temperature—are recommended because they leave the stomach more rapidly than warm fluids.[69] If it is cold outside, however, slightly warmer fluids (room temperature) are more suitable. *Note:* If you choose a temperature that is palatable to you, this will increase the likelihood of consuming adequate fluid amounts.

Fluid Delivery for Thirsty Athletes. Fashion and functionalism have merged in the sports water bottle, now a ubiquitous fixture carried by many exercisers. As a matter of fact, it is so "in" that it is not chic to be without one. However, for many engaged in outdoor sports, adequate hydration still remains a problem because water bottles can be an inconvenience. For example, when cycling, reaching for a water bottle while pedaling can be dangerous; long-distance runners need larger quantities than a single bottle holds.

A relatively new innovation, water packs, is now catching on. These water delivery systems are simple in design: a soft plastic bladder filled with water and ice fits inside an insulated nylon carrier, which is strapped on the back or around the waist. A long plastic tube is clipped to a convenient spot—usually the shoulder—so that wearers can grasp it and sip without fumbling for a bottle or taking their eyes off the road. There's no sloshing because the bladder contracts as the water is driven out and adjustable straps allow the water pack to be kept comfortably in place. These products are being adopted by many outdoor sports enthusiasts because they encourage frequent and easy sipping.

What We Know

The excess protein in a high-protein diet will just be an expensive source of fat and energy. Further, performance can actually be impaired on high-protein diets because they don't provide adequate amounts of carbohydrates.

Special Diets

Going Vegetarian. People give many reasons for adopting a vegetarian-based diet. These include religious, philosophical, and environmental concerns, and, of course, health considerations. There is evidence that a vegetarian diet reduces the risks of obesity, coronary artery disease, hypertension, and certain cancers such as colon and breast. Having said that, it must be noted that vegetarians also are more likely to exercise and not smoke, which makes definitive health comparisons with meat-eaters somewhat difficult.

Vegetarian diets may vary considerably. The ones that demonstrate the greatest health benefit include some dairy products. According to the American Dietetic Association, these diets should have up to three servings of low- or nonfat dairy foods per day and no more than three or four egg yolks per week. *Note:* Make sure you get adequate amounts of iron. Additionally, if you don't eat dairy products, you must find other sources to meet your requirements of calcium and vitamins B_{12} and D.

Increased Protein Diet Fad. If there's any nutrient besides fat that many Americans consume in excess, it's protein. Whether you are a vegetarian or not, you most likely will be eating more than enough protein. Yet, a new sports nutrition fad has sprouted, and it involves megadosing on proteins. The new fad's popularity owes much to *The Zone*, a book by Barry Sears, creator of *BioZone* nutrition bars. Much of Sears' theory of achieving the "Zone" relies on controlling eicosanoids—hormone-like compounds such as prostaglandins, thromoxanes, and leukotrienes. You gain control over them, according to Sears, by eating a diet of 30 percent protein, 40 percent carbohydrates, and 30 percent fat. While he presents lots of scientific-sounding information, real nutritional evidence does not support Sears' hypotheses and theories.[70]

Although Sears attempts to debunk accepted nutrition research, it is the double-blind, placebo-controlled, peer-reviewed published research that ultimately enables us to distinguish between hucksters peddling products and legitimate nutritional truths.

Energy Bars: Fast Fuel? Leafing through any sports magazine, you will see many ads for sports bars such as *PowerBar*, *Gatorbar*, or *PR*Bar*. You may wonder: Are they worth it? Will they provide more energy than other foods? Are they for me?

What We Know

If you've never used energy bars before, don't wait until the morning of an event to experiment. Try them while you are training to determine which, if any, is best for you—that is, which tastes good and agrees with your stomach.

To answer these questions we should look at two things: cost and effectiveness. Rest assured about effectiveness: Sports bars can enable athletes to perform better when they are eaten before exercise. They provide energy and usually don't upset finicky stomachs. Sports bars generally contain 100 to 300 calories, most of them from carbohydrates.

Sports bars are convenient, effective sources of energy, but they are not magic. They

What We Know

Danger: Because of their convenience, sports bars are often used as a substitute for breakfast or lunch. While it may be better than eating nothing, sports bars are not a complete meal, nor are they designed for that purpose. They generally are low in protein, fiber, calcium, and other nutrients found in a well-balanced diet. They are meant only as energy enhancers.

provide us with a fast way of getting lots of calories. However, we can get an equal number of calories from a bagel, banana, small bowl of cereal, or fruit yogurt.

Do you need the extra vitamins and amino acids provided by the bars? Most likely not. If you eat a well-balanced diet regularly, or take generic vitamin/mineral supplements, or eat cereal that is vitamin enriched, then the vitamins in the bar are wasted on you.

• **Now, About Costs . . .** Sport bars are an expensive source of calories. They cost approximately $1.50 to $2.50 per bar—that's about $.75 to $1.50 per 100 calories. Raisins cost about 25 cents for those same 100 calories; a breakfast of a low-fat granola bar comes in at about 40 cents for 100 calories.

Sometimes convenience overrides cost. Sports bars are easily carried, don't crush or spoil, and are easily digested. But raisins, granola bars, and fig bars also meet those criteria, and they are far less costly.

Vitamin and Mineral Supplements. In surveys of athletes, 53 to 80 percent use vitamin or mineral supplements.[71] With few exceptions, these pills are not necessary. As mentioned earlier, female athletes are rarely deficient in vitamins and minerals, except for iron.

Herbal Roulette. Americans spend almost a billion dollars a year on herbal supplements. Despite being the oldest, most popular of self-prescribed medications, not all of them help athletic performance, and some may even be harmful. For example, ginseng has been touted for its ability to increase work performance by enhancing the body's resistance to stress and fatigue. A recent study designed to test this claim found that dietary supplementation with a standardized extract of ginseng does not result in greater work performance, a change in energy metabolism, or improved recovery from maximal work.[72]

While quinine, aspirin, and digitalis were originally all derived from plants, and while certain herbs probably have been shown to help conditions ranging from headaches to high cholesterol, you may face problems if you decide to use herbs.

When Congress passed the Dietary Supplement and Health Education Act of 1994, it specified that any supplement (vitamin, mineral, herb, or amino acid) on the market before October 15, 1994 was, for the most part, beyond the rules and regulations of the FDA. As a result, these products went to market without testing for efficacy, nor do companies have to prove that those products are safe. Supplements, for the time being, do not have to be manufactured according to any standards. Because these products are beyond the FDA's jurisdiction, we are not protected when buying these products. Let the buyer beware!

Allergic reactions are one of the dangers. Unregulated, untested herbal substances might produce allergic reactions, but they won't carry an FDA warning. If you are taking any medications, herbs may interact with them. Consult your doctor or pharmacist about possible adverse interactions before taking herbs.

What We Know

Remember: In order to meet increased energy demands, consume enough calories through a well-balanced diet. That way you also get adequate amounts of vitamins and minerals.

What to Do

If you decide to use herbal preparations, you should do so cautiously.

• Make sure you know what the supplement is supposed to do. Don't just rely on the hype printed on the package or in pamphlets.

• Seek out other sources of information. Consumer Reports' November 1995 issue is a good place to start.

• Choose herbs with the words "standardized" on their labels—you are more likely to get consistency and quality from those products.

• Start with low doses and call your doctor if you have a problem (allergic reaction, abdominal pain, or darkened urine).

• Take only one herb at a time, and save the packaging with the label to provide information in case you have a problem.

With unregulated herbs, you do not know exactly what you are getting. Besides possible contamination and incorrect or varying formulations (remember, they are not under FDA control), many herbal supplements mix a variety of ingredients and there is no guarantee that what's on the label is what's inside the package. *Up Your Gas*, a supplement touted to be an energy-booster, contains among other things, ginseng, spirulina, bee pollen, royal jelly, wheat grass, ma huang (also known as ephedra), and cayenne pepper. Ephedra is an herb that can be harmful—even deadly—and its use has been restricted in some states.

Grazing Tips for Hikers. As hiking's popularity has grown, so has the variety of food available for munching in the great outdoors. The amount of fuel a hiker needs depends on the difficulty and length of the hike, the weather, and the hiker's fitness. Generally, the longer and harder the hike, the more calories and water needed.

While we may nourish ourselves for a short hike in the same way we would eat for a regular daily workout, a longer hike takes a little more preparation and thought. Of course, some foods make for better eating than others, but we should mix simple and complex carbohydrates. For a hike of several hours, a carbohydrate breakfast is essential. Eating styles during the hike itself vary from person to person. Some people prefer walking until lunchtime; others prefer eating small bits every 90 minutes or so. This latter grazing style keeps energy high and doesn't produce the drowsiness that sometimes follows a large lunch.

Carrying a bag of gorp—traditionally a mix of "good old raisins and peanuts"—is a matter of pride among many seasoned hikers. But, with a little imagination, mountain munching can be taken beyond the merely functional. For example, gourmet gorp can contain oat granola, nuts, dried fruit, and coconut. But gorp is not the only option, and hikers are experimenting with all kinds of foods to fill their packs and stomachs.

Long-Distance Mountain Munching. Food for backpackers—people taking a long hike with all their worldly needs on their backs—requires a different approach. Not only must you be concerned about the quantity and quality of food, but weight now becomes a crucial factor. Your backpack should weigh no more than a third of your body weight. Keeping the pack weight down to a quarter of your body weight, while difficult to do, will make the hike even more pleasant. That weight usually includes: tent, sleeping and cooking equipment, clothes, and first aid supplies. The weight of those items adds up quickly and food supplies suddenly can seem like a luxury item—something to skimp on. A study of Appalachian Trail backpackers found that only 53 percent of the backpackers questioned could provide an accurate estimate of the number of calories they needed to eat each day (3000 to 4000). However, 68 percent took multivitamins intentionally as a nutritional supplement in case they were not eating properly.[73] Skimping on food often results in a less-than-enjoyable backpacking experience. With the many freeze-dried and dehy-drated foods now on the market, a well-rounded diet can easily be maintained. Dried foods are a boon to backpackers, enabling them to carry sufficient nourishment without adding a lot of weight to their packs. A fairly balanced meal can be found in some packets of freeze-dried food. Check the labels.

Tip: Often supermarkets have dehydrated foods that are cheaper than similar products from camping supply stores.

Nutrition, Energy, and Our Periods. Our eating patterns change over the course of a monthly menstrual cycle. Reports indicate that most women's caloric intake is greatest during the six to eight days premenstrually and lowest six to eight days after our periods. Our reproductive hormones seem to be responsible for this by altering either our basal metabolic rate[74] or our total 24-hour energy expenditure.[75] These natural variations in our eating patterns mean that we do not need to do anything special. Our bodies are doing what they have to do in order to meet our requirements.

Periods, Problems, and Food: Iron-Deficiency Anemia. One area calls for special attention—iron-deficiency anemia. Iron combines with protein to make hemoglobin, the red substance in the blood that carries oxygen from the lungs to cells, and myoglobin, which stores oxygen in our muscles. Some symptoms of iron deficiency are: weakness and fatigue, headaches, and shortness of breath.

Iron deficiency occurs in three stages, and only in the last stage is it clinically called **anemia**. While 30 percent of adult women and 39 percent of adolescent girls may cyclically have depleted iron, only 6 percent are actually anemic.[76]

The preeminent cause of iron deficiency is an inadequate intake of iron. The recommended iron dietary allowance (RDA) for women is 15 mg per day. The average U.S. diet contains 5 to 7 mg of iron per 1,000 calories; therefore, exercising women need to eat 2,500 to 3,000 well-balanced calories per day to get enough iron.

While inadequate intake is the primary cause of iron deficiency, menstruation is the primary source of iron loss in females. Iron-deficiency anemia, due to heavy menstrual blood losses, is estimated to occur in about 6 percent of women between the ages of 18 and 44.[77] Menstrual blood loss varies significantly from individual to individual. Those women who lose large amounts through heavy periods are at greatest risk of becoming iron deficient.

Whether female athletes are more apt to be iron deficient than their non-athletic counterparts is still unclear.[78] Some women, especially those in vigorous activities and sports that place a premium on thinness, do not consume enough calories. In addition, modified vegetarian diets, which are low in iron content, can aggravate the condition.

- **Recommendation.** It makes sense to be medically screened if you are at risk with more than one of these factors:
  1. excessive menstrual flow (because of length, frequency, or amount),
  2. low body weight,
  3. intense and/or prolonged endurance training,
  4. a low caloric intake or trying some fad or weight loss diet,
  5. a vegetarian diet, or
  6. personal or family history of anemia or bleeding disorders.

Treatment. Iron-deficiency anemia is usually treated by iron supplements prescribed by a doctor. However, whether your physician opts to use supplementation for non-anemic iron deficiency is a medical judgment call. In this latter case, the possible benefits must be weighed against costs of supplements (versus dietary changes) and risks of gastrointestinal distress. *Note:* Although anemia clearly will impair your physical performance, it is unclear whether iron deficiency without anemia impairs performance. Thus, iron supplements should not be administered as a way to improve athletic performance in non-anemic iron-deficient women.[78]

Prevention Is Better Than Treatment. It's easy to avoid iron deficiency—meet the RDA allowance recommendations. To do that, emphasize iron-rich foods in your daily diet.

Tips to Boost Dietary Iron
- If you are a meat eater, remember that your body is more efficient at absorbing the iron in meat than that in vitamin supplements. Eat lean beef, lamb, or pork three to four times per week as described in the food pyramid.
- If you are a vegetarian, some good sources of iron include enriched breads and cereals, dried fruits, beans, tofu, and spinach.
- Whether you are a vegetarian or a meat eater, you can enhance iron absorption from food or supplements by combining them with foods containing vitamin C.
- On the other hand, when you are consciously eating to maximize your iron, avoid taking it with foods that inhibit its absorption, such as coffee or tea.
- Cook in iron skillets—iron from the pan is absorbed by the foods cooked in it.

Eating For Success. In closing, remember: To do no harm, the most effective approach to nutrition is simply to eat a balanced diet. Beyond any supplement, healthful varied meals are most effective in helping us achieve peak performance.

ENDNOTES

1. Baron, R. B. Nutrition. In L. M. Tierney, Jr., S. J. McPhee, & M. A. Papadakis, (eds.). *Current Medical Diagnosis and Treatment*, 33rd ed. Norwalk, CT: Appleton & Lange, 1994, 1025–1052.

   Berning, J. R. Eating on the road. In J. R. Berning, & S. N. Steen, (eds.). *Sports Nutrition for the 90s*. Gaithersburg, MD: Aspen Publishers, 1991, 63–74.

2. Short, S. H., & Short, W. R. Four-year study of university athletes' dietary intake. *Journal of the American Dietetic Association*, 1983, 82, 632–645.

3. Baron, R. B. Nutrition. In L. M. Tierney, Jr., S. J. McPhee, & M. A. Papadakis, (eds.). *Current Medical Diagnosis and Treatment*, 33rd ed. Norwalk, CT: Appleton & Lange, 1994, 1025–1052.

4. Christian, J. L. & Greger, J. L. *Nutrition for Living*, 4th ed. Redwood City, CA: Benjamin/Cummings Publishing Co., 1994.

5. Subar, A. S., Heimendinger, J., Grebs-Smith, S. M., et al. *Five a Day for Better Health*. Bethesda, MD.: National Cancer Institute, 1992.

6. *Dietary Guidelines for Healthy American Adults: A Statement for Physicians and Health Professionals*. Dallas: American Heart Association, 1991.

7. Gerster, H. The role of vitamin C in athletic performance. *Journal of American College of Nutrition*, 1989, 8, 636–643.

8. Buzina, R., & Sobuticanec, K. Vitamin C and physical working capacity in adolescents. *International Journal of Vitamin Nutrition Research*, 1985, 27(suppl), 157–166.

9. Howald, H., & Segesser, B. Ascorbic acid and athletic performance. *Annals of the New York Academy of Science*, 1975, 258, 458–464.

10. Karpovich, P., & Millman, N. Vitamin B and endurance. *New England Journal of Medicine*, 1942, 226, 881–882.

    Archdeacon, J., & Murlin, J. The effect of thiamine depletion and restoration on muscular efficiency and endurance. *Journal of Nutrition*, 1944, 28, 241–254.

11. National Research Council Committee on Dietary Allowances. *Recommended Dietary Allowances*. Washington, DC: National Academy of Sciences, 1989.

12. Bergstromm, J., Hultman, E., Jorfeldt, L., et al. Effect of nicotinic acid on physical working capacity and on metabolism of muscle glycogen in man. *Journal of Applied Physiology*, 1969, 26, 170–176.

13. Williams, M. H. Vitamin and mineral supplements to athletes: Do they help? *Clinics in Sports Medicine*, 1984, 3, 623–637.

14. Tin-May-Than, Ma-Win-May, Khin-Sann-Aung, et al. The effect of vitamin B_{12} on physical performance capacity. *British Journal of Nutrition*, 1978, 40, 264–273.

15. Keith, R. E. Vitamins in sport and exercise. In I. Wolinsky, & J. F. Hickson, (eds.). *Nutrition in Exercise and Sport*. Boca Raton, FL: CRC Press, 1989, 233–278.

16. Shephard, R. J., Campbell, R., Pimm, P., et al. Vitamin E, exercise, and the recovery from physical activity. *European Journal of Applied Physiology*, 1974, 33, 119–126.

17. Williams, M. H. *Beyond Training: How Athletes Enhance Performance Legally and Illegally*. Champaign, IL: Human Kinetics, 1989.

18. Nelson, R. A. Preventing and treating dehydration. *Physician and Sportsmedicine*, 1985, 13, 176 & 178.

19. Consumer Reports. Iron in the diet: Do you need supplements? *Consumer Reports*, March, 1996, 62–63.

20. Grandjean, A. The vegetarian athlete. *Physician and Sportsmedicine*, 1986, 14, 122–125, 129–130.

21. Williams, M. H. Vitamin and mineral supplements to athletes: Do they help? *Clinics in Sports Medicine*, 1984, 3, 623–637.

22. Krause, M. V., & Mahan, L. K. (eds.). *Food, Nutrition and Diet Therapy*, 7th ed. Philadelphia: Saunders, 1984.

23. Williams, M. H. *Beyond Training: How Athletes Enhance Performance Legally and Illegally*. Champaign, IL: Human Kinetics, 1989.

24. Slavin, J. L., Lanners, G., & Engstrom, M.A. Amino acid supplements: Beneficial or risky? *Physician and Sportsmedicine*, March 1988, 16 (3), 221–223.

25. Wesson, M., McNaughton, L., Davies, P., et al. Effects of oral administration of aspartic acid salts on the endurance of trained athletes. *Research Quarterly for Exercise and Sport*, 1988, 59, 234–239.

26. Mirkin, G. Can bee pollen benefit health? *Journal of the American Medical Association*, 1989, 262, 1854.

27. Williams, M. H. Ergogenic Aids. In J. R. Berning, & S. N. Steen, (eds.). *Sports Nutrition for the 90s*. Gaithersburg, MD: Aspen Publication, 1991, 101–127.

28. Yocum, L. Carnitine toxicity. *Sports Medicine Digest*, 1986, 8, 4.

29. Brody, J. E. Chromosome damage in the lab is tied to a chromium supple-

ment. *New York Times*, October 25, 1995, c8.

30. Williams, M. H. Ergogenic aids. In J. R. Berning, & S. N. Steen, (eds.). *Sports Nutrition for the 90s*. Gaithersburg, MD: Aspen Publishers, 1991, 101–127.

31. Klaas, R., & Saris, W. M. Limits of energy turnover in relation to physical performance: achievement of energy balance on a daily basis. *Journal of Sports Science*, 1991, 9, 1–15.

32. Lemon, P. W. Protein requirements of soccer. *Journal of Sports Science*, 1994, 12(special issue), 517–522.

33. Grandjean, A. What are the protein requirements for athletes? *Food and Nutrition News*, 1993, 65(2), 11.

34. Mirkin, G. Nutrition for sports. In M. M. Shangold, & G. Mirkin, (eds.). *Women and Exercise: Physiology and Sports Medicine*, 2nd ed. Philadelphia: F. A. Davis Company, 1994, 102–125.

35. Horton, E. S. Metabolic fuels, utilization, and exercise. *American Journal of Clinical Nutrition*, 1989, 49, 931–937.

36. McArdle, W. D., Klatch, F. I., & Klatch, V. L. *Exercise Physiology: Energy, Nutrition, and Human Performance*. Philadelphia: Lea & Febiger, 1981.

37. Ahlborg, G., Felig, P., Hagerfeldt, L., et al. Substrate turnover during prolonged exercise in men. *Journal of Clinical Investigation*, 1974, 53, 1080–1090.

38. Tremblay, A., & Buemann, B. Exercise-training, macronutrient balance, and body weight control. *International Journal of Obesity*, 1995, 19, 79–86.

39. Martin, W. H., Dalsky, G. P., Hurley, B. F., et al. Effect of endurance training on plasma free fatty acid turnover and oxidation during exercise. *American Journal of Physiology*, 1993, 265, E708–E714.

40. Cohen, J. C., Noakes, T. D., & Spinnler Benade, A. J. Postprandial lipemia and chylomicron clearance in athletes and in sedentary men. *American Journal of Clinical Nutrition*, 1989, 49, 443–447.

41. Coyle, E. F. Substrate utilization during exercise in active people. *American Journal of Clinical Nutrition*, 1995, 61(suppl), 968S–979S.

42. Coleman, E. Carbohydrates: The master fuel. In J. R. Berning, & S. N. Steen, (eds.). *Sports Nutrition for the 90s*. Gaithersburg, MD: Aspen Publishers, 1991, 31–62.

43. Phinney, S. D., Bistrian, B. R., Evans, W. J., et al. The human metabolic response to chronic ketosis without caloric restriction: Preservation of submaximal exercise capacity with reduced carbohydrate oxidation. *Metabolism*, 1983, 32, 769–776.

44. Coyle, E. F. Substrate utilization during exercise in active people. *American Journal of Clinical Nutrition*, 1995, 61(suppl), 968S–979S.

45. Costill, D. L. Carbohydrate for exercise: Dietary demands for optimal performance. *International Journal of Sports Medicine*, 1988, 9, 1–18.

46. Coyle, E. F. Substrate utilization during exercise in active people. *American Journal of Clinical Nutrition*, 1995, 61(suppl), 968S–979S.

   Sherman, W. M., Brodowicz, G., Wright, D. S., et al. Effects of 4–hour preexercise carbohydrate feedings on cycling performance. *Medicine in Sports and Exercise*, 1989, 12, 598–604.

47. Coleman, E. Carbohydrates: The master fuel. In J. R. Berning, & S. N. Steen, (eds.). *Sports Nutrition for the 90s*. Gaithersburg, MD: Aspen Publishers, 1991, 31–62.

48. Fruth, J. M., & Gisolfi, C. V. Effects of carbohydrate consumption on endurance performance: Fructose versus glucose. In *Nutrient Utilization During Exercise*. Columbus, OH: Ross Laboratories, 1983, 68–77.

49. Coyle, E. F. Substrate utilization during exercise in active people. *American Journal of Clinical Nutrition*, 1995, 61(suppl), 968S–979S.

50. Coleman, E. Carbohydrates: The master fuel. In J. R. Berning, & S. N. Steen, (eds.). *Sports Nutrition for the 90s*. Gaithersburg, MD: Aspen Publishers, 1991, 31–62.

51. Montain, S. J., Hopper, M. L., Coggan, A. R., et al. Exercise metabolism at different time intervals following a meal. *Journal of Applied Physiology*, 1991, 70, 882–888.

52. Neufer, P. D., Costill, D. L., Flynn, M. G., et al. Improvements in exercise performance: Effects of carbohydrate feedings and diet. *Journal of Applied Physiology*, 1987, 62, 983–988.

53. Horowitz, F. F., & Coyle, E. F. Metabolic responses to preexercise meals containing various carbohydrates and fat. *American Journal of Clinical Nutrition*, 1993, 58, 235–241.

54. Coyle, E. F. Substrate utilization during exercise in active people. *American Journal of Clinical Nutrition*, 1995, 61(suppl), 968S–979S.

55. Coggan, A. R., & Coyle, E. F. Carbohydrate ingestion during prolonged exercise: Effects on metabolism and performance. *Exercise Sport Science Review*, 1991, 19, 1–40.

56. Below, P. R., & Coyle, E. F. Fluid and carbohydrate ingestion individually benefit intense exercise lasting one hour. *Medicine and Science in Sports and Exercise*, 1995, 27, 200–210.

57. Coyle, E. F., & Montain, S. J. Carbohydrate and fluid ingestion during exercise: Are there trade-offs? *Medicine and Science in Sports and Exercise*, 1992, 24(6), 671–678.

58. Ivy, J. L., Katz, A. L., Cutler, C. L., et al. Muscle glycogen synthesis after exercise: Effect of time of carbohydrate ingestion. *Journal of Applied Physiology*, 1988, 65, 1480–1485.

59. The American Dietetic Association. *Journal of the American Dietetic Association*, 87, 933–929,1087.

60. Maughn, R. J. Fluid and electrolyte loss and replacement in exercise. In C. Williams, & J. T. Devlin, (eds.). *Food, Nutrition, and Sports Performances: An international scientific consensus.* London: E & F N Spon, 1992, 19–33.

61. Greenleaf, J. E. The body's need for fluids. In W. Haskel, J. Scala, & J. Whittam, (eds.). *Nutrition and Athletic Performance: Proceedings of the Conference on Nutritional Determinants in Athletic Performance.* Palo Alto, CA: Ball, 1982, 34–50.

62. American College of Sports Medicine. Position stand: Exercise and fluid replacement. *Medicine and Science in Sport and Exercise*, 1996, 28(1), i–vii.

63. Willimans, M. H. *Nutrition for Fitness and Sport.* Dubuque, IA: William C. Brown Publishing, 1992.

64. Lyle, B. J., & Forgac, T. Hydration and fluid replacement. In J. R. Berning, & S. N. Steen, (eds.). *Sports Nutrition for the 90s.* Gaithersburg, MD: Aspen Publishers, 1991, 175–196.

65. Nose, H., Mack, G. V., Shi, X., et al. Role of osmolality and plasma volume during rehydration in humans. *Journal of Applied Physiology*, 1988, 65, 325–331.

66. Okano, G., Takeda, H., Morita, I., et al. Effect of pre-exercise fructose ingestion on endurance performance in fed men. *Medicine and Science in Sports and Exercise*, 1988, 20, 105–109.

67. Longman, J. Jones trying to break 26.2 mile jinx. *New York Times*, November 3, 1996, B3.

68. Williams, M. H. Ergogenic aids. In J. R. Berning, & S. N. Steen, (eds.). *Sports Nutrition for the 90s.* Gaithersburg, MD: Aspen Publishers, 1991, 101–127.

69. Costill, D. L. Water and electrolyte requirements during exercise. *Clinical Sports Medicine*, 1984, 3, 639–648.

70. Coleman, E. The BioZone Nutrition System: Dietary panacea or myth. *Sports Medicine Digest*, December 1995, 6–7.

71. Belko, A. Z. Vitamins and exercise—an update. *Medicine and Science in Sports and Exercise*, 1987, 19, S191–S196.

72. Engels, H. J., Said, J. M., & Wirth, J. C. Failure of chronic ginseng supplementation to affect work performance and energy metabolism in healthy adult females. *Nutritional Research*, 1996, 16, 1295–1305.

73. Puretz, S. L. Health problems of the long-distance backpacker. *The Australian Journal of Science and Medicine in Sport*, 1992, 24(2), 55–59.

74. Solomon, S. J., Kurzer, M. S., & Calloway, D. H. Menstrual cycle and basal metabolic rate in women. *American Journal of Clinical Nutrition*, 1982, 36, 611–616.

75. Webb, P. 24-hour energy expenditure and the menstrual cycle. *American Journal of Clinical Nutrition*, 1986, 44, 614–619.

76. Summary of a report on assessment of the iron nutritional status of the United States population: Expert scientific working group. *American Journal of Clinical Nutrition*, 1985, 42(6), 1318–1330.

77. Consumer Reports. Iron in the diet: Do you need supplements. *Consumer Reports*, March 1996, 62–63.

78. Harris, S. S. Helping active women avoid anemia. *The Physician and SportsMedicine*, 1995, 23(5), 35–46.

11

Menstrual Matters: Cycles Through Life

SUSAN L. PURETZ, ED.D.

Things have really changed nowadays. I remember when I was in high school, you could always tell who had her period. Girls were excused from gym when it was their time of month. I used to take advantage of that opportunity to sit on the bleachers and do homework for other classes. I didn't take gym seriously, but I also didn't really understand why we were automatically not expected to exercise when we were menstruating. —Ruth, age 59

From about the time we reach age 12, our hormones control our menstrual periods and make us biologically, uniquely women. As exercising women, we have questions about whether our menstrual periods influence our physical performance, and if so, how? We also question whether exercise affects the menstrual cycle. Folk remedies and advice abound, but it is only recently that enough scientific evidence has been accumulated to debunk some as myth and substantiate others as fact. Even when menstruation stops, and we are post-menopausal, hormones continue to have an impact on our bodies.

WHY IS THIS HAPPENING TO ME?

Puberty: The Start

In order to conceive and give birth, our bodies have to be hormonally primed. In days of old, societies celebrated this transition from girl to woman with ritual and celebration. Some societies still do. While it is difficult to say exactly when a boy becomes a man, an obvious marker for a woman is her first period. But the appearance of blood only heralds the fact that the possibility of reproduction is imminent. Approximately a year passes before a ripe egg is actually produced and **puberty**—the ability to conceive—occurs.

Although we think of puberty as the start of our sexual being, it is actually the second time that our bodies come under the influence of sexual hormones. The first occurs during fetal development. Both males and females begin with the potential to become female. Testosterone in prenatal boys prompts the development of masculine organs. The lack of testosterone in females permits the structures to remain female. The sexual hormones affect not only the reproductive organs in utero, but they also act in the developing brain to cause its sexual differentiation.

Puberty, then, is a reawakening for the hormones. The terms puberty and **pubescence** are often used interchangeably; however, pubescence technically refers to the period of time and concomitant physiological changes leading to puberty. Puberty is the point when we are actually able to reproduce, that is, to produce viable sperm or eggs. To be precise, pubescence—during which the first period takes place—culminates in puberty.

Menarche: The First Time.   **Menarche**, the first menstrual period, occurs because of hormonal changes influenced by the hypothalamus of the brain. Girls, usually between the ages of 9 and 12 (about two years before boys), begin a series of physiological and anatomical changes including obvious external transformations such as breast "budding"; broadening of the pelvic area; and hair growth in the vulvar and underarm regions. Most American girls experience menarche during their twelfth year, although the range is from 9 to 17. However, as previously mentioned, ovulation will not occur until about a year or so later. Growth and maturation will continue for the next several years. At the time of menarche the ovaries are one-third their adult size, reaching maximum size and weight by the time a woman is 19 or 20 years of age.

Fat vs. Thin.   The average age for menarche among American girls has dropped from about age 15 a century and a half ago to approximately age 12½ today (although there is a broad range). Accepted theory has it that the better the nutrition, the earlier the age of menarche. While nutrition may be associated with an earlier age of onset, very thin girls (especially those who exercise intensely) often have a delayed age of menarche—sometimes as late as age 20.[1] That observation led Rose Frisch, in the 1970s, to hypothesize that menarche is influenced by the ratio of a girl's lean body mass to her body fat. She observed that fatter girls have menarche earlier than do thinner girls, and postulated the onset of menarche requires at least 17 percent body fat by weight.[2] Frisch noted that since ancient times, female fertility symbols have always been fat; she believes this makes biological sense because she contends that body fat has a regulatory role in reproduction.[3]

Critics of Frisch's theory maintain that no one has been able to replicate her research, and that her data are unreliable because, among other reasons, accurate body fat measurements are difficult to obtain.[4] Researchers also point to studies showing that body fat loss from intensive training does not consistently induce loss of menstruation in runners.[5]

In summary: There is no conclusive proof that body fat and menarche are related, yet Frisch's work will not go away, as we shall see later in this chapter.

Exercise and Menarche. According to numerous studies, strenuous exercise seems to retard menarche.[6] For example, in a Harvard University study, runners and swimmers whose training had begun prior to their menarche began menstruating at an average age of 15. In contrast, those who had begun training after puberty began their periods at an average age of 13.[7] Similarly, data from a 1995 study of swimmers found a delayed age of menarche among the competitive swimmers compared to girls of the same age who were not athletes.[8] It has been suggested by one research study that for every year of strenuous exercise—more than one hour daily—a girl's menarche may be delayed by approximately five months.[9]

• **Hypotheses.** Some researchers point to the number of hours spent daily in exercise[10]; others cite the number of years spent in formal sports or dance training before menarche[11] as possible reasons for the later onset. A psychosocial explanation, also proposed, posits a preselection of athletics by girls with certain body characteristics.[12] For example, a girl with long legs and narrow hips—sometimes indicative of a late maturer—may be attracted to and successful in certain sports because of her physique. Menarche, according to this theory, would have been delayed whether or not she participated in sports. Frisch and her associates, however, maintain that it is the intense physical activity that retards the acquisition of a critical fat mass and thereby delays menarche. Problems with methods and statistics in these studies have cast doubt upon their conclusions.

• **Questioning Previous Studies.** To demonstrate how some studies can come up with absurd conclusions about the relationship between exercise, age at which training began, and delayed menarche, a group of researchers intentionally did a "study" using only numbers—not people.[13] The researchers created 30,000 imaginary athletes and then manufactured statistics for these imaginary athletes. One set of numbers represented when these girls started their athletic training (the average was 10 years of age) and another set of numbers represented when these imaginary athletes started their periods (the average was 13.4 years). When the researchers analyzed the relationship between these fictitious sets of numbers, there was no relationship—that is, age of initiation of training had no effect on menarche.

The authors then played with their imaginary athletes by rearranging them into two groups. One group had the imaginary athletes who began training prior to menarche, while those in the other make-believe group had begun training after their menarche. The authors then reanalyzed their data, and lo and behold, there was now a relationship. Remember, these are imaginary athletes.

The authors of this study conjectured that the type of data analysis used by most researchers to show that menarche is delayed by prepubertal physical activity probably would be sensitive to an inherent bias. The results of their experimental manipulation of made-up numbers confirmed this hunch. The authors went so far as to state that studies, using this traditional design, will yield a "a significant relationship between the age at which athletes begin training and the age at which they reach menarche . . . regardless of whether or not a true relationship exists."[13]

• **Delayed vs. Later.** Another problem with drawing conclusions from some research studies is that many studies automatically assume that if a woman does not have her period by age 17, she has a delayed menarche. In fact, these young women may represent the group whose periods begin "later"—remember, the range for first menses is 9 to 17 years of age. While the term "later" falls within a normal range of ages, "delayed" connotes pathology. Once something is defined as pathologic, it's a small step to link it to problems of female athletes.[14]

In Summary: When researchers say that premenarcheal training causes delayed menarche, they are basing their statements on data that can't be checked for its accuracy and reliability. For example, any comparison of age of menarche in dancers and non-dancers will be biased because most dancers begin training before menarche and there is no way of proving that these dancers would have begun their periods in a normal way but for the dance training. Reliable and accurate information is very important because of the large number of prepubertal girls engaging in athletics and dance each year, and their parents, coaches, and health care professionals, who are trying to assess potential long-term risks associated with early and intense training in these activities. While it may be correct to say that the average age of menarche is later in athletes than non-athletes, thus far, there has been no valid experimental evidence to support the statement that athletic training delays menarche.[15]

What We Know

The average age of menarche is later in athletes than non-athletes; however, it has not been proven that athletic training causes pathologically delayed menarche.

MENSTRUATION

According to a New Guinean legend, in ancient times the moon lived on earth in the form of a handsome young man, who made repeated attempts to seduce innocent young maidens. One day, a young wife succumbed to his pleas, but unfortunately, her husband discovered them and set fire to the house in anger.

The young man was trapped and killed; his blood spurted to the heavens in a great stream and there it became the moon. His revenge was to cause young women to suffer a loss of blood, whenever he, the moon, appeared.

What Causes the Monthly Period?   The brain's hypothalamus controls our periods through a system of hormonal feedback with the ovaries and the pituitary gland. The menstrual cycle involves maturation of the egg-containing follicles in the ovary (**the follicular phase**), ovulation, preparation of the uterus for implantation of a fertilized egg (**the luteal phase**), and menses (or menstrual flow).

   The Follicular Phase. A woman's cycle is described as beginning on the first day of her menstrual flow. At that time, levels of the hormones estrogen and progesterone are at their lowest. The hypothalamus responds by secreting **Gonadotropin Releasing Hormone (GnRH)**, which in turn stimulates the pituitary gland to secrete **Follicle Stimulating Hormone (FSH)**.

   As a result of FSH secretion, several follicles in the ovary start to mature. As they develop, they begin to secrete estrogen. The rising level of estrogen in the blood makes the hypothalamus stop producing GnRH; in turn, that causes the pituitary to stop releasing FSH. With the shutdown of hormone production, all but one follicle stops growing (why one follicle continues to grow is unknown). Estrogen levels drop slightly with the decrease in the number of follicles; however, that is compensated for as the one follicle (known as the graffian follicle) continues to mature and secrete greater quantities of estrogen.

   Although it is the most variable part of the cycle, the events up to this point take approximately 12 days (but can range from 11 to 23 days and still be considered normal).[16] During this time, the effects of the increased quantities of estrogen have caused the endometrium of the uterus to start to proliferate. Changes in other reproductive organs, for example, the vagina, are also noticeable as a result of increased levels of estrogen.

   • **Ovulation.** Rising amounts of estrogen and progesterone (produced by the ovary) are detected by the hypothalamus, which causes GnRH to be secreted, which, in turn, stimulates the pituitary to release **Luteinizing Hormone (LH)**. This may sound confusing because you just read that in the follicular phase, high levels of estrogen cause the hypothalamus to inhibit FSH. But, estrogen's relationship to LH works the opposite way; high levels of estrogen cause the release of LH. LH has a rapid effect on the ovaries, causing ovulation to occur within 16 to 24 hours. Ovulation involves the rupture of the ovarian wall by the graffian follicle, which has now grown so large that it takes up approximately one-third of the ovary. This rupture allows the egg contained within the follicle to be released and begin its journey into and through the fallopian tubes.

   Some women can tell when they are ovulating because they suffer from Mittel-

schmerz, a German term for pain in the middle (of the monthly cycle). The pain is on one side of the abdominal region and the ovary on that side may be very tender to touch. Some women experience breakthrough bleeding, while others can judge when they're starting to ovulate by the changed consistency of their mucosal discharge. It becomes very thick and viscous. This condition is known as **spinbarkeit**, and under the microscope the mucous exhibits a beautiful branching pattern known as **ferning**. Finally, women who have been monitoring their temperatures with a special thermometer know when they have ovulated because their basal body temperature rises at least four-tenths of a degree Fahrenheit.

The Luteal Phase. Once ovulation has occurred, the cells of the graffian follicle (under the influence of LH) change and begin producing progesterone in large quantities. This transformed graffian follicle is now known as the **corpus luteum** (Latin for body and yellow, respectively). If fertilization occurs, progesterone will continue to be produced, the uterine lining is not shed, and the embryo has a place in which to develop.

If the egg is not fertilized, the corpus luteum starts to regress and ceases production of progesterone and estrogen approximately eight to ten days after ovulation. The corpus luteum becomes inactive and white, and it is now called the **corpus albicans**. The uterus responds to this hormonal deprivation by sloughing off its currently unneeded, enlarged endometrial lining. The superficial two-thirds of the endometrium is almost all sloughed off as part of the menstrual flow. The discharge is a combination of uterine blood and dead tissues and is the equivalent of approximately two to four ounces.

The Menstrual Cycle

While I'm used to the fact that my cycle is somewhat irregular, it doesn't keep me from being embarrassed in certain situations. For example, in a recent aerobics class, I suddenly felt that I was bleeding heavily. When I looked at my groin in the mirror I noticed a stain on my light blue spandex pants. I quickly grabbed my gym bag and headed for the bathroom so I could change. I hoped that nobody had noticed, especially not the two men who were in the class. —Heidi, age 27

The onset of bleeding or menses (Latin for month) is the start of the new cycle, which will be approximately 28 days in length. Within the 28 days, the follicular and luteal phases are each approximately 14 days. However, a normal cycle can be anywhere from 23 to 35 days—resulting in 10 to 13 cycles per year. **Eumenorrheic** is the term used to describe cycles that fall within this range on a regular basis.

Accompanying the follicular and luteal development are concomitant hormonal changes in the levels of estrogen, progesterone, LH, and FSH. While these can be monitored with frequent sampling of either blood or urine, there is no reason to do so unless medically required.

There's More to the Cycle Than Blood. Despite the increasing frankness with which Americans discuss sexuality, a survey conducted for the manufacturer of Tampax tampons as recently as 1981 found that many people are still uncomfortable discussing the topic of menstruation.[17]

In the survey, only 35 percent said that it was an appropriate subject to discuss at the office; and fewer, 33 percent, thought it fitting to mention in social situations. More than a third of the respondents said that, even at home, women should conceal the fact that they are menstruating. Further, 56 percent of the women in the survey agreed that women should abstain from intercourse during menstruation, while 8 percent believed that women should avoid contact with others during this time. Those beliefs are based on religious convictions and old myths.

It is also well substantiated that women experience physical and emotional changes during their cycles. Yet the perceptions of these alterations are very individual and may even vary within the same person. Symptoms include: breast tenderness, abdominal cramping or discomfort, fatigue, moodiness, edema, lower back pain, tension, general joint aches, shoulder or knee pain, headache, nausea, irritability, and depression.[18]

Typically, symptoms occur either premenstrually or during the time of menstrual flow. The term **dysmenorrhea** (painful menstruation), while sometimes used to generally describe all of the above problems, technically refers to the wave-like cramping pelvic pain.

While most women experience some premenstrual symptoms, a small proportion of women experience them so severely that their lives are disrupted. Those women are said to be suffering from **premenstrual syndrome** (**PMS**)—a diagnostic term used by psychologists and medical professionals. Scientists believe the syndrome is caused by hormonal changes, but they have been unable to document any differences in quality and types of hormones between women with true PMS and those who experience "normal" symptoms.

Our Data

I am quite aware of my body and my feelings, and how they change over the course of the month. —Judy, age 33

In our survey, 63 percent of the women said that they had physical discomfort during their periods and 58 percent reported physical discomfort prior to their periods. Of the 228 women who offered explanations about their physical discomfort, 138 cited cramps

TABLE 11.1

Physical Discomfort Associated with Menses

	Number of Women Reporting		
Symptoms	Prior to Menses	During Menses	Total
Cramps	35	138	173
Bloating (Water Retention)	51	27	78
Pain	23	20	43
Breast Tenderness	26	1	27
Headaches	14	7	21
Tiredness	12	7	19
Premenstrual Syndrome	13	NR	13
Heavy Flow	NR	5	5

NR—not relevant
Sample Size = 228
Note: Women gave multiple responses.

during their periods and 35 women experienced cramps prior to their periods. Bloating was the second most cited factor causing physical discomfort during menses. For a comparison of the problems identified as being associated with menses, see Table 11.1.

Almost 60 percent of the women we surveyed experienced premenstrual psychological tension. Phrases that were used to describe that tension included: "I get emotional and cry easily"; "I'm moody"; "depressed"; "anxious and feeling stressed"; "irritable and grouchy"; "short tempered"; "nervous"; "tense and edgy." This is not just a phenomenon experienced by American women. Researchers at State University of New York, Buffalo recently found that women in Italy and Bahrain experienced similar symptoms.[19]

Although many theories and remedies have been advanced for treating premenstrual symptoms, no one therapy has yet proven effective in treating the constellation of problems. Probably, awareness that these symptoms exist and are commonplace is the single most helpful measure; we can then try to keep this time as stress-free as possible, as well as treat some of the more annoying symptoms.

Help for Period Problems

If I haven't been exercising regularly my period can be quite painful because of cramping. With regular exercise, I experience minimal discomfort. —Alice, age 35

Until fairly recently, it was assumed that 70 to 80 percent of the cause of painful menstruation was due to faulty living habits, including poor posture, lack of exercise, fatigue, and tension.[20] The result of one survey from that former era indicated that college women need "to acquire more knowledge and understanding about menstruation, to develop a wholesome attitude toward menses, to enhance their pride in a healthy feminine body, to improve their postures, and to assume responsibility for preventing their own menstrual problems."[21] We have come a long way since that time and attitude!

Today, two avenues of approach are recommended: exercise and medication. Whether regular and ongoing exercise alleviates premenstrual and menstrual symptoms is still unclear. In a 1985 study evaluating whether 12 weeks of aerobic training would alleviate menstrual symptoms, one group of women was assigned to aerobics while a second (control) group was told not to exercise.[22] Both groups reported similar levels of symptoms before the experiment began, but afterwards menstrual symptoms were markedly reduced in the experimental group that underwent the 12 weeks of aerobic training. Other studies concur that regular conditioning exercise decreases premenstrual symptoms.[23]

As for exercise helping premenstrual syndrome, the current medical literature lacks scientific support for the widely held belief that exercise improves PMS symptoms.[24] No well-designed studies either prove or disprove this hypothesis. If exercise does help relieve some PMS symptoms, it may be as a result of its tranquilizing effect through the release of endorphins.[25]

For women who find exercise does not help, **anti-prostaglandin** medication—ibuprofen or even aspirin—has been shown to be very effective in relieving both PMS and menstrual symptoms.

MENSTRUATION AND PHYSICAL PERFORMANCE

Performance-Related Questions

I seem to perform better when I have my period because instead of focusing my energy on my period, I focus it on my performance. —Diane, age 28

I run badly right before I get my period. —Louise, age 33

I don't feel as good during the first couple of days of my period, but I run the same.

—Carol, age 35

Research Dilemma. Three women, three different perceptions: So what's the story—can we make any general statements? A body of literature is beginning to accumulate documenting the menstrual cycle's effect on exercise performance. The majority of the earlier research supports the belief of many individual athletes and coaches that menstruation impairs performance, with poorest performance prior to and during one's period.[26] Although some studies have reported an improvement during menstruation,[27] most pinpointed best performances as occurring in the days immediately after menstruation.[28] Interestingly, variations seem to be somewhat dependent upon the sport: rowers[29] and cross-country skiers[30] reported poor performance during menstruation, while swimmers reported fewer cycle-related influences.[31]

• **Possible Solutions.** The reason for such conflicting results in these studies can perhaps be found in the methods of gathering information. Many studies relied on memory of performance long since past (which can be faulty); others did not precisely identify cycle phases, and this failure colored results.

Not surprisingly, the results from research using actual performance measurements and/or hormonal levels contradict earlier findings. In one study, swimmers who had their times recorded showed no difference in performance during any of the three phases of their cycles.[32] The same investigators obtained similar results for strength performance in weight lifters, that is, the phase of the cycle did not affect performance. Likewise, a study of the dynamic strength and work capability of untrained, normally menstruating women during various stages of the menstrual cycle showed no discernible change in performance on a leg machine.[33]

In another study, researchers examined 16 women on four indices of athletic performance—aerobic capacity, anaerobic capacity, isokinetic strength, and high intensity endurance—during the early follicular and midluteal phases of the menstrual cycle.[34] The only significant finding was that aerobic capacity was slightly lower during the midluteal phase (a few days after ovulation). Despite this finding, the researchers concluded that no overall important variations in physical performance occur during the cycle. Other research concurs with this finding.[35]

Menstruation: A Help or a Hindrance?

Our Data. In answer to the question: "Is your performance affected by your menstrual cycle?," 64 percent of the women said "No," thus concurring with other surveys, which indicate that from 37 to 63 percent of athletes do not report any detrimental effects over the course of their cycles.[36] Of the 161 women in our study who indicated that their performance was affected, approximately half said it happened during their period, and the rest said prior to their period. One hundred and twenty-six women took the opportunity to explain how their performance was impacted. The explanations overwhelmingly described negative performance effects with words like: tired, no energy, fatigued, lethargic, hard to get going. One respondent indicated that she was aware that her performance was poor during her period and this made her psychologically upset as well—a self-fulfilling prophecy?

There were a handful of women who reported being energized prior to their periods. One said she performed better on the first day of her period and another went as far as saying, "some of my best races are during my period." One respondent said she didn't feel like exercising, but once she decided to, there wasn't a difference in her performance. When the data for the effect of menstruation on performance were analyzed comparing competitors with what we classified as hobbyists (women who participated in exercise for a variety of reasons other than competition), 45 percent of the competitors felt their performance was affected, compared with 33 percent of the hobbyists.

Sixty-nine women answered that they had objective evidence to support observations that their performance was affected by their periods. Of that group, 31 explained further what they meant. For example, 14 women kept calendars, charts, and logs of their performance times. Several women indicated that their spouses or significant others could predict their periods by looking at their performance and their times.

Of the 69 women who indicated that they had objective evidence, women who were actively competing in sports were proportionally more aware of performance differences and had objective evidence (logs or performance times) to support their feelings.

Exercise / Training and Hormonal Changes

Short-Term Effects. Just as hormonal variations associated with menstruation may influence athletic capability, exercise itself may alter hormonal function. Researchers have found the following transient blood level changes associated with exercise: an increase in prolactin,[37] estradiol,[38] progesterone,[39] testosterone,[40] cortisol,[41] and LH.[42]

That being said, it is no easy task to find out if exercise actually causes short-term hormone level fluctuations. For example, our level of fitness affects the way our bodies physiologically respond to an activity's demand. Other factors possibly affecting short-term fluctuations include: nutritional state, temperature, and stress level. It is not enough to know all these other possible influences; researchers must also be able to separate and measure them independently in order to say definitively that hormonal changes result from exercise regimens.[43]

Long-Term Changes. While the effects just discussed are short-lived, some researchers believe that daily training will cause some of the transient changes to persist. Several researchers provide excellent overviews of the various studies documenting

What We Know

Does having your period affect your performance? Probably not!

chronic hormonal alterations with training.[44] The studies they cite have looked at the "stress" hormone (cortisol) and the gonadotropins (LH, FSH), as well as the releasing factor GnRH.

All the technical data aside, it should be noted that it is not yet clear whether menstrual irregularities should be viewed as an adverse effect of exercise. Just the reverse, they may be a natural reaction aiding our body's adaptation to strenuous exercise.[45]

MENSTRUAL IRREGULARITIES

My periods come when they feel like it. —Joan, age 29

When I started running, my periods became shorter and lighter. —Trudy, age 33

I was without my period for a long time, but I've always been somewhat irregular.
—Denise, age 26

Almost everyone is aware of the positive physical and mental aspects of exercise, both at the recreational and competitive levels. Fewer of us recognize that apart from those benefits, there may be negative consequences as well: menstrual irregularities, eating disorders, and osteoporosis—known collectively as the Female Athlete Triad—not to mention the usual strains, sprains, and broken bones (See Chapter 18: Beware of the Danger Zones for more information). Menstrual dysfunction is recognized as a common problem in some exercising women—especially runners, dancers, gymnasts, rowers, and cyclists.[46] Swimmers, too, are not exempt. A recent study found that 82% of the 69 competitive swimmers surveyed had menstrual irregularities.[47] Although menstrual dysfunction is recognized as a distinct medical entity and is experienced by many exercising women, unanswered questions still remain.

The Spectrum

I'm glad I had my experience as an athlete—but I paid for it dearly. During the prime childbearing years, I could not consider having children because I had menstrual problems—I was amenorrheic. —Jane, age 49

The normal (**eumenorrheic**) menstrual cycle is commonly defined by the presence of more or less regular menstrual bleeding every 23 to 35 days.[48] In addition, to fully qualify as a "normal" cycle, hormonal levels appropriate to each phase must also be present.

The absence or cessation of menses is known as **amenorrhea**. Amenorrhea is characterized by fewer than two menstrual cycles per year, with none in the previous three to six months. Women who have not begun their menstrual periods by age 17 are defined as having **primary amenorrhea**. Women who have had a normal menarche and regular

The spectrum of menstrual cycles goes from:

• *Eumenorrhea ("regular" or "cyclic"). Menstrual cycles that recur consistently at regular intervals.*

• *Luteal Phase Disturbances. Problems that usually produce so subtle an abnormality that they escape detection unless a specific reason, for example, infertility, has prompted a medical consultation.*

• *Oligomenorrhea ("irregular"). Menstrual cycles that occur inconsistently at intervals from 39 to 90 days.*

• *Amenorrhea ("absence of periods" or "acyclic"). Menstrual cycles that occur at intervals of longer than 90 days. This includes primary (delayed menarche beyond age 17) and secondary (absence of menstruation in women who previously were regular).*

menstrual cycles and who then miss three to twelve consecutive menstrual periods have **secondary amenorrhea.**

According to some researchers, the route from normal menstruation to amenorrhea is a continuum, leading progressively from one to the other with **luteal phase disturbances** and **oligomenorrhea** as intervening intermediary menstrual problems.[49]

Types of Menstrual Dysfunction

Luteal Phase Disturbances. "Luteal phase disturbance" means that either the hormone level (specifically progesterone) or the normal length of the luteal phase (approximately 14 days) are not as expected. Some researchers have suggested that there is a continuum of luteal phase problems ranging from inadequate progesterone secretion—the earliest and most subtle type—to shortened luteal phases, which are more serious.[50]

A woman diagnosed as having a luteal phase disturbance either may menstruate regularly or more frequently than every 23 days.[51] Keep in mind that having your period does not always mean that your periods are "normal," nor does having your period frequently (every 23 or less days) mean that you are abnormal. Researchers have documented that some women may have frequent menses and yet have normal luteal function[52]; conversely, some exercising women with normal cycles may have luteal phase alterations.[53]

• **Luteal Phase Suppression.** A shortening of the luteal phase (less than ten days from ovulation to the start of menstrual flow) accompanied by decreased levels of progesterone is known variously as luteal phase suppression, deficiency, or short luteal phase. This condition can only be determined by hormonal measurements, since it is not uncommon for women to continue to menstruate. One researcher reported this condition in intensely training athletes who had their periods, and noted that these athletes regarded themselves and their periods as being perfectly regular and normal.[54] *Note:* Women with either luteal phase disturbance or irregular periods (the next condition to be discussed) may also not ovulate, that is, they can be **anovulatory.**

Oligomenorrhea (Infrequent Periods). Infrequent menses (**Oligomenorrhea**) is when a woman has three to six cycles per year inconsistently at intervals ranging from 36 to 90 days. Infrequent menses may be the result of either low levels of estrogen and progesterone or they may be because of not ovulating.[55] A woman who does not ovulate has normal estrogen levels but abnormally low progesterone levels, as well as cycles that are irregular. When the irregular periods are the result of not ovulating, the low progesterone production and the abundance of estrogen in the system (estrogen is considered to be "unopposed") can possibly lead to increased growth of the uterus's endometrial layer and possibly endometrial cancer.[56] When infrequent periods do come, they come at unpredictable times, and heavy bleeding is common.[57] This bleeding can be inconvenient—especially for competitive athletes—and may occasionally cause iron deficiency, which may impair performance.

Amenorrhea. Amenorrhea is now believed to originate in the brain's hypothalamus; it results in low estrogen levels (a **hypoestrogenic** state). Although the exact mechanism remains unclear, amenorrhea typically indicates suppression by the hypothalamus of the LH stimulating messenger—GnRH, the Gonadotropin Releasing Hormone. As previously mentioned, GnRH ordinarily causes the pituitary to release the hormone LH—which in turn further stimulates the ovaries to produce additional estrogen and progesterone. Without that stimulation, we get low levels of both hormones.

While only 2 to 5 percent of all women suffer from amenorrhea, estimates of the prevalence of amenorrhea in athletes range anywhere from 3.4 to 66 percent, depending on which study you read.[58] This type of amenorrhea is known as **exercise-associated amenorrhea**. The highest incidence occurs in long-distance runners.[59]

Although amenorrhea is not limited to any particular sport, most of the research has been done on runners and dancers, who typically exhibit low estrogen levels. One study of swimmers found that their hormonal patterns were quite distinct from the low estrogen levels described for runners and dancers.[60] Their data indicate that swimmers have mild hyperandrogenism (elevated levels of adrenal androgens). The researchers conjecture that this distinct hormonal profile in swimmers might be a result of a different mechanism than the one that causes menstrual irregularities in runners and dancers. Women who swim are not as thin as runners and dancers because they are participating in a sport where thinness is not essential to performance or aesthetics. The study's authors recommend that clinical distinctions be made among the various types of athletic amenorrhea, based on hormonal profiles with attention to weight and body type. *Note:* A hormonal profile is necessary not only for accurate treatment of individual athletes, but also would be helpful for use in research—to standardize definitions of menstrual irregularities in the groups of athletes being studied.

Why Me?

FLASH: *Uta Pippig wins the 1996 Boston Marathon. Pippig came in first despite being plagued by menstrual cramps the entire race.*

Why do some athletes lose their periods and others, like Uta Pippig, do not? A Chinese study of the menstrual cycle in 199 female Olympic-style weightlifters, with an average age of 16 years, reported 75 percent were regular in their menses and 25 percent were

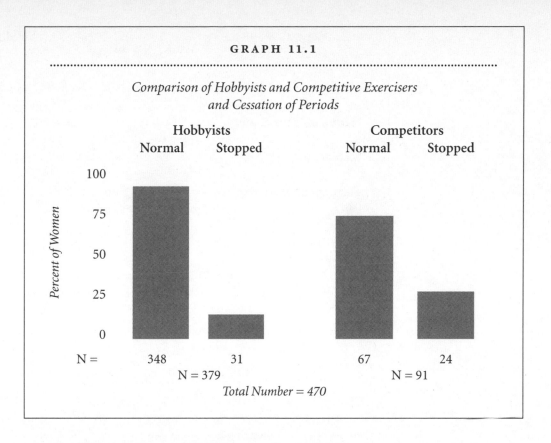

GRAPH 11.1

*Comparison of Hobbyists and Competitive Exercisers
and Cessation of Periods*

	Hobbyists		Competitors	
	Normal	Stopped	Normal	Stopped
N =	348	31	67	24
	N = 379		N = 91	

Total Number = 470

irregular. The authors concluded that female weightlifters have fewer problems with regular menses than female swimmers or long distance runners.[61]

While regular, particularly intense exercise is associated with changes in reproductive hormones, the majority of female athletes menstruate normally.[62] Later in this chapter, we provide suggestions for women who exercise and have menstrual problems.

Our Data. In our study, 12 percent (55 women) indicated they stopped menstruating as a result of their participation in exercise/sports (See Graph 11.1). Of the 55 women who stopped menstruating, 31 (56 percent) defined themselves as recreational exercisers and 24 (44 percent) described themselves as competitors.

However, of the 91 women in our study who defined themselves as competitors, a significantly higher number (26 percent versus 8 percent of all recreational exercisers) said they had stopped having periods because of their exercise/sports.

TABLE 11.2

....

Profile of Exercising Women Whose Periods Stopped

Frequency of Exercise:	1–2 days per week	3–4 days per week	5 or more days per week
Percent	4%	23%	73%

Time Spent Exercising:	Under 1 hour	Over 1 hour
Percent	19%	81%

Intensity of Exercise:	Mild	Moderate	Intense
Percent	3%	53%	44%

....

*Percentages are based on a total of 55 women representing 12 percent of the study's sample.

TABLE 11.3

....

Comparison of Age when Training Began and Cessation of Periods

Age at Start of Training	Number in Study	Number and Percent Developing Amenorrhea
Under 12	49	7 (14 percent)
In Teens	69	14 (20 percent)
In Twenties	147	22 (5 percent)
In Thirties	104	9 (2 percent)
In Forties	73	3 (.06 percent)
Total	442	55 (12 percent)

Other interesting findings from our study include data regarding the relationship between frequency, intensity, time, and menstrual periods. For example, as frequency of exercise increased from once a week to every day, the number of women who stopped menstruating increased. Eighty-one percent of the women who experienced cessation of their periods were serious exercisers, that is, they spent an hour or more per workout, and 97 percent of them classified their workout as moderate or intense (See Table 11.2).

One last observation from our study was the relationship between cessation of menstruation as a result of exercise and the age at which women began exercising. Although only 5 percent of the women who began exercising in their twenties developed amenorrhea, they represent 40 percent of the 55 women who experienced menstrual difficulties (See Table 11.3).

Exercise-Associated Amenorrhea: Theories and Research. The observation that menstrual irregularities don't happen to all exercising women has led researchers to investigate many aspects of athletic training as well as individual characteristics of female athletes. Following are various theories on the causes of exercise-associated amenorrhea. Table 11.4 presents an overview.

• **Predisposition.** Some researchers suggest that severe menstrual dysfunction occurs only in predisposed women athletes.[63] Women who develop menstrual irregularities after starting a training regimen are more apt to have had a history of menstrual problems before they began training.[64] In fact, one study found that the best predictor of each woman's menstrual pattern during training was her pre-training menstrual status.[64] Several other studies of runners,[65] ballet dancers,[66] and ultramarathon runners[67] found similar results. The research seems to suggest that whatever caused the athlete's prior menstrual problems is very likely involved with the current problems.

• **Hypothalamic Immaturity.** Some researchers have studied the possibility that age is associated with menstrual dysfunction. Many young women engage in vigorous training programs before they have reached complete reproductive status, including full maturation of the nerves in the hypothalamic-pituitary-ovarian axis. This may make them more susceptible to menstrual irregularities. Menstrual problems are also more likely in athletes under 30 years of age. These findings have been questioned, however, because in order to reliably demonstrate an age association, it is necessary to study a population of athletes that varies widely in age. This condition has not been met by the research so far.[68]

• **Training Intensity.** While it may appear that an increase in exercise intensity also causes an increase in amenorrhea, research does not always support such an unqualified conclusion. At a first, fast glance, most studies, including ours, support the association of increased training intensity with a greater likelihood of menstrual dysfunction.

Although the preponderance of studies demonstrate this relationship—as intensity

TABLE 11.4

....

Possible Causes of Exercise-Associated Amenorrhea

Predisposition (previous history of menstrual dysfunction)

Hypothalamic Immaturity

Training Intensity

Low Percentage Body Fat

Caloric Drain

Nutritional Deficiency

Reproductive Protection

Emotional Factors

Psychological Stress

increases, so does amenorrhea—many of these studies may have design faults. For example, no standard definition of training regimen exists. Since training includes frequency of exercise, duration of practice sessions, intensity of practice (distance, time, speed), and level of performance, it is difficult to equate results from various studies using different definitions of training.

Illustrating this difficulty is a study where previously untrained women abruptly started a high-intensity training program. A significant proportion of the subjects suffered some type of menstrual dysfunction within the first two months.[69] While it may be tempting to uncritically accept the results, the data make it possible to say only that the abrupt start of such a regimen (as distinct from the intensity of the training) disrupts the reproductive system in some women.

It is worth noting a study presenting a different interpretation of the link between training and menstrual problems.[72] The authors decided to reanalyze some of their data from an earlier study. Their original research had supported the association between menstrual irregularities and intensity of training. They observed menstrual problems more often among high-mileage runners than among low-mileage runners. In their reanalysis, the investigators controlled for menstrual cycle irregularities that were present before individuals started their running programs. They found that when prior cycle irregularities were factored out, increased mileage was no longer a significant cause of menstrual problems.

Looking at the available data leads us to conclude that, before a link between exercise intensity and menstrual dysfunction can be established, more standardized research is necessary. Factors such as type of training and training intensity, prior gynecological problems, and definitions of gynecological problems based on hormonal levels need to be incorporated into research designs.

• **Low Percentage Body Fat.** Earlier in this chapter, we cited Frisch's theory that body fat is associated with the age of menarche. Frisch also found that higher fat percentages (22 percent) were necessary to maintain regular ovulatory cycles in mature women (women over 18).[71] Body fat composition has been suggested as a possible explanation for maintenance of menstrual function because fat tissue is a site for converting the hormone androgen to estrogen. An alteration in body fat composition may change the level of estrogen. Studies have shown that amenorrheic runners and dancers have body fat levels below 22 percent while those athletes with normal periods as well as sedentary women tend to be above that level.[72]

However, menstruation may depend on a combination of factors instead of the amount of body fat alone. A study of ballet dancers found that amenorrheic dancers whose injuries halted their exercising, had a resumption of their periods in the absence of any change in weight or change in percent body fat.[73] Another study of 24 athletes, half with normal and half with absent periods, showed no difference between the two groups in percentage of body fat.[74] And finally, recreational athletes in a recent study were reported to have normal menstrual cycles even though each had a lower relative fat content than Frisch's critical 22 percent.[75]

Given all these confusing results, there seems to be no conclusive evidence that percentage of body fat alone is associated with menstrual dysfunction.

• **Caloric Drain.** Fuel availability, rather than some critical body weight or percentage of body fat, may be a prerequisite for normal menstrual cycles. Some researchers claim that the cause of abnormal hormonal secretions is not exercise, per se, but rather, the energy deficit that results from an imbalance between calories consumed and calories burned.[76] These investigators hypothesize that the increase in caloric energy requirements because of strenuous exercise is not being met in some women. That is, these women are not adequately increasing their caloric intake, thereby predisposing them to energy drain.

The idea of constant energy drain was hypothesized by Warren in 1980, after she observed the high incidence of amenorrhea in ballet dancers who were constantly striving to be thin.[77] Since that time, some researchers have focused on energy requirements. A recent study of four moderately trained, normally menstruating women supports this hypothesis.[78] The investigators found that an abrupt increase in training led to disruption in LH (Luteinizing Hormone) secretion *only* when caloric intake was insufficient to meet the caloric drain. Low energy availability produced a significant loss of weight. The authors conjecture that there might be a specific threshold of energy availability below which occurs an inhibition of GnRH (Gonadotropin Releasing Hormone) release by the hypothalamus. More studies are necessary to explore the role of metabolism in causing exercise-induced menstrual dysfunction.

• **Nutritional Deficiency.** While no published evidence relates a single nutritional deficiency to menstrual dysfunction in exercising women, it is commonly acknowledged that long-distance runners are more likely to be vegetarians and eat less lean red meat than sedentary individuals.[79] Differences in diet between normal and abnormally menstruating runners have also been demonstrated.[80] One study found that although amenorrheic runners consumed more calories, their daily protein intake was significantly less than that of either normally menstruating runners or a non-running control group.[81] But the jury is still out: The causal link between dietary changes and menstrual abnormalities has not been clearly established.

• **Reproductive Protection.** One hypothesis views amenorrhea as a biologically protective mechanism that occurs in response to elevated stress levels. It is conjectured that the extra energy that strenuous exercise demands can be viewed as a threat to energy reserves that may be necessary for the life of the woman. Accordingly, to protect itself, the body directs energy away from the demands of menstruation (and possible reproduction) and toward the demands of the exercise. Thus, this temporary form of infertility (that is, no periods) can be viewed as a health-protecting response to a reproductive stress challenge.

• **Emotional Factors.** A group of researchers found that emotional disorders may be involved in menstrual cycle problems.[82] The investigators studied 13 amenorrheic runners, 11 of whom reported major emotional disorders in themselves or close relatives. Of particular note: 8 of the subjects also reported eating disorders (eating disorders are addressed more fully in Chapter 18, Beware of the Danger Zones). But whether emotional disturbance caused the amenorrhea or vice versa is unknown.

• **Psychological Stress.** Stress has been proposed as a possible cause of reproductive disruptions. Stress may affect neurotransmitters, such as dopamine, and circulating levels of the adrenal hormone cortisol, both of which are involved in reproductive system regulation.[83]

One researcher reported that of the first women cadets at the U.S. Military Academy—certainly a stressful environment—almost half were amenorrheic after their first six months of classes and endurance training.[84] However, these women were probably more physically active than they had been previously and may have lost weight since their civilian days.

If stress is defined by the level of cortisol, then there is a strong relationship between stress and menstrual dysfunction, according to several studies.[85] On the other hand, if only psychological tests are used as criteria, the association between stress and menstrual problems is much less certain. Of the several studies using runners as subjects, no important differences were found in scores on a number of psychological tests between sedentary women and either runners with or without their periods. The amenorrheic runners, however, subjectively reported significantly more stress than did runners with normal periods.[86]

Problems Associated with Amenorrhea. Because of the importance of estrogen in the maintenance of bone density,[87] athletes with low estrogen levels may be especially vulnerable to osteoporosis.[88] Of particular concern is the long-term effects of prolonged low estrogen and the possibility that if one waits for symptoms and signs of osteoporosis, it is conceivable that irreversible damage has already been done.

Catch-22. Exercise works to maintain healthy bones by increasing bone density.[89] However, not all kinds of exercise are equally beneficial to bone strength. For example, weight-bearing exercise is more helpful than non-weight-bearing exercise. Additionally, the beneficial effects of exercise on bone density seem to be specific to that part of the body receiving the greatest activity.[90] Runners and cyclists have denser bones in their legs and hips than in their arms or spines; tennis players tend to have denser bones in their arms and shoulders than in their legs.[91]

• **Here's the Catch.** The beneficial relationship may not exist for those athletes who develop amenorrhea; these women may have decreased bone density. As a result, those who suffer from amenorrhea and have low estrogen levels are possibly susceptible to an increased risk of skeletal injuries due to reduced bone density.[92] Stress fractures among athletes and dancers are more likely in those with low bone density, lower caloric intake, and current menstrual irregularities.[93] So women with intense exercise routines and low body weight who have stopped menstruating may actually have less bone density than those who are sedentary. The benefits of exercise have vanished.

One research group observed menstrual patterns and bone density in 97 athletes.[94] Those having regular cycles had the highest vertebral bone mineral density and those with a history of amenorrhea had the lowest. Two years after their original study, the authors retested nine previously amenorrheic runners.[95] Surprisingly, seven of those runners had spontaneously regained their periods and also had an increase in bone mineral density. Interestingly, those seven had decreased their training mileage by 10 percent and increased their body weight by approximately four pounds each. Left unanswered was what caused the recurrence of their periods and increased bone density: Was it decreased exercise intensity, increased body weight, a combination of the two, or some other unknown factor?

Contradictions. While almost all studies agree that amenorrhea is associated with low estrogen levels and low bone mineral density, one study presented some important contradictory findings. The authors examined the relationship between running intensity, sex hormone disturbances, and bone mass of females who were running at recreational and competitive levels.[96] Unlike other studies, theirs found no basic difference in bone mass between amenorrheic runners and those runners menstruating normally. The researchers also found no statistically significant association between training regimens (for example, amount of miles run per week) and bone density measurements. Based on their findings, they concluded that the potential positive skeletal side effects of long-distance running have been previously overestimated.

Furthermore, in contrast to most previous studies, which document a bone density increase with weight-bearing exercise, the researchers found that moderate levels of exercise had no positive effect on spinal bone density. They concluded that although running was related to sex hormone changes significant enough to affect menstrual regularity, bone metabolism was not affected in the large majority of female runners. Their bottom line recommendation is that research results obtained from highly selected groups of super elite athletes should not be extrapolated to the average female runner in general.

In Summary: Although this last cited study may presage things to come, the problem of bone loss is still of concern. Our recommendation is to seek a consultation with a physician if you are experiencing menstrual irregularity.

Treatment of Menstrual Dysfunction

First Things First.   Before proceeding with any treatment regimen, expect your physician to have done a:

1. Complete medical history (family history, medications, menstrual history, exercise patterns), as well as obtaining past and current dietary intake information. Your medical history will indicate any predisposing factors, such as genetics or lifestyle patterns, while your dietary history is important to determine if there are any unrecognized caloric, vitamin, or iron deficiencies.

TABLE 11.5

....

Blood Tests to Rule Out Pathologies

For:	Test:
Hypothyroidism	Thyroid Stimulating Hormone (TSH)
Hyperprolactinemia	Serum prolactin*
Hyperandrogenism	Dehydroepiandrosterone Sulfate (DHEAS)
	Testosterone
Hypoestrogenism	Serum estradiol
Hypothalamic / Pituitary Problems	Follicle Stimulating Hormone (FSH)
	Luteinizing Hormone (LH)
To rule out pregnancy	β-human chorionic gonadotropin(β-HCG)

....

* Radiographic assessment (skull x-ray) of the sella turcica may be called for if FSH and LH levels are very low despite normal serum prolactin levels.

2. Physical examination, including a pelvic examination.
3. Blood workup, to include tests to rule out pathological conditions such as pituitary tumors, thyroid dysfunction, polycystic ovary disease, and premature ovarian failure (see Table 11.5).
4. Bone Mineral Density Test (dual photon densitometry) to assess the current status of your skeletal bones.
5. Progestin Challenge Test to determine estrogenic stimulation of the endometrium.

Some additional screening tests, such as a complete blood count, measurement of electrolytes and liver enzymes, and urinalysis, may also be done. One prominent physician, Mona Shangold, who specializes in the area of sports medicine and menstrual dysfunction, finds that it has not proven cost-effective to do the latter tests and does not routinely perform them.[97]

What We Know

After reviewing your history, performing an examination, and evaluating laboratory tests, expect that your physician will most likely begin treatment appropriate to your diagnosis.

General Treatment Recommendations

Luteal Phase Disorder.   If you are diagnosed as having a luteal phase disorder, the current recommendation is to treat for this condition only if you desire to become pregnant. If so, then your physician will probably prescribe clomiphene citrate in varying dosages.

Anovulatory Oligomenorrhea.   Because women who are diagnosed as having irregular periods are at a higher risk of developing endometrial hyperplasia, the recommendation by many physicians is for treatment with progestin on a monthly basis. This can be accomplished through either oral contraceptive pills (which contain estrogen and progestin) or medroxyprogesterone acetate (which contains progestin only). The oral contraceptives may serve the secondary function of protection against pregnancy.

Exercise-Associated Amenorrhea.   The treatment options are varied because there can be several causes for exercise-associated amenorrhea. The logical first line of treatment would be to recommend decreased physical activity and/or increased caloric intake. However, a recent study indicated that sports medicine specialists are more likely to prescribe hormone therapy as the first line of treatment rather than activity or calorie recommendations.[98] While that may seem extreme, it reflects the difficulty of getting exercising patients to follow an optimum treatment program. Many athletes do not want to gain weight or back off from their activity. The study's authors recommend that all women be fully informed about treatment options and risks, whether they are willing to accept those treatments or not. We agree with that recommendation.

If your amenorrhea is caused by too little estrogen in your system, several possible treatments are currently available. Historically, many physicians treated patients with menstrual dysfunction conservatively, that is, with no treatment unless pregnancy was desired.[99] This approach has changed because of the concern, discussed previously, that menstrually dysfunctional athletes had decreased bone mineral content and increased frequency of stress fractures.[100]

Unfortunately, even when menses return because of intervention, some athletes who had irregular periods or amenorrhea continue to have a reduced bone mineral level when compared with the menstrually normal athletes.[101] Early intervention may be key. Physicians are now more inclined to intervene soon after diagnosing the problem by prescribing hormone therapy. In 1995, a study by researchers from Baylor College of Medicine reported significant increases in spine bone mass after four amenorrheic women took oral hormone therapy for six months. Especially noteworthy, and surprising, is the improvement in bone mass that occurred independently of weight change and caloric or calcium intake, lending additional support to the importance of estrogen.[102] Note that this last study had only four subjects and thus needs to be replicated with a larger sample.

If you are low in estrogen and do not desire pregnancy, the treatment recommendation may be hormone therapy with either:

- conjugated estrogens and medroxyprogesterone acetate pills,
- transdermal (skin patch) estradiol and medroxyprogesterone acetate pills, or
- oral contraceptives.

An advantage of using the first two methods is that dose levels are lower and more natural. A disadvantage is that they do not provide contraceptive protection. An advantage of using the third hormone therapy method, oral contraceptives, is that it also provides contraceptive protection. However, oral contraceptives may be a good option, regardless of whether you're sexually active. Disadvantages of oral contraceptives include the two most common side effects: breakthrough bleeding (which occurs spontaneously during the days that you take the pill), and lack of withdrawal bleeding, the bleeding that should occur at the end of each pill cycle.[103] Both side effects, however, can be controlled by changing dosage levels.

If you have any risk factors that would make you vulnerable to problems associated with hormonal therapy, then it should be avoided. You should discuss this with your physician. Risk factors include:

- a history of thromboembolic (blood clotting) disorders,
- vascular disease,
- known or suspected cancer of the breast or reproductive organs (or a family history of these cancers), and
- impaired liver function.

Note: Although researchers have demonstrated that exercise-associated amenorrhea is often reversible, there is no guarantee that it will be reversible in all cases.

Primary Amenorrhea. Delayed menarche may have several causes. Lack of breast development and the absence of a uterus could indicate a genetic cause. Women with undeveloped breasts but a normal uterus may have a congenital defect or hypogonadotropic problem; women with normal breasts and no uterus very likely have testicular feminization or a mullerian anatomy problem; and women with normal breasts and normal uterus may have either hypothyroidism or a hypothalamic-pituitary-ovarian axis disorder.[104]

If you have been diagnosed as having primary amenorrhea, then you should expect that treatment will begin as soon as a determination is made as to the cause of your problem. If you have a hypothalamic-pituitary-ovarian axis disorder, then the recommended

*The treatment options for
amenorrhea include:*

*1. Reduction of exercise
regimen—by as much
as 10 percent*

*2. Weight gain—by as
much as 5 percent*

*3. Correcting dietary
deficiencies—usually by
adding vitamins and
minerals, including calcium*

*4. Hormonal therapy—
usually estrogen
supplementation*

treatment is the same as for exercise-associated amenorrhea.

Dietary Treatment Recommendations. While exercise promotes bone formation and retards bone loss, inadequate calcium or estrogen levels may counteract this effect. Although estrogen may be more effective than dietary calcium in maintaining bone density, calcium supplements are often more acceptable.[105] For example, you may already take vitamin and mineral pills; calcium is cheap compared to estrogen therapy; and calcium seems less threatening, more natural.

In a recent one-year study, 61 women with menstrual dysfunction were assigned to four different treatment therapies.

- Group 1 had cyclic hormones plus calcium carbonate,
- Group 2 had cyclic hormones with a calcium placebo,
- Group 3 had a placebo hormone and active calcium, and
- Group 4 had a placebo for both hormone and calcium.

While initial spinal bone density tests did not differ among the groups, one year later, bone density had increased in group 1 and 2, did not change in group 3, and decreased in group 4.[106] The results point to the importance of estrogens in bone maintenance.

For amenorrheic women who lack estrogen and do not want to use hormone replacement therapy, increasing dietary calcium may improve calcium balance.[107] The amount recommended for hypoestrogenic women is 1,500 mg of calcium per day, compared to 1,000 mg for normally menstruating women and 1,200 mg for those over 50 years of age. Non-hormonal options are also available (see pages 352–353).

Note: If the initial diagnostic evaluation points to vitamin or iron deficiency or a caloric deficit, then nutritional counseling also makes sense.

The Athletes's (and Physician's) Dilemma. Many respondents in our survey indicated discomfort, stained clothes, heavy bleeding, and poor performance at competitions related to their periods. Some were relieved not to have their periods at the time of an athletic event. It seems likely, nevertheless, that if there were a choice between never menstruating or the inconvenience and problems associated with bleeding, few women would take the first choice. However, menstrual dysfunction presents problems and dilemmas not just for the athlete, but also for the physician.

If you have menstrual irregularities and are competing in activities placing a premium on thinness and calling for a high-intensity exercise regimen, you may be reluctant to eat more or exercise less. This can be a stumbling block to treatment. If you also have an aversion to taking hormones, then the resolution is especially complex.

Because significant amounts of bone loss may occur within the first three years of low estrogenism, some sports medicine physicians prescribe hormone replacement

What to Do

If you are significantly delayed in menstruating, try reducing your exercise pattern and eating a bit more. If this does not help, see your physician and consider hormonal treatment.

within the first year[108]—without trying non-hormonal treatment alternatives.

Perhaps the answer to the dilemma is improved communication between doctor and athlete.

We've Come a Long Way

In closing, although "we've come a long way," many questions still remain about our periods. The good news is that symptoms seem to be alleviated by regular exercise and that performance does not, in general, seem to be affected by the menstrual cycle. Although excessive weight loss and very heavy exercise routines may cause menstrual irregularities and possibly lead to osteoporosis, prompt attention can usually correct the situation.

ENDNOTES

1. Frisch, R. E. Fatness and fertility. *Scientific American*, 1988, 258(3), 88–95.

2. Frisch, R. E., & McArthur, J. W. Menstrual cycles: Fatness as a determinant of minimum weight for height necessary for their maintenance or onset. *Science*, 1974, 185, 949–951.

3. Frisch, R. E. Fatness and fertility. *Scientific American*, 1988, 258(3), 88–95.

4. Stager, J. M., Wigglesworth, J. K., & Hatler, L. K. Interpreting the relationship between age of menarche and prepubertal training. *Medicine and Science in Sports and Exercise,* 1990, 22(1), 54–58.

5. May, M. Battles over body fat. *Science*, 1993, 260, 1592–1593.

6. Malina, R. M. Menarche in athletes: A synthesis and hypothesis. *Annals of Human Biology*, 1983, 10, 1–24.

   Merzenich, H., Boeing H., & Wahrendorf, J. Dietary fat and sports activity as determinants for age at menarche. *American Journal of Epidemiology*, 1993, 138(4), 217–224.

7. Golub, S. Exercise and late menstruation. *Science News*, 1981, 120(16), 249.

8. Constantini, N. W., & Warren, M. P. Menstrual dysfunction in swimmers: A distinct entity. *Journal of Clinical Endocrinology and Metabolism*, 1995, 80(9), 2740–2744.

9. Frisch, R. E., Gotz-Welbergen, A. B., McArthur, J., et al. Delayed menarche and amenorrhea of college athletes in relation to onset of training. *Journal of the American Medical Association*, 1981, 246(14), 1559–1563.

10. Warren, M. P. The effects of exercise on pubertal progression and reproductive function in girls. *Journal of Clinical Endocrinology and Metabolism*, 1980, 51(5), 1150–1157.

11. Hamilton, L. H., Brooks-Gunn, J., Warren, M. P., et al. The role of selectivity in the pathogenesis of eating problems in ballet dancers. *Medicine and Science in Sports and Exercise,* 1988, 20(6), 560–565.

12. Malina, R. M. Menarche in athletes: A synthesis and hypothesis. *Annals of Human Biology*, 1983, 10, 1–24.

13. Stager, J. M., Wigglesworth, J. K., & Hatler, L. K. Interpreting the relationship between age of menarche and prepubertal training. *Medicine and Science in Sports and Exercise,* 1990, 22(1), 54–58.

14. Sanborn, C. F., Albrecht, B. H., & Wagner, W. V. Athletic amenorrhea: Lack of association with body fat. *Medicine and Science in Sports and Exercise*, 1987, 19(3), 207–212.

    Stager, J. M., Ritchie-Flanagan, B., &. Robertshaw, D. Reversibility of amenorrhea in athletes (Letter). *New England Journal of Medicine*, 1984, 310(1), 51–52.

    Wakat, D. K., Sweeney, K. A., & Rogol, A. D. Reproductive system function in women cross-country runners. *Medicine and Science in Sports and Exercise*, 1982, 14(4), 263–269.

15. Loucks, A. B. Effects of exercise training on the menstrual cycle: Existence and mechanisms. *Medicine and Science in Sports and Exercise*, 1990, 22(3), 275–280.

16. Vollman, R. F. *The Menstrual Cycle.* Philadelphia: Saunders, 1977.

17. Brozan, N. Menstruation: Survey finds it's still uneasy subject. *New York Times*, June 22, 1981, c8.

18. Puretz, S. L. Menses and exercise: Attitudes and actions. *Journal of Sports Medicine and Physical Fitness*, 1986, 26(2), 140–145.

19. Brody, J. PMS is a worldwide phenomenon. *New York Times*, November 11, 1992, c10.

20. President's Council on Physical Fitness and Sports. Physical activity during menstruation and pregnancy. *Physical Fitness Research Digest*, 1978, 8(3).

21. Nolan, J. Problems of menstruation. *Journal of Health, Physical Education and Recreation*, 1965, 36(8), 65.

22. Israel, R. G., Sutton, M., & O'Brien, R. F. Effects of aerobic training on primary dysmenorrhea symptomatology in college females. *Journal of American College Health*, 1985, 33, 241–244.

23. Prior, J. C., Vigna, Y. M., & Alojads, N. Conditioning exercise decreases premenstrual symptoms: A prospective controlled six months trial. *Fertility and Sterility*, 1987, 47, 402–408.

24. Gannon, L. The potential role of exercise in the alleviation of menstrual disorders and menopausal symptoms: A theoretical synthesis of recent research. *Women & Health*, 1988, 14(2), 105–127.

25. Shangold, M. M. Menstruation and menstrual disorders. In M. M. Shangold, & G. Mirkin (eds.). *Women and Exercise: Physiology and Sports Medicine*, 2nd ed. Philadelphia: F. A. Davis Company, 1994, 152–171.

26. Bale, P., & Davies, J. A. Effect of menstruation and contraceptive pill on the performance of physical education students. *British Journal of Sports Medicine*, 1983, 17(1), 46–50.

    Corcoran, T. The influence of four phases of the menstrual cycle on selected motor abilities of high school girl athletes and non-athletes. *Disser-*

tation Abstracts, 1969, 31(1), 198.

Puretz, S. Menses and exercise: Attitudes and actions. *The Journal of Sports Medicine and Physical Fitness*, 1986, 26(2), 140–145.

Rougier, G., & Linquette, Y. Menstruation and physical exercise. *Presse Medicale*, 1962, 70, 1921–1923.

Wearing, M. P., Yuhosz, M., Campbell, R., et al. The effect of the menstrual cycle on tests of physical fitness. *The Journal of Sports Medicine and Physical Fitness*, 1972, 12, 38–41.

27. Kral, J., & Markalous, K. The influence of menstruation on sport performance. In A. Mollwitz (ed.). *Proceedings of the 2nd International Congress on Sports Medicine*. Leipzig: Thiene-Stratton, 1939.

Ingman, O. Menstruation in Finnish top-class sportswomen. In A. Karvonen (ed.). *Sports Medicine*. Helsinki: Finnish Association of Sports Medicine, 1953, 96–99.

Erdelyi, G. J. Gynecological survey of female athletes. *Journal of Sports Medicine and Physical Fitness*, 1962, 2, 174–179.

28. Lebrun, C. M. Effect of the different phases of the menstrual cycle and oral contraceptives on athletic performance. *Sports Medicine*, 1993, 16(6), 400–430.

29. Erdelyi, G. J. Gynecological survey of female athletes. *Journal of Sports Medicine and Physical Fitness*, 1962, 2, 174–179.

30. Fomin, S., Pivovarova, V., & Vornova, V. Changes in the special working capacity and mental stability of well trained woman skiers at various phases of the biological cycle. *Sports Training and Medical Rehabilitation*, 1989, 1, 89–92.

31. Erdelyi, G. J. Gynecological survey of female athletes. *Journal of Sports Medicine and Physical Fitness*, 1962, 2, 174–179.

32. Quadagno, D., Facquin, L., Lim, G. N., et al. The menstrual cycle: Does it affect athletic performance? *The Physician and Sportsmedicine*, 1991, 19(3), 121–124.

33. Dibrizzo, R., Fort, I. L., & Brown, B. Dynamic strength and work variations during three stages of the menstrual cycle. *Journal of Orthopaedic and Sports Physical Therapy*, 1988, 10(4), 113–116.

34. Lebrun, C. M., McKenzie, D. C., Prior, J. C., et al. Effects of menstrual cycle phase on athletic performance. *Medicine and Science in Sports and Exercise*, 1995, 27(3), 437–444.

35. DeSouza, M. J., Maguire, M. I., Rubin, K. R. et al. Effects of menstrual phase and amenorrhea on exercise performance in runners. *Medicine and Science in Sports and Exercise*, 1990, 22(5), 575–580.

36. Lebrun, C. M. Effect of the different phases of the menstrual cycle and oral contraceptives on athletic performance. *Sports Medicine*, 1993, 16(6), 400–430.

37. Shangold, M. M., Gatz, M. L., & Thysen, B. Acute effects of exercise on plasma concentrations of prolactin and testosterone in recreational women runners. *Fertility and Sterility*, 1981, 35(6), 699–702.

38. Bonen, A., Ling, W., MacIntyre, K., et al. Effects of exercise on the serum concentrations of FSH, LH, progesterone and estradiol. *European Journal of Applied Physiology*, 1979, 42(1), 15–23.

39. Bonen, A., & Keizer, H. A. Pituitary, ovarian and adrenal hormone responses to marathon running. *International Journal Sports Medicine*, 1987, 8, 161–167.

40. Shangold, M. M., Gatz, M. L., & Thysen, B. Acute effects of exercise on plasma concentrations of prolactin and testosterone in recreational women runners. *Fertility and Sterility*, 1981, 35(6), 699–702.

41. Hartley, L. H., Mason, J. W., Hogan, R. P., et al. Multiple hormonal responses to prolonged exercise in relation to physical training. *Journal of Applied Physiology*, 1972, 33, 607–610.

42. Cumming, D. C., Vickovic, M. M., Wall, S. R., et al. The effect of acute exercise on pulsatile release of luteinizing hormone in women runners. *American Journal of Obstetrics and Gynecology*, 1985, 153, 482–485.

43. Shangold, M. M. Exercise and the adult female: Hormonal and endocrine effects. *Exercise and Sports Sciences Reviews*, 1984, 12, 53–79.

44. Arena, B., Maffulli, N., Maffulli, F., et al. Reproductive hormones and menstrual changes with exercise in female athletes. *Sports Medicine*, 1995, 19(4), 278–287.

Keizer, H. A., & Rogol, A. D. Physical exercise and menstrual cycle alterations: What are the mechanisms? *Sports Medicine*, 1990, 10(4), 218–235.

45. Arena, B., Maffulli, N., Maffulli, F., et al. Reproductive hormones and menstrual changes with exercise in female athletes. *Sports Medicine*, 1995, 19(4), 278–287.

46. Loucks, A. B., & Horvath, S. M. Athletic amenorrhea: A review. *Medicine and Science in Sports and Exercise*, 1985, 17(1), 56–72.

47. Constantini, N. W., & Warren, M. P. Menstrual dysfunction in swimmers: A distinct entity. *Journal of Clinical Endocrinology and Metabolism*, 1995, 80(9), 2740–2744.
48. Noakes, T. D., & Van Gend, M. Menstrual dysfunction in female athletes. A review for clinicians. *South African Medical Journal*, 1988, 73(6), 350–355.
49. Shangold, M. M. Menstruation and menstrual disorders. In M. M. Shangold, & G. Mirkin (eds.). *Women and Exercise: Physiology and Sports Medicine*, 2nd ed. Philadelphia: F. A. Davis Company, 1994, 152–171.
50. Daly, D. C., Walters, C. A., Soto-Alberes, C. E., et al. Endometrial biopsy during treatment of luteal phase defects is predictive of therapeutic outcome. *Fertility and Sterility*, 1983, 40, 305–310.
51. Noakes, T. D., & Van Gend, M. Menstrual dysfunction in female athletes. A review for clinicians. *South African Medical Journal*, 1988, 73(6), 350–355.
52. Shangold, M. M. Menstruation and menstrual disorders. In M. M. Shangold, & G. Mirkin (eds.). *Women and Exercise: Physiology and Sports Medicine*, 2nd ed. Philadelphia: F. A. Davis Company, 1994, 152–171.
53. Rebar, R. W. Exercise and the menstrual cycle. In *Current Topics in Obstetrics and Gynecology*, New York: Elsevier Science Publishing Company, 1991, 59–75.
54. Loucks, A. B. Effects of exercise training on the menstrual cycle: Existence and mechanisms. *Medicine and Science in Sports and Exercise*, 1990, 22(3), 275–280.
55. Shangold, M. M., Rebar, R. W., Weentz, A. C., et al. Evaluation and management of menstrual dysfunction in athletes. *Journal of the American Medical Association*, 1990, 263(12), 1665–1669.
56. Putukian, M. The female triad. *Sports Medicine*, 1994, 78(2), 345–356.
57. Shangold, M. M. Menstruation and menstrual disorders. In M. M. Shangold, & G. Mirkin (eds.). *Women and Exercise: Physiology and Sports Medicine*, 2nd ed. Philadelphia: F. A. Davis Company, 1994, 152–171.
58. Loucks, A. B., & Horvath, S. M. Athletic amenorrhea: A review. *Medicine and Science in Sports and Exercise*, 1985, 17(1), 56–72.
59. Feicht, C. B., Johnson, T. S., Martin, B. J., et al. Secondary amenorrhea in athletes. *Lancet*, 1978, 2, 1145–1146. Sanborn, D. F., Bartin, B. J., & Wagner, W. W. Is athletic amenorrhea specific to runners? *American Journal of Gynecology*, 1982, 143, 859–863.
60. Constantini, N. W., & Warren, M. P. Menstrual dysfunction in swimmers: A distinct entity. *Journal of Clinical Endocrinology and Metabolism*, 1995, 80(9), 2740–2744.
61. Liu, H., Liu, P., & Qin X., et al. Investigation of menstrual cycle in women weightlifters. Cited in Hollaway, J. B., & Baechle, T. R. Strength-training for female athletes: A review of selected aspects. *Sports Medicine*, 1990, 9(4), 216–228.
62. Loucks, A. B. Effects of exercise training on the menstrual cycle: Existence and mechanisms. *Medicine and Science in Sports and Exercise*, 1990, 22(3), 275–280.
63. Noakes, T. D., & Van Gend, M. Menstrual dysfunction in female athletes. A review for clinicians. *South African Medical Journal*, 1988, 73(6), 350–355.
64. Shangold, M. M., & Levine, H. S. The effect of marathon training upon menstrual function. *American Journal of Obstetrics and Gynecology*, 1982, 143, 862–869.
65. Schwartz, B., Cummings, D. R., Riordan, E., et al. Exercise-induced amenorrhea: A distinct entity? *American Journal of Obstetrics and Gynecology*, 1981, 141, 662–670.
66. Abrahams, S. F., Beaumont, P. J. V.., Fraser, I. S., et al. Body weight, exercise and menstrual status among ballet dancers in training. *British Journal of Obstetrics and Gynecology*, 1982, 89, 507–510.
67. Van Gend, M. A., & Noakes, J. D. Menstrual patterns in ultramarathon runners. *South African Medical Journal*, 1987, 72, 789–793.
68. Loucks, A. B., & Horvath, S. M. Athletic amenorrhea: A review. *Medicine and Science in Sports and Exercise*, 1985, 17(1), 56–72.
69. Bullen, B. A., Skrinar, G. S., Beitins, I. Z., et al. Induction of menstrual disorders by strenuous exercise in untrained women. *New England Journal of Medicine*, 1985, 312, 1349–1353.
70. Cokkinades, V. E., Macera, C. A., & Pate, R. R. Menstrual dysfunction among habitual runners. *Women & Health*, 1990, 16(2), 59–69.
71. Frisch, R. E. Fatness and fertility. *Scientific American*, 1988, 258(3), 88–95.
72. Frisch R. E., Wyshak, G., & Vincent, L. Delayed menarche and amenorrhea in ballet dancers. *New England Journal of Medicine*, 1980, 303, 17–19. Schwartz, B., Cumming, D. C., Riordan, E., et al. Exercise-associated

amenorrhea: A distinct entity? *American Journal of Obstetrics and Gynecology*, 1981, 141, 662–670.

73. Warren, M. P. The effects of exercise on pubertal progression and reproductive function in girls. *Journal of Clinical Endocrinology and Metabolism*, 1980, 51(5), 1150–1157.

74. Loucks, A. B., Horvath, S. M., & Freedson, P. S. Menstrual status and validation of body fat prediction in athletes. *Human Biology*, 1984, 56(2), 383–392.

75. Broocks, A., Pirke, K. M., Schweiger, U., et al. Cyclic ovarian function in recreational athletes. *Journal of Applied Physiology*, 1990, 68(5), 2083–2086.

76. Williams, N. I., Young, J. C., McArthur, J. W., et al. Strenuous exercise with caloric restriction: Effect on luteinizing hormone secretion. *Medicine and Science in Sports and Exercise*, 27(10), 1390–1398, 1995.

77. Warren, M. P. The effects of exercise on pubertal progression and reproductive function in girls. *Journal of Clinical Endocrinology and Metabolism*, 1980, 51(5), 1150–1157.

78. Williams, N. I., Young, J. C., McArthur, J. W., et al. Strenuous exercise with caloric restriction: Effect on luteinizing hormone secretion. *Medicine and Science in Sports and Exercise*, 27(10), 1390–1398, 1995.

79. Noakes, T. D., & Van Gend, M. Menstrual dysfunction in female athletes. A review for clinicians. *South African Medical Journal*, 1988, 73(6), 350–355.

80. Duester, P.A., Kyle, S. B., Moser, P. B., et al. Nutritional intakes and status of highly trained amenorrheic and eu-menorrheic women runners. *Fertility and Sterility*, 1986, 46, 636–643.

81. Schwartz, B., Cumming, D. C., Riordan, E., et al. Exercise-associated amenorrhea: A distinct entity? *American Journal of Obstetrics and Gynecology*, 1981, 141, 662–670.

82. Gadpaille, W. J., Sanborn, C. F., & Wagner, W. W. Jr. Athletic amenorrhea, major affective disorders, and eating disorders. *American Journal of Psychiatry*, 1987, 144(7), 939–942.

83. Rebar, R. W. Exercise and the menstrual cycle. In *Current Topics in Obstetrics and Gynecology*. New York: Elsevier Science Publishing Company, 1991, 59–75.

84. Anderson, J. L. Women's sports and fitness programs at the U.S. Military Academy. *Physician and Sportsmedicine*, 1979, 7, 72–78.

85. Rebar, R. W. Exercise and the menstrual cycle. In *Current Topics in Obstetrics and Gynecology*. New York: Elsevier Science Publishing Company, 1991, 59–75.

86. Schwartz, B., Cumming, D. C., Riordan, E., et al. Exercise-associated amenorrhea: A distinct entity? *American Journal of Obstetrics and Gynecology*, 1981, 141, 662–670.

87. Christiansen, C., & Lindsay, R. Estrogen, bone loss and preservation. *Osteoporosis International*, 1990, 1, 7–13.

88. Nattiv, A., Agostini, R., Drinkwater, B., et al. The female athlete triad: The inter-relatedness of disordered eating, amenorrhea, and osteoporosis. *Clinics in Sports Medicine*, 1994, 13(2), 405–418.

89. Lanyon, L. E. Functional strain in bone tissue as an objective, and controlling stimulus for adaptive bone modeling. *Journal of Biomechanics*, 1987, 20, 1083–1093.

90. Nattiv, A., Agostini, R., Drinkwater, B., et al. The female athlete triad: The inter-relatedness of disordered eating, amenorrhea, and osteoporosis. *Clinics in Sports Medicine*, 1994, 13(2), 405–418.

91. Smith, E. L., & Gilligan, C. Bone concerns. In M. M. Shangold, & G. Mirkin (eds.). *Women and Exercise: Physiology and Sports Medicine*, 2nd ed. Philadelphia: F. A. Davis Company, 1994, 89–101.

92. Lloyd, T., Triantafyllou, S. J., Baker, E. R., et al. Women athletes with menstrual irregularity have increased musculoskeletal injuries. *Medicine and Science in Sports and Exercise*, 1986, 18(4), 374–379.

93. Myburgh, K. H., Hutchins, J., Fataar, A. B., et al. Low bone density is an etiologic factor for stress fractures in athletes. *Annals of Internal Medicine*, 1990, 113, 754–759.
   Bennell, K. L., Malcolm, S. A., Thomas, S. A. Risk factors for stress fracture in female track-and-field athletes: A retrospective analysis. *Clinical Journal of Sports Medicine*, 1995, 5(4), 229–235.
   Warren, M. P., Brooks-Gunn, J., Hamilton, L. H., et al. Scoliosis and fractures in young ballet dancers. *New England Journal of Medicine*, 1986, 314(21), 1348–1353.

94. Drinkwater, B. L., Nilson, K., Ott, S., et al. Bone mineral density after resumption of menses in amenorrheic athletes. *Journal of the American Medical Association*, 1986, 256, 380–382.

95. Drinkwater, B. L., Bremner, B., & Chestnut III C. H. Menstrual history

as a determinant of current bone density in young athletes. *Journal of the American Medical Association*, 1990, 263, 545–548.

96. Hetland, M. L., Haarbo, J., Christiansen, C., et al. Running induces menstrual disturbances but bone mass is unaffected, except in amenorrheic women. *The American Journal of Medicine*, 1993, 95(1), 53–60.

97. Shangold, M. M. Menstruation and menstrual disorders. In M. M. Shangold, & G. Mirkin (eds.). *Women and Exercise: Physiology and Sports Medicine*, 2nd ed. Philadelphia: F. A. Davis Company, 1994, 152–171.

98. Haberland, C. A., Seddick, D., Marcus, R., et al. A physician survey of therapy for exercise-associated amenorrhea: A brief report. *Clinical Journal of Sports Medicine*, 1995 (4), 246–250.

99. Myburgh, K. H., Watkin, V. A., & Noakes, T. D. Are risk factors for menstrual dysfunction cumulative? *Physician and Sportsmedicine*, 1992, 20(4), 114–125.

100. Shangold, M. M. Hormone therapy and the female athlete triad. *Physician and Sportsmedicine*, 1996, 24(7), 76.

101. Micklesfield, L. K., Lambert, E. V., Fataar, A. B., et al. Bone mineral density in mature, premenopausal ultramarathon runners. *Medicine and Science in Sports and Exercise*, 1995, 27(5), 688–696.

102. Hergenroeder, A. C. Bone mineralization, hypothalamic amenorrhea, and sex steroid therapy in female adolescents and young adults. *Journal of Pediatrics*, 1995, 126(5 Part 1), 683–689.

103. Shangold, M. M. Menstruation and menstrual disorders. In M. M. Shangold, & G. Mirkin (eds.). *Women and Exercise: Physiology and Sports Medicine*, 2nd ed. Philadelphia: F. A. Davis Company, 1994, 152–171.

104. Roberts, W. O. Primary amenorrhea and persistent stress fracture: A practical clinical approach. *The Physician and Sportsmedicine*, 1995, 23(9), 33–43.

105. Riis, B., Thomsen, K., & Christiansen, C. Does calcium supplementation prevent post- menopausal bone loss? A double-blind, controlled clinical study. *New England Journal of Medicine*, 1987, 316, 173.

Smith, E. L., & Gilligan, C. Bone concerns. In M. M. Shangold, & G. Mirkin (eds.). *Women and Exercise: Physiology and Sports Medicine*, 2nd ed. Philadelphia: F. A. Davis Company, 1994, 89–101.

106. Prior, J. C., Vigna, Y. M., Barr, S. I., et al. Cyclic medroxyprogesterone treatment increases bone density: A controlled trial in active women with menstrual cycle disturbances. *American Journal of Medicine*, 1994, 96(6), 521–530.

107. Recker, R. R., Saville, P. D., & Heaney, R. R. Effect of estrogen and calcium carbonate on bone loss in postmenopausal women. *Annals of Internal Medicine*, 1977, 87(6), 649–655.

108. Shangold, M. M. Menstruation and menstrual disorders. In M. M. Shangold, & G. Mirkin (eds.). *Women and Exercise: Physiology and Sports Medicine*, 2nd ed. Philadelphia: F. A. Davis Company, 1994, 152–171.

12 Fitness for Two: Pregnancy & Exercise

DONNA I. MELTZER, M.D.

My mother told me that when she was pregnant with me she was warned against exerting herself and especially against stretching. But I just became pregnant and want to keep working out. My doctor said it's up to me but I should be careful. I don't know what that means. —Sara, age 30

As more and more women of childbearing age participate in recreational and competitive athletic events, a growing need exists to consider questions raised about pregnancy and exercise. As in Sara's case, your physician or health care provider may be unsure how to respond to such questions because few guidelines can be found in the medical literature. Recommendations may be based on myths, misperceptions, and seeming common sense, but not current research.

How will pregnancy affect athletic performance? More importantly, how will exercise affect you, the pregnant woman, and your passenger, the developing baby? Can exercise and pregnancy co-exist safely? Are you risking a premature delivery if you exert yourself? Will the course of labor be altered by physical exercise? What about resuming exercise after delivery? Can you breastfeed your newborn and continue to exercise? This chapter will address these questions and discuss some of the risks and benefits of exercise during pregnancy. Suggestions for a healthy exercise program during pregnancy and the postpartum period will also be presented.

ONE BODY — TWO LIVES

The body undergoes a multitude of changes and adaptations during pregnancy. Some of these alterations are subtle and may go undetected by the pregnant woman. Other body changes can be a cause of concern and discomfort. Just as all pregnancies are different, so are some of the changes and adaptations. Physiological and anatomical alterations occur during all three trimesters. Although nearly all organ systems in the body can be affected by pregnancy, we will focus primarily on changes involving the cardiovascular, respiratory, and musculoskeletal systems.

The Maternal Heart

In the first trimester of pregnancy, maternal blood volume and oxygen consumption increase. Additional demands for oxygen are made by both the developing infant and the maternal organs, including the uterus, heart, respiratory muscles, and kidneys. As a result, oxygen consumption rises gradually throughout the pregnancy until it is approximately 36 percent greater in the last trimester than it was before you became pregnant.[1] Your heart rate also gradually increases by 15 to 20 beats per minute above pre-pregnancy resting values. The increases in stroke volume and heart rate subsequently lead to a 30 to 50 percent increase in cardiac output.[2]

Early in pregnancy, some women report they feel stronger and better able to exercise than ever before. This is probably due to the increased cardiac output.[3] Later in pregnancy, as fetal needs increase, this maximization in cardiac output is put to good use in supplying the placenta with additional blood flow that is rich in oxygen and nutrients.

A Fresh Look at Heart Rate.   Heart rate is influenced by both exercise and pregnancy. You must evaluate it very carefully. If you are physically fit, you probably have a lower resting heart rate compared to a sedentary person. It is therefore important to consider pre-pregnancy fitness levels before making any estimate of your target maximum heart rate.[4] (See Chapter 4, Focus on Fitness.) The formula you may have used to estimate your target heart rate before pregnancy [(220 − age) × 80%] may not be applicable or safe to employ during pregnancy. Since this needs to be individualized, you should discuss your target heart rate range with your health care provider. We recommend that this topic be reviewed at different times during your pregnancy because your body undergoes so many adaptations during the 40-week gestational period. Another simpler and perhaps more practical approach to monitoring exertional stress is to tone down your workout so you can exercise and simultaneously carry on a conversation without undue breathlessness.

Changes in Blood Pressure

As a rule, blood pressure drops during pregnancy, reaching its lowest value in the second trimester. Blood pressure tends to normalize back to the baseline prepregnancy level as the pregnancy nears term. Blood pressure often varies with changes in body position in both men and women, pregnant or not. However, when you are pregnant and lie on your back, the enlarged uterus can compress the inferior vena cava, the large vein that carries blood back to the heart. This results in a decrease in cardiac output and a subsequent drop in blood pressure.[5] It is therefore not uncommon for a pregnant woman near term to feel lightheaded when lying flat on her back. This phenomena has prompted the recommendation that women avoid exercising in the supine position after the first trimester of pregnancy.

Catching Your Breath

As gestational age advances, the enlarging uterus pushes upward and raises the diaphragm, which often makes pregnant women feel short of breath. Also, while pregnant, you are carrying around a fair amount of added weight. Remember how winded you felt the last time you lugged a heavy bag of groceries up a flight of stairs and you weren't even pregnant? Imagine doing this all day long. Since each breath you take supplies the developing baby with oxygen, it is important for you not to overexert yourself to the point of gasping for air. Shortness of breath could be serious and may be a warning sign to ease up on your exercise regime.

Weight Gain

During pregnancy, approximately 300 extra calories are required daily. Very active women, whether pregnant or not, obviously need more calories than sedentary women. If you are

---

TABLE 12.1

Recommended Weight Gain in Pregnancy

Prepregnant	Weight Gain Total (lb)	Rate (lb/month) (2nd, 3rd trimesters)
Underweight	28–40	5
Normal weight	25–35	4
Overweight	15–25	2.6
Obese	15	2

Adapted from American College of Obstetricians and Gynecologists. Nutrition during pregnancy. *ACOG Bulletin*, April 1993 (179), 1–7.

---

near your ideal body weight, you can expect to gain between 22 and 27 pounds by term.[6] The weight gain recommended by ACOG is between 25 and 35 pounds (see Table 12.1), but many fit and athletic women gain less than that without any ill effects on the baby or the pregnancy. Most maternal weight gain occurs in the latter half of pregnancy. In fact, near term, you may find yourself gaining one or more pounds per week.

The specifics of diet and appropriate weight gain in pregnancy are beyond the scope of this book. As proper nutrition is so important to your health and that of your developing baby, it is a good topic to discuss individually with your health care provider. Table 12-1, outlining recommended weight gain in pregnancy, is included here as a reminder to prompt you to raise this discussion on your next prenatal visit.

Hormonal Changes

Shortly after conception, lots of different hormones kick in and do their thing to support a pregnancy. Most of the organs in your body are affected in some way by these hormonal changes. For example, elevated levels of certain hormones during pregnancy are thought to produce joint and ligament laxity,[6] thereby changing the way the body responds to exercise.

The Pelvic Connection

The hip bones form most of the bony pelvis. They are joined in the front at an area referred to as the **pubic symphysis** and, behind, are united by the lower part of the spine, or sacrum. The **sacroiliac joint** is the connection between the hips and the sacrum. Widening and increased mobility of the pubic symphysis in the front and the sacroiliac joints of the back may occur by the late first trimester. Occasionally, there is also a partial or complete separation of the pubic symphysis. When either happens, a significant amount of lower back or pelvic pain can occur as these pain-sensitive structures are stretched. This pain is usually worsened with simple activities of daily living, such as walking and bending.

While research is limited, it has been theorized that this hormonally mediated increased joint mobility and relaxation may predispose pregnant women to sports-related injuries like sprains and strains. Restriction of activity and use of a pelvic girdle or binder may help to remedy some of this pelvic joint discomfort.

Maintaining New Balance

The changes in your muscles and bones that occur during pregnancy have some important implications, even if you decide not to continue your exercise program. As the fetus grows and the uterus enlarges, curvature of the lower spine (lumbar lordosis) increases. These alterations, along with breast enlargement, can adversely affect balance because they change your center of gravity. This is especially true as the pregnancy advances and your belly protrudes even more. Consequently, you may want to avoid physical fitness activities that involve sudden changes in balance and body position. For example, taking some of the step out of step aerobics helps to lessen the chance that your equilibrium will be upset, thus reducing the risk of tripping or falling.

Oh, My Aching Back

As your pregnancy advances and your abdominal girth increases, you may tend to lean forward. This new posture often stresses the spinal muscles and ligaments, resulting in lower back discomfort. In fact, low back pain is one of the most common physical complaints voiced during pregnancy.

Low back pain usually begins in the first trimester and has a tendency to worsen as the pregnancy nears term. Unfortunately, back soreness does not always spontaneously resolve with the delivery of the newborn—in fact, it may linger for up to six months. Women with pre-existing back pain and those who have been pregnant before may be more predisposed to developing this discomfort. Older women may be at higher risk of developing increased back pain during pregnancy.[7] This is especially relevant as many of today's baby boomers have delayed their childbearing and are now giving birth at older ages.

Back Pain and Weight Gain.   No correlation between back pain and maternal weight gain has been reported. There is also no relationship demonstrated between the pregnant woman's weight or the weight of the newborn and lower back discomfort. In other words, moms who gain less than 25 pounds during a pregnancy may have as much discomfort as those who put on triple that weight. Similarly, a mom whose newborn has a birth weight of five pounds may complain of as much low back pain as another mom delivering a nine-pound bundle of joy. Although these findings do not explain why back pain is so prevalent during pregnancy, it may be reassuring for lean and overweight moms-to-be alike to learn that they do not suffer alone.

Help for Your Back.   Lower back pain may be remedied by performing abdominal strengthening exercises, wearing a corset, sleeping on a firm mattress, and by restricting activities that seem to make the pain more intense.

During the day, try keeping the pelvis in a neutral position (not tipped forward) in order to prevent the back muscles from being strained. Pelvic tilt, or leaning forward, can be minimized by strengthening the abdominal muscles and hip extensors (hamstrings), along with relaxation or stretching of the erector spinae (iliopsoas) and hip flexors (erector femoris muscles).[8] This can be accomplished by standing straight and keeping your back against the wall while slowly bending the knees. (See Diagram 12.1.) Alternatively,

What to Do

- *Maintain good posture.*
- *Avoid excessive pelvic tilt.*
- *Wear low-heeled shoes.*

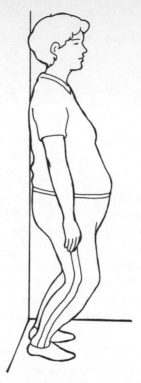

Diagram 12.1
Maintaining Good Posture

Strengthening and stretching the muscles that support your back and legs will help you maintain better posture. Stand with your back to a wall, keeping your legs straight. Distribute your weight evenly so it is not just on your heels. Slowly bend your knees while keeping your shoulders, back, and buttocks against the wall. Hold this position for a count of 10. Repeat 10 times.

the hip flexors can be stretched by kneeling with one foot flat on the floor while leaning forward. Hold these positions for a count of ten seconds, several times a day throughout your pregnancy. These stretches are easy to perform and should not be painful. If you experience any discomfort, seek the advice of your physician before proceeding with any more of these strengthening exercises.

Pay close attention to your posture and body mechanics throughout the day. Practice good posture by remembering to keep your ear, shoulder, and hip in a straight line while standing and sitting. When it comes to lifting, squat and bend the knees, not the waist. Keep your feet spread apart and hold the item you are lifting close to your body. Also, try to avoid sudden twisting motions, which may strain your back.

In order to lessen the stress on your lower back, wear low-heeled shoes. Wearing shoes with flat or low heels will help to normalize your center of gravity and minimize your risk of losing your balance. Avoid prolonged standing or sitting; change positions frequently.

Another suggestion is to always sit with your knees higher than your hips. This position will help lessen the curvature and stress on your lower back. You may also try placing a pillow in the small of the back to support the natural curve of the spine while sitting.

NIGHTTIME SUGGESTIONS

As your pregnancy advances, you will probably be told over and over again by your health care specialist to try to sleep on your side. (The left-sided position helps to promote good circulation to the placenta by making sure the weight of the fetus does not compress the blood vessels returning blood to your heart.) Some women have found that sleeping on their side with a pillow between the legs can help to relieve back pain. Others have alleviated pregnancy-related night pain by placing a small, soft pillow under the abdomen. If you are still plagued by pelvic or low back pain, your physician may suggest that you try wearing a lightweight, stretchy uterine support garment to bed.

A movement as simple as getting out of bed is often taken for granted. It shouldn't be, especially when you are in the later stages of pregnancy. When you get out of bed, be sure to roll to one side and swing your legs over the side. Sit up and use your arms to push yourself off the bed. Hopefully, some of our recommendations will help you to alleviate or prevent backache during and after pregnancy.

IS EXERCISE DANGEROUS TO MY UNBORN CHILD?

I had already had two first-trimester miscarriages when I became pregnant again. Naturally I was concerned that I might not carry this baby to term. I didn't know whether it was my advancing age or some other factor that contributed to this problem. Since I normally led a very active life, including swimming and jogging, I wondered if I should stop exercising this time. —Helen, age 35

Given the number of changes and discomforts occurring to the mother during pregnancy, one may wonder what risks exercise might pose to the unborn child. Specifically, what are the risks of early miscarriage, preterm labor, fetal distress, and changes in fetal growth and birth weight?

Researchers have found it difficult to answer a lot of these questions because so many factors need to be evaluated. Women would have to be entered into a study protocol before they became pregnant in order to accurately assess the effects of exercise on early pregnancy and miscarriage rates. Finding a control group to study is difficult because many pregnancies end in miscarriage even before a woman has been diagnosed as being pregnant. For example, an irregular period or spotting may simply have been a very early unrecognized pregnancy that became nonviable. In addition, women would have to be entered into a standard exercise regimen so that all the different physiological responses to that program could be measured.

Limited scientific consensus exists as to whether there are serious risks associated with exercising at the time of conception or several weeks thereafter. However, current

What We Know

Moderate exercise in healthy pregnant women is probably safe for both mom and baby.

research studies are beginning to reinforce the safety of recreational exercise in healthy females. In one study, pregnant women who ran or performed aerobic exercise were compared to a group who did not exercise. No difference in the incidence of congenital or placental abnormalities was reported in this study. The incidence of spontaneous miscarriages was 15 percent in the exercisers, compared to 17 percent in the matched control group, which is not a statistically significant difference.[9]

Will I Go to Term If I Exercise?

A full-term pregnancy is anywhere between 37 and 42 weeks of gestation, with 40 weeks considered the average and used as the "due date." At one time, it was reported that exercise during pregnancy was associated with prematurity (birth before 37 weeks). Subsequent studies, however, have not supported this claim.

James F. Clapp III, M.D., who has extensively researched the interactions of exercise and pregnancy, observed that physically active pregnant women delivered their babies at term but, on the average, about five days earlier than non-exercisers.[10] Dr. Clapp also reported that 72 percent of pregnant exercisers delivered on or before their due date, compared to 50 percent of the control subjects. Fortunately, there was not an association between continued exercise and premature labor. Patients and their health care providers looked upon this earlier labor as beneficial.[11]

Fetal Health

When a pregnant women exercises, there are potential risks to the baby. Inadequate oxygen supply, elevated body temperature, and adverse heart rate changes in the fetus are some possible concerns. However, when a woman is physically fit, physiological adaptations seem to prevent these conditions from developing. For example, when physically fit expectant mothers exercise, blood flow may not be excessively diverted from the placenta to feed other maternal organs.[12] Let's examine how some of our fears about pregnancy and physical activity developed.

Early research on exercise during pregnancy was conducted on animal models. For example, studies on pregnant sheep who were exercised on a treadmill to near exhaustion prompted some concerns about low blood oxygen levels.[13] Since the fetus relies on maternal circulation for its oxygen and nutrients, maternal blood flow is of paramount importance. The data from some of these studies should be interpreted with caution since we now know that not all animal-based research is applicable to humans. It should also be noted that follow-up animal studies have not confirmed these earlier findings about uterine blood flow.

Watch Your Temperature!   When you exercise, heat is produced by skeletal muscles. Therefore, increases in body temperature are directly related to the intensity and duration of your exercise routine. Body temperature can also be influenced by environmental conditions and your fluid level. Remember how uncomfortable you might have felt on a hot, humid day when you failed to drink plenty of fluids before and during a long, hard workout! We also know that trained athletes are better adapted to dispose of heat compared to unconditioned individuals.

The effects of maternal temperature elevation become an important issue when discussing exercise during pregnancy since the fetus is totally dependent on the mother's ability to dispose of excess heat. As noted earlier, the expectant mother's blood flow increases, which appears to help transfer some heat away from the fetus.[14] This is probably a built-in protective mechanism.

Paying attention to your body temperature is crucial. Some studies on animals have suggested an association between increased maternal temperatures and fetal malformations. Although many of the animal studies have been retrospective and otherwise criticized, they still raise concerns. So, should a pregnant woman avoid all exercise that may raise her body temperature? Probably not, although avoiding extreme body temperature elevations makes sense. Perhaps a good piece of advice, whether you're pregnant or not, is to listen to your body cues. If you feel you are overdoing it, slow down or take a breather. As has been emphasized before, you should discuss your exercise activities with your health care provider.

WARNING SIGNS TO STOP EXERCISING

- Feeling dizzy or lightheaded
- Vaginal bleeding or spotting
- Leakage of fluid from the vagina
- Regular uterine contractions
- Heart palpitations
- Chest pain
- Feeling breathless

Fetal Heart Rate.   One fetal response that has been carefully analyzed is heart rate. Physicians often use a hand-held doppler to measure fetal heart rates during routine office visits. Your unborn baby should normally have a heart rate between 120 to 160 beats per minute. Just as your heart rate may increase with physical activity or stress, so may that of your baby.

Fetal movements are often associated with a transient increase in heart rate, which normally is not alarming. On the other hand, **fetal bradycardia** (baby's heart rate less than 120 beats per minute) may indicate some problem or stress, such as oxygen deprivation. This is in contrast to adults, in whom a low heart rate is often a sign of athleticism and correlates well with conditioning.

When a pregnant woman exercises, her baby's heart rate may increase 10 to 30 beats per minute.[15] While maternal exercise may result in increased fetal movements, sustained exercise-induced **fetal tachycardia** (baby's heart rate greater than 160 beats per minute) and fetal bradycardia have not been reported by researchers.[16]

In another study comparing cyclists and swimmers, Dr. William Watson and colleagues demonstrated a transient fetal bradycardia in 15 percent of pregnant women performing vigorous exercise. Curiously, this drop in fetal heart rate was noticed more often with cyclists than swimmers.[17] The importance and long-term significance of these temporary changes is currently not clear. Perhaps the fundamental concept associated with these heart rate changes is the term "temporary." That is, when you exert yourself, your baby acknowledges the exercise and responds with a heart rate change that normalizes when the workout is terminated.

IS EXERCISE A HEALTH HAZARD FOR BOTH OF YOU?

Recent studies indicate that both mother and fetus tolerate exercise better than previously thought. It is also important to realize that the response of both the mother and her

---

TABLE 12.2

....

Excercise Recommendations During Pregnancy

- Make sure you have a comprehensive prenatal evaluation
- Monitor your heart rate so that it is less than or equal to 70 percent of maximum
- Take frequent rest periods
- Make sure that your heart rate and respiratory rate return to resting values within 15 minutes after stopping exercise
- Sweating is okay, but be sure to maintain a normal body temperature

....

Adapted from: Jarski, R. W., & Trippett, D. L. The risks and benefits of exercise during pregnancy. *The Journal of Family Practice*, 1990, 30 (2), 185–89.

---

fetus to exercise will depend on the stage of pregnancy, factors complicating the pregnancy, and the mother's level of fitness prior to pregnancy. One thing is for sure—there are various forms of exercise, and all exercise regimens need to be individualized. The woman training for the Olympics is quite different from the individual who is challenged by climbing a flight of stairs. This reinforces the importance of discussing your exercise routine with your physician. Additionally, following the guidelines below should help promote a safer pregnancy.

BIRTH WEIGHT

My first baby weighed over eight pounds at birth. During my second pregnancy, I began an exercise program and gave birth to a full-term baby girl who weighed just five pounds, two ounces. My newborn was healthy, but I have always wondered whether my workouts contributed to this low birth weight. —Michelle, age 38

Several studies have examined the relationship between women who exercise during pregnancy and their baby's birth weight. Again, the data have been difficult to interpret because women engage in various forms and intensities of exercise training. Also, some women may modify their exercise regimens and workouts during the different stages of pregnancy. One physician has reported that well-conditioned athletes who continued aerobic exercise at or above minimum training levels gave birth to newborns who had a lower fat mass—that is, they were lean like their mothers! It's interesting that the lower birth weights in the exercisers were restricted to less body fat and not other bodily differences like length and head circumferences.[18] In other words, if you exercise near your training level (of course, this will be different for everyone), your newborn may just have a lower percentage of baby fat.

EXERCISE AND LABOR

What is the relationship between physical fitness and the course of labor? Do aerobic instructors and Olympic athletes have faster and easier childbirths than couch potatoes? What about the well-conditioned athlete who decides to decrease or stop exercising during pregnancy? Let's see if we can answer some of these questions.

In 1990, Dr. James Clapp III studied two groups of pregnant athletes, two-thirds of whom continued to exercise regularly, and one-third of whom decided to stop their aerobic training before the end of the first trimester. In addition to the birth weight differences noted earlier, the researchers found that the exercisers had shorter active labor and less evidence of fetal stress. The group who continued to exercise also experienced fewer obstetrical interventions: a lower number of caesarean sections, fewer deliveries requiring the use of forceps, less use of epidural anesthesia, and a decreased number of episiotomies.[19]

An additional benefit to exercising during pregnancy is supported by research that demonstrates increased blood levels of β-endorphin and decreased pain perception during labor in a group of pregnant aerobic exercisers.[20] Although we cannot be completely certain, it appears likely that a well-conditioned body is an asset during pregnancy as well as during childbirth.

GUIDELINES FOR THE PREGNANT ATHLETE

Overall, the benefits and risks of exercise need to be evaluated in terms of both the mother and the fetus. One view of exercise during pregnancy is provided by the guidelines originally published by the American College of Obstetricians and Gynecologists [ACOG] Technical Bulletin in 1985 and revised in 1994.[21] The 1985 guidelines are invaluable because they were a beginning and served as a foundation for many of the exercise programs designed specifically with the pregnant woman in mind. Finally, doctors who prescribed exercise during pregnancy could do so with some backing from the medical literature.

The 1994 ACOG exercise update emphasizes that no human studies show that pregnant women should limit exercise intensity because of potential adverse effects. Instead, the bulletin advocates that healthy pregnant women should continue to exercise during pregnancy. The document recommends that women maintain adequate nutritional and fluid intake, wear appropriate clothing, avoid abdominal trauma, and modify the intensity of a workout according to maternal symptoms.

Activity Considerations

With the exception of starting a walking or yoga routine, pregnancy is not always the time to try out a more strenuous exercise program. On the other hand, pregnancy is also not a time to allow yourself to get out of shape. If you are already exercising and then become pregnant, perhaps the following guidelines will help you stay fit and have a healthy pregnancy and baby.

Walking: Walking is one of the best exercises for normal pregnant women, even for those who lived a sedentary lifestyle prior to pregnancy. As with all exercise programs, be sure to wear proper clothing and footwear and keep yourself well-hydrated. (Carry a water bottle.) Your clothing and shoes should be comfortable and keep you from getting overheated or from being too cold.

Jogging/Running: Some authorities advise women who did not engage in jogging or running prior to pregnancy not to take it up during pregnancy. Others feel it is safe,

What We Know

• *Water workouts are ideal for many pregnant women.*

• *Low-impact activities may be safer than high-impact aerobics.*

What to Do

• *Do not lie flat on your back in the last two trimesters.*

• *Avoid sudden and rapid changes of direction while exercising.*

provided you begin slowly. As with walking, pay close attention to your body temperature and fluid intake. The running surface should be smooth and free of obstacles. Mileage and speed need to be individualized. A competitive marathoner will have a different regimen than the recreational jogger and for both it may need to be modified in the latter half of pregnancy.

Bicycling: Recommendations concerning cycling need to be tailored to the individual and to the stage of the pregnancy. With later stages of pregnancy, balance is affected and you could be at an increased risk of falling. Some pregnant women find a stationary bicycle an acceptable and safer alternative. Switching to a bicycle that has fat tires should also be considered. A larger and well-cushioned bike seat and upright handlebars may make cycling more comfortable.

Swimming: Swimming is considered by many to be an ideal aerobic activity provided the water temperature is neither too hot nor too cold. Water's natural buoyancy helps to reduce musculoskeletal stresses, while its temperature-regulating property transfers excess heat away from the body. One study has even shown that immersion in a water bath may help to mobilize fluid and decrease swelling more rapidly than bed rest.[22]

Pay attention to your footwear if you are likely to walk on a slippery, wet pool deck. If you normally dive into the water, you should consider modifying this activity, because a high-velocity impact could traumatize the placenta. This is especially important with high diving boards and during the latter half of pregnancy.

Yoga: This is a nonaerobic exercise that may enhance flexibility and has been known to promote relaxation. It is also an activity that you can safely begin during pregnancy.

Aerobics: As a rule, sudden jerking and jarring movements should be avoided during pregnancy, especially in the later stages, because of possible damage to the placenta. A low-impact (as opposed to high-impact) aerobic routine is usually better tolerated. Proper clothing and footwear may help reduce injuries. Try to avoid exercising on hard surfaces. Care should be taken with deep bends and stretches in order to avoid upsetting your balance and increasing the risk of falling or adding too much stress to your joints and ligaments.

Weight Lifting: Weight lifting may help to maintain your strength during pregnancy, but you should be careful when lifting heavy weights, especially ones that require straining and squatting. The supine (on your back) position should probably be avoided in the later stages of pregnancy because it may reduce blood supply back to the heart. Pay special attention to your breathing. You should exhale while lifting a weight—do not hold your breath. (Holding your breath while bearing down is called a **Valsalva maneuver**, and should be avoided as it could cause you to faint.)

It has been suggested that low weight, high repetition exercises are preferable to

What to Do

- *Avoid jarring movements.*
- *Refrain from activities that have an inherent risk of falling.*

heavy weight exercises.[23] Extra care must be taken to eliminate any risk of dropping weights on the pregnant abdomen. You should also probably seek the approval of your health care provider if you plan to lift weights throughout your pregnancy.

Racket Sports: Racket sports are generally considered safe during pregnancy; however, your intensity of play may need to be modified. Be careful to avoid sudden movements and rapid changes in direction as this may harm the placenta. Remember to drink plenty of water while playing.

Ballet/Dance: Musculoskeletal injuries, especially of the ankle and knee, may be more prevalent in women who dance while pregnant. You may wish to modify movements to lessen any risk of losing your balance while dancing.

Contact Sports: The major risk associated with contact sports such as soccer is the chance that a collision may occur, simply because of the unpredictability of an opponent's movements. Since contact sports also carry an inherent risk of abdominal trauma and musculoskeletal injury (such as sprains and strains), you may want to refrain from these activities during your pregnancy.

Skiing: Both downhill and cross-country skiing carry the risk of falling, although the former is inherently more dangerous due to speed and terrain factors. Familiarity with snow conditions and the topography along with a conservative skiing style may all help to lessen the peril. The risk of abdominal trauma associated with falling needs to be taken into consideration if you decide to ski while pregnant. One authority has noted fewer fractures among pregnant skiers because they seem to adapt toward a less aggressive style.[23]

Gymnastics: The concern here is again with the risk of falling and subsequent abdominal trauma or musculoskeletal injury. As noted earlier, sudden jerking movements should be avoided, especially in the later stages of pregnancy.

Horseback Riding: This is an activity that should either be modified or avoided due to the jarring movements that may occur while riding on uneven terrain. Horseback riding also carries a risk of falling because of the animal's unpredictable behavior.

Waterskiing and Jetskiing: Case reports describing "vaginal douches" and injuries and "rectal enemas" after high speed water sport accidents have prompted some concern with these activities.[24] If pregnant jetskiers or waterskiers fall at high speed on the surface of the water, there may be a risk of miscarriage. Wearing a wetsuit or other protective clothing could help to prevent injury, whether you are pregnant or not. Respect for the elements is also important—take care to avoid sunburn, windburn, and exposure to extremes in water and air temperature.

Scuba Diving/Snorkeling: Few studies have considered women who continued to scuba or deep sea dive while pregnant. No scientific consensus exists about an increased

What to Do

Pregnancy and
Exercise Limitations

• *Avoid high-impact sports*

• *Avoid high-acceleration sports*

• *Avoid high-load sports*

• *Avoid high-intensity workouts*

• *Avoid exercise that requires balance or sudden twisting movements*

• *Avoid exercising flat on your back*

• *Avoid exercising to lose weight, but rather to control weight gain*

risk of **decompression sickness** if you continue to dive while pregnant. Healthy, experienced divers should probably limit dives to 30 minutes or less and not exceed one atmosphere in pressure (approximately 33 feet).[25]

If you are pregnant and want to continue to dive, we recommend that you discuss this activity with your health care provider. On the other hand, provided you avoid extremes in body temperature and listen to your body cues, snorkeling during pregnancy probably carries no unique risks.[26]

Exercise Tips For Pregnant Women

- Choose a form of exercise you can enjoy
- Exercise regularly
- Maintain good nutrition
- Get adequate rest
- Drink plenty of fluids
- Wear comfortable clothing
- Be aware of medical conditions that may complicate pregnancy
- Recognize warning signs to stop exercising
- Do adequate warm-up and cooldown exercises
- Lower the exercise intensity as pregnancy progresses
- Shorten the exercise sessions as pregnancy progresses
- If you did not exercise before pregnancy, begin with walking or water aerobics

Don't Dry Up!

Of paramount importance is the risk of dehydration with exercise. Dehydration can lead to false labor and temperature elevation, and may also adversely affect your developing baby. The amount of fluid that you must drink to stay well hydrated will vary from day to day. It depends on the amount of fluid your body excretes as waste and how much you sweat, among other factors. A good rule of thumb is to "pee light." In other words, your urine should be light in color. If it's concentrated and dark, you probably aren't drinking enough water. Don't rely on thirst to be your indicator as to the amount you need to drink. (By then, you probably are already a bit dehydrated.) Always carry a water bottle and remember to drink before, during, and after you exercise. This also holds true for the postpartum period and is especially important for the breast-feeding mom.

Exercise Is Not for Every Pregnant Woman

Should every pregnant woman exercise? Probably not! There are several contraindications to exercise during pregnancy. Some of these guidelines are noted in the ACOG

Technical Bulletin.[27] If you have a pre-existing medical problem or a complicated pregnancy, it is important to have your physician give you specific instructions. Even if you are healthy and have always exercised, it would be prudent to discuss your sporting activity and fitness goals with the medical provider overseeing your pregnancy. Good judgment needs to prevail at all times!

As alluded to earlier, many medical schools and allied health training centers do not have formalized instruction in sports medicine. As a result, your health care provider may not be well versed on the subject of exercise during pregnancy. Others may not share your interest in staying fit during pregnancy and thus refrain from discussing the topic. So what do you do? Be an informed consumer. Go to your prenatal doctor visits with specific questions in mind. You may want to bring some of the information offered in this chapter and discuss it with your health care provider.

If you are pregnant and are continuing an exercise regime or want to start to exercise, you should be aware of signals to either slow down or stop exercising. If you feel short of breath, become dizzy, or develop heart palpitations or any pain, you should stop exercising. If you experience leakage of fluid or have vaginal bleeding or spotting, you should contact your physician. Decreased sensation of fetal movements and the presence of uterine contractions are also indications that you should stop your workout and seek medical advice.

AFTER THE BABY IS BORN

You may be surprised to read that no specific medical guidelines for postpartum exercise are available. There is also a good reason—exercise after childbirth needs to be individualized. A woman who was restricted to bed rest for weeks because of a complicated high-risk pregnancy that ended in a caesarean section is very different from a woman who ran a 10K race three days before a vaginal delivery. A woman who has a 24-hour labor and ends up with an episiotomy will probably be more fatigued and more uncomfortable than a woman who only labors two hours and delivers her baby over an intact perineum that does not require any stitches.

The American College of Obstetricians and Gynecologists recognizes that some of the bodily changes occurring during pregnancy may persist for four to six weeks postpartum. However, recent studies published by family physician Dwenda Gjerdingen, M.D. challenge the traditional six-week recovery period and suggest that many pregnancy-related physical changes do not return to "normal" in that time frame.[28] Your doctor can give guidance, but only you know how you feel. Some women may feel like exercising a few days after childbirth, but others may take longer before they are ready to undertake a fitness program.

What We Know

Postpartum exercise routines should be tailored to each individual.

Getting Back in Shape

Exercise prescriptions for the postpartum woman have usually focused on back, abdominal, and pelvic strengthening routines. These are usually worthwhile, but individual factors also need consideration.

After giving birth, you need to listen to your body and its signals. You should also heed the advice of your health care provider. Common sense makes good sense!

Nursing

When it comes to breastfeeding, myths abound. Will a vigorous exercise program affect the amount of milk produced or its content? Does breastfeeding promote weight loss? Is it safe to resume a fitness program while breastfeeding?

Registered Dietician Cheryl A. Lovelady and her colleagues at the University of California studied two groups of well-nourished postpartum women who were breastfeeding their newborns.[29] One group performed vigorous exercise, while the control group remained sedentary. Analysis showed no difference in plasma hormones in breast milk from the two groups. The fat and protein content of milk from the exercisers and sedentary controls were also similar. The exercisers, however, tended to produce more milk daily and their milk had more calories. To date, the evidence suggests that vigorous exercise has no adverse effect on lactation.

Before or After Exercise?   In general, you probably do not have to wait any specified time before or after nursing to exercise.[30] Your individual preferences will determine your best time to exercise. Many nursing moms find that morning is a good time to exercise because that's when they feel more energetic. If you always pick a time when you are sapped for energy, you will probably abandon the exercise routine. You may also be more prone to injury if you exercise when fatigued. Remember, exercising should be fun and relaxing!

Eating for Two.   The postpartum period tends to be a time when many women, whether or not they exercised during their pregnancies, would like to shed extra body fat. In fact, a desire for weight reduction often motivates mothers to begin an exercise program.

Lactating women require about 400 to 600 additional calories per day.[30] Opinions are mixed as to whether breastfeeding, with its extra caloric requirements, actually promotes weight loss or gain. While most authorities agree that pregnancy is not a good time to go on a weight reducing diet, it is, however, an ideal time to pay appropriate attention to overall nutritional needs. (See Chapter 10, Food for Fitness.) The same thoughts hold for the postpartum period.

The nursing mom should not attempt to go on an extreme weight reduction diet, but should take special care to provide herself and her baby with proper nourishment. The adage "you are what you eat" has important ramifications for both the pregnant woman and the new mother. It is also important to keep yourself well hydrated. The water bottle you should have carried while pregnant should continue to be your partner once the baby is born.

Finding the Time

I didn't exercise when my children were young. I was working part-time and my husband was working more than 12 hours a day, six days a week. Even if I had the time, we could not have afforded to pay for a baby-sitter. —Nina, age 45

In addition to postpartum physical discomforts, other obstacles to exercise are often quickly apparent. Finding time for exercise can be a major hurdle. The issue of babysitters and child care takes on new meaning after the birth of a child. While some gyms provide babysitting services, many parents do not feel comfortable leaving their precious newborns with a stranger or in the company of other children.

Women who replied to our questionnaire concurred that finding time was often a major deterrent to exercise. Many of their responses revealed conflict when it came to juggling schedules and struggling with childcare. Several have reported feeling guilty about not having enough time with their children.

One Mom's Solution.   We interviewed 35-year-old Michelle, who gave birth to her third child nearly two years ago. She gained 20 pounds after her second pregnancy and due to time constraints and a complicated third pregnancy could not exercise. Now that her older two children were enrolled in school and her youngest, Emily, was nearly two years old, she decided to join a gym that had baby-sitting services. Unfortunately, Emily suffered from separation anxiety and cried when her mother headed off to the stair climbers and treadmills. Michelle felt guilty about leaving her toddler in tears and proceeded to have a miserable workout. The baby-sitters at the gym also made it clear that they did not want to look after a "crybaby." Still wanting to exercise, Michelle now gets up at 5:30 A.M. and goes to the gym while her husband and children sleep. Not exactly an ideal time, but well worth it, says Michelle, who has lost several pounds in the last few months.

You Are Important Too!   Most mothers need some personal time away from their daily routines, whether they work in the home or an office. An exercise program often provides them with that freedom. Whether it is a few minutes every day or an hour several times a week, you may find it healthy and useful to establish an exercise routine as high priority. You should not feel guilty about investing time in a fitness program—it's important from both physical and emotional standpoints.

Some moms may decide to take on an exercise routine that allows their baby to travel alongside them. Activities that lend themselves to this include biking and jogging with a special child seat or carrier. (See Chapter 13, Starting Early.) If your work load is such that your time with your new baby is limited or if baby-sitting services are scarce, this may be an ideal setup for you. You may also want to swap baby-sitting and exercise times with a neighbor who also has children. While one exercises, the other tends to the children, and then you switch roles. If you are enterprising with your time and resources, you may find that you can raise a family and still exercise. Be creative and be fit!

The Rewards of Exercise

This chapter has examined concerns about exercising while pregnant. Perhaps, in closing, some of the benefits of exercise during pregnancy should be repeated (see below). Aside from maintaining fitness and controlling excess weight gain, there are very important psychological perks.[31] Exercise helps to improve your self-image and gives a sense of increased control. What better time than pregnancy to reap these benefits? Exercise during pregnancy can also help relieve tension, increase energy levels, and help to improve sleep. In addition, it may hasten the postpartum recovery period by boosting energy levels and reducing fatigue, stress, and depression.

Benefits of Exercise During Pregnancy

- Maintenance of maternal fitness
- Control of weight gain
- Improvement in mental outlook
- Increased energy
- Relief of tension
- Less backache

THE FINISH LINE

The interaction between exercise and pregnancy is just beginning to be better understood. Research investigating the short- and long-term effects of exercise on mother and fetus is under way. Different routines, various intensities of exercise, and previous levels of fitness are also being considered.

Pregnancy is no longer considered such a dangerous or delicate state. Instead, it is becoming clearer that exercise and pregnancy can and should co-exist. Your exercise prescription should be individualized and flexible. You need to be an informed consumer, and at the same time health care providers need to continue to keep women informed. Listen to your body cues carefully. Be sure to discuss your fitness goals and expectations with your health care specialist. While pregnant, exercise your body—and be sure to exercise common sense.

ENDNOTES

1. Bell, R., & O'Neill, M. Exercise and pregnancy: A review. *BIRTH*, June 1994, 21, 85–95.
2. Leaf, D. A. Exercise during pregnancy: Guidelines and controversies. *Postgraduate Medicine*, January 1989, 85 (1), 233–234, 237–238.
   Bell, R., & O'Neill, M. Exercise and pregnancy: A review. *BIRTH*, June 1994, 21, 85–95.
3. Paisley, J. E., & Mellion, M. B. Exercise during pregnancy. *American Family Physician*, November 1988, 38 (5), 143–150.
4. Kulpa, P. J. Exercise during pregnancy. *Family Practice Recertification*, January 1989, 11 (1), 35–56.
5. Leaf, D. A. Exercise during pregnancy: Guidelines and controversies. *Postgraduate Medicine*, January 1989, 85 (1), 233–234, 237–238.
6. Paisley, J. E., & Mellion, M. B. Exercise during pregnancy. *American Family Physician*, November 1988, 38 (5), 143–150.
7. Artal, R. Exercise and pregnancy. *Clinics in Sports Medicine*, April 1992, 11 (2), 363–377.
   Heckman, J. D., & Sassard, R. Musculoskeletal considerations in pregnancy. *Journal of Bone and Joint Surgery*, November 1994, 76–A (11), 1720–1730.
8. Artal, R., Friedman, M. J., & McNitt-Gray, J. L. Orthopedic problems in pregnancy. *The Physician and Sportsmedicine*, September 1990, 18 (9), 93–100, 105.
9. Clapp, J. F. 3rd. A clinical approach to exercise during pregnancy. *Clinics in Sports Medicine*, April 1994, 13 (2), 443–458.
10. Clapp, J. F. 3rd. The course of labor after endurance exercise during pregnancy. *American Journal of Obstetrics and Gynecology*, 1990, 163, 1799–1805.
11. Clapp, J. F. 3rd. A clinical approach to exercise during pregnancy. *Clinics in Sports Medicine*, April 1994, 13 (2), 443–458.
12. Jarski, R. W., & Trippett, D. L. The risks and benefits of exercise during pregnancy. *The Journal of Family Practice*, 1990, 30 (2), 185–189.
13. Paisley, J. E., & Mellion, M. B. Exercise during pregnancy. *American Family Physician*, November 1988, 38 (5), 143–150.
14. Jarski, R. W., & Trippett, D. L. The risks and benefits of exercise during pregnancy. *The Journal of Family Practice*, 1990, 30 (2), 185–189.
15. Artal, R. Exercise and pregnancy. *Clinics in Sports Medicine*, April 1992, 11 (2), 363–377.
16. Jarski, R. W., & Trippett, D. L. The risks and benefits of exercise during pregnancy. *The Journal of Family Practice*, 1990, 30 (2), 185–189.
17. Watson, W. J., Katz, V. L., Hackney, A. C., Gall, M. M., & McMurray, R. G. Fetal responses to maximal swimming and cycling exercise during pregnancy. *Obstetrics & Gynecology*, 1991, 77, 382–386.
18. Clapp, J. F. 3rd, & Capeless, E. L. Neonatal morphometrics after endurance exercise during pregnancy. *American Journal of Obstetrics and Gynecology*, 1990, 163, 1805–1811.
19. Clapp, J. F. 3rd. The course of labor after endurance exercise during pregnancy. *American Journal of Obstetrics and Gynecology*, 1990, 163, 1799–1805.
20. Varrassi, G., Bazzano, C., & Edwards, W. T. Effects of physical activity on maternal plasma B-endorphin levels and perception of labor pain. *American Journal of Obstetrics and Gynecology*, 1989, 160, 707–712.
21. American College of Obstetricians and Gynecologists. Exercise during pregnancy and the postnatal period. *ACOG Home Exercise Programs*, May 1985, 1–6.
   American College of Obstetricians and Gynecologists. Exercise during pregnancy and the postpartum period. *ACOG Technical Bulletin*, February 1994 (189), 1–5.
22. Katz, V. L., Ryder, R. M., Celfalo, R. C., Carmichael, S. C., & Goolsby, R. A comparison of bed rest and immersion for treating the edema of pregnancy. *Obstetrics and Gynecology*, February 1990, 75 (2), 147–151.
23. Artal, R., Friedman, M. J., & McNitt-Gray, J. L. Orthopedic problems in pregnancy. *The Physician and Sportsmedicine*, September 1990, 18 (9), 93–100, 105.
24. Wein, P., & Thompson, D. J. Vaginal perforation due to jet ski accident. *Australia New Zealand Journal of Obstetrics and Gynaecology*, 1990, 30 (4), 384–385.
25. Bergfeld, J. A., Martin, M. C., Shangold, M. M., & Warren, M. P. Women in athletics: Five management problems. *Patient Care*, February 28, 1987, 21, 60–82.
26. Jarski, R. W., & Trippett, D. L. The risks and benefits of exercise during

pregnancy. *The Journal of Family Practice*, 1990, 30 (2), 185–189.

27. American College of Obstetricians and Gynecologists. Exercise during pregnancy and the postnatal period. *ACOG Home Exercise Programs*, May 1985, 1–6.

28. Gjerdingen, D. K., Froberg, D. G., Chaloner, K. M., & McGovern, P. M. Changes in women's physical health during the first postpartum year. *Archives of Family Medicine*, March 1993, 2, 277–283.

29. Lovelady, C. A. Lactation performance of exercising women. *American Journal of Clinical Nutrition*, 1990, 52, 103–109.

30. Schelkun, P. H. Exercise and breast-feeding mothers. *The Physician and Sportsmedicine*, April 1991, 19 (4), 109–109–116.

31. Jarski, R. W., & Trippett, D. L. The risks and benefits of exercise during pregnancy. *The Journal of Family Practice*, 1990, 30 (2), 185–189.

13 *Starting Early: A Family Affair*

ADELAIDE HAAS, PH.D.

DOING IT ALL

While I was pregnant I continued to exercise, although I modified my routine some-
what. But once my first child was born, my exercise life changed more dramatically.
I was no longer free to go off and run or work out. I needed to plan whether to try to
take the baby with me or arrange for childcare or just not exercise. Fortunately
a good friend, another exercise nut, had a child a few months older than mine so
together we worked out some solutions. —Maureen, age 36, mother of two

Women today want it all—and why shouldn't we? But it often requires massive juggling. Many of us want a career as well as a life-partner and children. We also want to take care of ourselves, exercise, feel fit, and enjoy our personal lives. In fact, more than simply wanting these things, most have become necessary. One salary may no longer be enough for a family, and so work outside the home by two adults may be essential. Good health, too, is not a luxury, and we recognize the role of regular exercise. Researcher Patrice Heinz, for example, reports the results of several studies that show that resuming exercise after childbirth helps to give mothers increased energy and may also prevent postpartum blues.[1] But how do we do it all?

More than two-thirds (68 percent) of the women in our study who had children reported that having children affected their exercise routines. The major concern that these women reported was a lack of time. Many indicated that their children's needs came first, and they had to plan around these priorities. Just how women with children organize their exercise lives is the topic of the next several pages. Further on we address the exercise needs of children and adolescents. We consider some of the problems associated with organized and competitive athletics as well as the benefits. In keeping with the theme of this book, our focus is primarily female.

EXERCISING WITH CHILDREN

How do you continue working out when your time, now that you are a parent, is even more limited? Some new mothers don't even try. Others, however, are taking advantage of innovative ways to stay fit, have fun, and enrich the lives of their offspring.

Taking Them Along

It is remarkable how many ways children, even as young as infants, can participate in your fitness life. Some of our respondents noted that the situation was easiest before their children started to walk—when they were "tote-able." The toddler period was more challenging, because children are too heavy and independent to simply be carried. With flexibility, however, both parents and children can find ways to stay fit. As children get older, they can often participate in your physical activities and you can join them in theirs.

> *I never thought I'd want to take up roller-blading, but when Sally came home from third grade desperately wanting to skate, we decided that this was something both of us could do.* —Peggy, age 41

> *My exercise routine changed considerably after the children were born. But I think it is for the better. I sometimes play tennis with my daughter after school, and weekends we often get together with family and friends for backyard sports. But things continue to evolve; no life stage is like another.* —Virginia, age 37

Equipment Is Available

Tote-able Tots.   Manufacturers have recognized that many parents do not want to change their lifestyle with the advent of children. From front-packs to backpacks, bicycle seats to jog-strollers, more and more infants today are joining their parents in exercise and adventure.

Gwynn Press recently evaluated baby carriers for *Parents* magazine.[2] She suggests that slings are most useful for infants who can't hold their heads up yet. If you are nursing, the baby can be positioned at breast level for easy access. Front carriers with stiff head support are an option to the sling, especially for an older baby who can be faced away from you to see the passing scenery. As the child gets bigger and heavier, backpack-type carriers make the load easier on you. With this equipment, also, children get to see where they are going. Some makes of back carriers can be converted to strollers, for variety and the next phase in a child's life. Whichever type of carrier you use, it is essential to fasten your child in securely, and to check periodically to assure that she or he remains in a safe position.[2]

Preschoolers Plus.   Too big to be toted, preschoolers and older children can often participate in biking by taking advantage of tandems designed for youngsters. The parent rides in front, and the child in back. The child's wheels are smaller, and the seat is adjustable so that she or he can pedal.

Warnings!

Watch the temperature.   While you are running and hot, your baby in the jog-stroller is sitting or lying still. The little one feels the wind and is not getting any exercise. This holds true for baby carriers as well. Be sure that the infant is adequately warm and protected from the elements. It is also possible for your child to become overly warm. Too heavy bundling and a direct sun can create heat problems that may be just as serious as excessive cold.

Use well-fitting safety helmets.   If you are biking, place your young passenger securely on the bicycle and obtain an appropriately sized helmet. Children in jog-strollers need helmets, too; they can be moving pretty fast!

Day Care at the Gym

Most "Ys" and Health Clubs have day care facilities for young children. While mothers and dads engage in grown-up workouts, children receive care. The quality of these programs varies, and it is worthwhile to investigate the child-care provisions before committing yourself to a program. Gyms at "Ys" are often family oriented; adults and children of various ages play and exercise near one another. A few minutes of observation and conversation with other parents can help you make an informed decision.

Buddy Systems

Many of our respondents noted the value of a friend or partner with similar exercise interests. Two children can often be watched as easily as one. A trade-off system with a like-minded adult can provide each of you with freedom to exercise. This requires planning and accommodation, but it can be beneficial to all concerned.

> *I want my children to know at an early age the importance of taking care of their bodies. Both my husband and I set the example for regular exercise throughout life.*
> —Donna, age 35

Adjust Your Routine

In addition to taking children along, or leaving them with a friend, you can plan your exercise routine with your children's needs in mind. You may not realistically be able to work out in the same place or in the same way as before you became a parent. Be ready to make some modifications.

Work Out at Home. Home videos and exercise equipment provide a way to stay fit without leaving your home. You can work out after the children are asleep. But this may not be necessary; children as young as two and three will often join in by jumping around to music. This is not only fun, but it is a great way to teach the pleasure and importance of exercise. (See Chapter 4, Focus on Fitness, and Chapter 9, Gearing Up, for more information on videos and home equipment.)

Keep the Space Restricted. If your pleasure has been to hike, run, or bike long distances, you may find that little legs can't keep up with you. When your children can no longer be transported by you, and they are still too young to be independent, exercise in a confined area may prove a useful solution. For example, many parents change the location of their workout to a track. There, the parent can run or walk, while the youngster plays within sight. As suggested earlier, cooperating with a like-minded parent is often helpful. One stays with the children, while the other exercises.

Consider the Interests and Abilities of Your Children. If you want your children to enjoy the exercise that you engage in, be sure to recognize their interests and abilities. Parents who like to hike may be disappointed that preschoolers and school-age children are not interested in joining them. However, when these youngsters are provided with age-appropriate motivators, they may eagerly participate. Rock crevices to climb through or over often delight children who are reluctant to just go for a walk— even if that walk is up a mountain to see a view.

STARTING YOUNG

What Do Infants Need?

Do infants need an exercise program? Some communities offer infant swimming classes or massage and exercise for babies. Are these worth the expense?

In New York City and elsewhere around the country, gym classes are available for babies as young as *three months*. These infants are not expected to pump iron or do push-ups; however, their arms and legs are moved in various ways and they get massaged by their parents.[3] While the value of these classes for developing physical fitness has not been demonstrated, the parent/child interaction promotes bonding and the sessions are usually pleasurable for both participants. However, it is likely that the normal bathing, stroking, and interplay between parents and infant yield similar benefits.

As children get older, other formal programs are available to provide instruction for two- to four-year-olds. In gymnastics, youngsters learn to hang from rings and to do log and forward rolls. Some programs teach the rudiments of climbing, balancing, and throwing and catching, while others stress rhythmic movement and "kinder" (pronounced as in kindergarten, meaning child) dance. Although certainly not a necessity, and generally quite costly (often $20 or so per 45-minute class), studies have shown that children who get instruction in physical activity tend to make more progress than those who simply play on their own.[3] The good news for the budget-minded, however, is that parents often can learn to be as effective as trained teachers in working with preschool youngsters.[3]

It is safe to say that during the first few years of life, children do not need a formal exercise program. However, they do need opportunity and freedom to move. Fortunately, most children will let their parents know what they need and will balk if confined excessively. Furthermore, children learn from example and from their parents' attitude. If you are physically active, chances are your children will be also.

The 1996 Surgeon General's report *Physical Activity and Health* recommends that "All people over the age of *two years* should accumulate at least 30 minutes of endurance-type physical activity, of at least moderate intensity, on most—preferably all—days of the week."[4] In addition, for optimal development, young children should engage in active play three to four hours each day.[5] Your positive attitude toward physical exercise should encourage this in your offspring.

Public Playgrounds.   Playgrounds are standard equipment in many parks, especially in cities. The newer ones tend to provide an excellent space for children to actively explore and play. But not all playgrounds are created equally, and some are blatantly unsafe. According to the U.S. Consumer Product Safety Commission, about 80,000 preschoolers are treated in emergency rooms each year due to playground accidents.[6]

Safety Check Your Local Playground. Evaluate your local playground. If it is unsafe, work with other parents and your city or town officials to rectify the situation. If you must answer "no" to any of the following questions, you would be wise to work to correct the problems.

- **Climbing Equipment**
  1. Is all climbing equipment less than five feet high?
  2. Do elevated platforms have guardrails?

3. Are climbing bars and handrails between one and two inches in diameter so they can be grasped easily by small hands?
4. Are spaces between bars and the like less than three or greater than nine inches, so that children will not get their heads caught?

- **Slides**
  1. Do slides have side guards at least four inches high to prevent children from falling off?
  2. Is there sufficient protective surfacing, such as rubber matting, to cushion falls? (Sand becomes hard and is less effective when wet, and therefore is not as good.)
  3. Are metal slides in a shady area so that children are not likely to get burned on hot metal?
- **Swings**
  1. Are swings sufficiently close to the ground to minimize the risk of falls from heights?
  2. Are swings made of lightweight material, such as rubber or plastic, so that collisions with them are less hazardous?
- **General Layout and Maintenance**
  1. Is equipment in good repair?
  2. Is the area free of broken glass and other hazardous litter?
  3. Are there separate areas of play for younger and older children?
  4. Is the area sheltered from car traffic, so that children are not tempted to run into a street while chasing balls?

Junior Athletes

The TV & Computer Generation.   Jamie Truscott, an observer of social trends, fears that we are raising "a nation of little butterballs."[7] Reports from the Federal Centers for Disease Control and Prevention confirm that more than 10 percent of all American children between the ages of 6 and 17 are overweight. In the 1970s the prevalence of overweight children was about 5 percent. Along with the increased poundage are the associated problems of high cholesterol and elevated blood pressure—all risk factors for coronary heart disease.[8]

While diet is a major culprit in producing overweight children, insufficient exercise is also partly responsible. Children do not engage in adequate physical activity for many reasons:

1. Television is an easy baby-sitter and diversion.

2. Computers have captured the imagination of many youngsters, and some children opt for computer sports over the real thing.
3. Streets and parks are not as safe as they were a generation ago. Parents are less comfortable about sending their children out to play.
4. Children today are required to do fewer physical chores around the house.
5. Many schools do not offer an adequate physical education program.[9]

Whatever Happened to Free Play? Many of us remember going into backyards or neighborhood parks to play while we were growing up. While some children do this today, unstructured physically active play may be less common than it once was. The reasons noted earlier—television, computers, safety—contribute to this reduction in activity. People living in regions with cold winters are also less likely to be active during that time of year.[9]

What Do Teenagers Want? A *New York Times* headline in the mid 1990s shouted, "Girls don't want to have gym." While 50 percent of high school boys exercise vigorously on a regular basis, only 25 percent of girls are similarly involved. The newspaper article quotes a 15-year-old sophomore saying, "When I was little, I used to love it. But most girls don't like to mess up their hair, to get changed or like, you know, be bothered." Other girls reported a lack of time: "When you go home from school at night, you have dishes to do, the house to clean, and you have homework. There really isn't time for anything else." Other teenage girls simply admitted to being "too lazy."[10] Many middle school girls admit they hate to get naked and take showers in the locker room.

Psychologists Erica Frydenberg and Ramon Lewis shed some light on the gender difference in athletic activities among teenagers. They studied coping behavior in Australian high school students and found that boys turned to sports and physical activity to improve their well-being, while girls tended to turn to other people.[11] Although these researchers studied Australian teens, the situation is likely similar in the United States and elsewhere.

Different attitudes toward exercise and play have resulted in two extremes emerging in our society. Some children do not exercise, and are therefore overweight and unfit. Inner city youths often fall into this category.[12] The other group comes from families who are more affluent and frequently better educated; these children are involved in organized athletics.

Organized Activities. While some children get little or no exercise, others take advantage of the wealth of organized physical activity options that exist in many communities. Some of these are free of charge, such as "Little Leagues"; others range from modest (usually those connected with municipalities or "Ys") to fairly expensive privately run programs.

For Fun and Fitness. If organized active recreation for grade school children is available in your geographical area, the evidence suggests that participation will enhance your child's level of fitness. Further, early participation often leads to a lifetime of good exercise habits. Dance and exercise classes are helpful for both girls and boys. They teach balance and poise as well as provide aerobic benefit. Swimming, skating, and soccer are also worthwhile activities for youngsters. They promote aerobic endurance and can be continued throughout life.

• **Emphasis on Fun.** Dr. Lawrence Kutner, author of several books on child-raising and an editor for *Parents* magazine, emphasizes that learning should be fun. Dr. Kutner notes a positive change in swimming instruction from when he was a child. Rather than focusing on strokes and form, children begin by playing water games. As children gain confidence, they are gradually challenged to engage in progressively more demanding activity. In selecting a program, Dr. Kutner suggests observing a class and then asking yourself:

1. Are the children having fun?
2. Is the instructor knowledgeable and well-qualified?
   (You should ask about his/her training and certification.)
3. Is the instructor supportive (doesn't demean or yell at children)?
4. Are multiple levels of instruction available as your child progresses?[13]

Selecting Your Child's Activity

It doesn't take long for parents to realize that children are people with very definite ideas and personalities. Even toddlers show preferences. So while you as the adult will make the final decision regarding your child's activity, you should take into consideration your child's interests and aptitudes. Provide your child with healthful options and then follow your child's lead.

> When I was eight years old, my mother enrolled me in a summer daycamp that my older cousin had attended for several years. My cousin loved it; I hated it. The camp's main focus was sports (softball and tennis), and my cousin enjoyed both games and was good at them. I was neither. My mother thought I was totally unathletic and that I was doomed to become fat and unfit. Fortunately, soon after that awful summer we learned about an after-school dance class. I was enrolled and flourished. In fact, I turned my aptitude and dance training into a part-time job. I now teach aerobics at a health club three evenings a week. —Delores, age 26

Getting Competitive

Physical activity may move quickly from where the objective is fun and fitness to competitive goals. Children who begin by taking swimming lessons may find that if they want to continue learning they must join a team. "Little League" soccer, softball, and basketball are all intrinsically competitive; confirmation is found in the adult audience. Running, dance, and gymnastics may also become competitive for those who stay with their programs. For many children as young as eight years of age, competition is a significant aspect of their physical activity. It is estimated that about one in four girls, and one in two boys, between the ages of eight and sixteen engage in some type of competitive athletics.[14]

Why Do Children Compete? Sports competition appears to have become a way of life for much of American society. This has stimulated researchers Darren C. Treasure and Glyn C. Roberts of the Department of Kinesiology at the University of Illinois at Urbana-Champaign to examine children's own motivation. They found two types of achievement motivators. Task orientation is "dependent on learning or improvement of the task," in other words, mastering a particular skill. Ego orientation, on the other hand, "is dependent on subjective assessment of one's ability relative to that of others."[15] When the two motivational factors were compared, it was found that children tend to work hard at sports because of ego orientation; they want to be better than their opponents. Mastering a skill, or task orientation, is a more important motivator in academic learning. Figure 13-1 shows a questionnaire used to measure children's motivations in sports.

As with most things, competition has both positive and negative features.

Caution! Don't be a pushy parent! Some parents, from the sidelines at athletic events, *demand* more from their children than they are capable of producing. These parents often measure their own adult success in their children's accomplishments. While encouragement is helpful, requiring sports victories of young children may damage morale and self-esteem.

Promote Personal, Not Competitive, Goals. Sadly, in much of our lives we compare ourselves to others. By its very nature, competitive athletics forces us to match our skills against those of someone else. While this can sometimes motivate improvement, other times it results in despair—especially when the contrast in skills is great. Let your child find her own athletic outlet. No one sport or activity is right for everyone.

In team sports, especially with young children, each child should be given appropriate turns and praised for efforts as well as accomplishments. Children should never be scolded or made to feel inadequate for poor performance. When this happens, sports stop being fun, and children are inclined to drop out.[16]

Athletic programs should focus on developing a child's "personal best." Children should work on mastering techniques and developing strength, speed, flexibility, and

FIGURE 13.1

....

Perception of Success Questionnaire (Children's Version)

What does success in sport mean to you?
There are no right or wrong answers.
We ask you to circle the number that best indicates how you feel.

When Playing Sports, I Feel Most Successful When:

		strongly disagree		neutral		strongly agree
a.	I beat other people	1	2	3	4	5
b.	I am the best	1	2	3	4	5
c.	I do better than others	1	2	3	4	5
d.	I show other people I am the best	1	2	3	4	5
e.	I accomplish something others cannot do	1	2	3	4	5
f.	I am clearly better	1	2	3	4	5
g.	I try hard	1	2	3	4	5
h.	I really improve	1	2	3	4	5
i.	I overcome difficulties	1	2	3	4	5
j.	I succeed at something I could not do before	1	2	3	4	5
k.	I perform to the best of my ability	1	2	3	4	5
l.	I reach a target I set for myself	1	2	3	4	5

....

Interpretation: Add your points from items a–f to obtain an "ego" score. Items g–l will yield your "task" score. Task orientation may be more important in academics, while ego orientation may be more significant in sports.
Adapted, and used with permission, from D. C. Treasure, Department of Kinesiology, University of Illinois at Urbana-Champaign.

endurance. Individual task goals can be developed for each child, so she or he can mark individual progress. With personal improvement the objective, every child can be a "winner."

Reviewing the Risks. Probably the most adverse publicity concerning the ill effects of competition involves young gymnasts. Joan Ryan, in her scathing indictment, *Little Girls in Pretty Boxes: The Making and Breaking of Elite Gymnasts and Figure Skaters*, details the horrors of overzealously pushing children to excel.[17] Problems reported by Ryan and others are described on the next few pages.

• **Injuries.** From sprained fingers in volleyball and tendinitis in tennis to broken legs in skiing, all sports put participants at risk of physical injury. Ryan reports a significant incidence of shin splints, stress fractures, sprained knees, hamstring pulls, broken ankles, and cracked vertebrae in gymnasts and ice-skaters.[17] Dental and facial injuries in children are also on the rise due to involvement in organized sports at increasingly younger ages.[18] Injuries of all types have similarly increased in frequency over the past 20 years, and when winning is everything, children are expected to compete even when injured.[19] Researchers are concerned about lifelong damage due to interference with normal growth mechanisms.[20]

Pediatric specialists at Albert Einstein College of Medicine in New York City analyzed the incidence of sports and recreation injuries in children and adolescents in the United States. Injuries related to falls from bicycles, horses, playground equipment, skates, skateboards, and in sports activities were tallied along with mishaps blamed on overexertion. More than four million children a year are hurt seriously enough to miss school or stay in bed for half a day or more. Over one million suffer critical injuries involving hospitalization and/or surgery. In all, more than one third of all injuries to children are sports related.[21]

In addition to acute, traumatic injury, children are especially prone to "overuse" microtrauma. Excessive repetition of any movement—whether throwing a ball, practicing a tennis serve, or reaching and stretching in swimming—can cause wear and tear on the muscles and tendons. These injuries may be as damaging as acute ones, especially since treatment is often delayed.

The reasons for sports accidents vary. Inappropriate or excessive training directed by unqualified adult leaders may result in acute trauma as well as overuse microtrauma. Faulty equipment and the absence of proper protective gear also contribute to injuries. Additionally, temperature and weather are often ignored by both youngsters and their supervisors. Children tolerate heat less well than adults, often do not drink enough, and may suffer from heat exhaustion. Finally, children may engage in activities without proper physical conditioning.[22]

FIGURE 13.2

....

The Bill of Rights for Young Athletes

- Right to participate in sports
- Right to participate at a level commensurate with each
  child's maturity and ability
- Right to have qualified adult leadership
- Right to play as a child and not as an adult
- Right of children to share in the leadership and decision-making
  of their sport participation
- Right to participate in safe and healthy environments
- Right to proper preparation for participation in sports
- Right to an equal opportunity to strive for success
- Right to be treated with dignity
- Right to have fun in sports

The Bill of Rights for Young Athletes is reprinted with permission from the National Association of Sport and Physical Education (NASPE), 1900 Association Drive, Reston, VA 20191-1599.

It is important to recognize that while younger athletes often suffer many of the same injuries as their adult counterparts, differences exist from an anatomical standpoint. The child's immature skeletal system may both contribute to and be adversely affected by sports injuries. Some writers go so far as to suggest that "parents and coaches must realize there may be little room for developing athletic prowess during that time when the so-called clumsy teenager is adjusting to body changes."[23]

• **Self-Image.** While sports and exercise improve self-perception for many children, this is not always the case. In one study, 42 boys and 32 girls from economically disadvantaged backgrounds participated in a month-long sports camp. These children's self-concept was measured utilizing the *Self-Perception Profile for Children* at the beginning and end of the camp program. The girls' scores showed a decline in five of the six sub-scales. Boys' scores did not decline. The end effect was that girls' scores dropped below those of boys. The researchers, psychologists J. M. Kishton and A. C. Dixon, attributed this decline in self-concept to the stresses of competition and an initially overly positive self-perception. Why the camp experience was negative only for girls is open to speculation.[24]

• **The Female Triad.** A particular combination of problems associated with athletics pertains only to females. This constellation has been dubbed "the female athlete triad." The triad consists of eating disorders, menstrual dysfunction, and osteoporosis. Although these concerns are not unknown among non-athletes, their prevalence is substantially greater in the athlete population.[25] For additional information on this important issue, see Chapter 18, Beware of the Danger Zones.

Preventing Problems. Lyle J. Micheli, M.D., of Harvard Medical School, blames most injuries on "inappropriate and excessive training by inexperienced or unqualified adult supervisors."[26] "Children are not small adults," emphasize orthopedic surgeons P. C. Cook and M. E. Leit; but, according to the doctors, proper training practices can help avoid injuries.[27]

• **Pre-Sports Medical Examination.** Although pre-participation sports examinations find most children medically sound, early identification of risk factors can often prevent later problems. Medical authorities recommend that children be evaluated about a month before the initial start of the athletic program and once every two years thereafter.[28] Some school districts mandate an evaluation prior to permitting youngsters to engage in physical exercise or sports.[29] If an exam is not required by the school, parents should independently have their children assessed.

The health care provider should speak separately, if possible, to the parents and to the young athlete to explore both physical and psychological factors related to safely participating in recreational and competitive sports. When talking to the youngster, the medical specialist should take the opportunity to provide counseling about injury risk and prevention, body function, and nutrition. The primary goal of the examination is to detect potentially dangerous medical conditions. Secondarily, the health care provider engages in general health counseling, maturity assessment, and fitness evaluation.[30]

Note: The medical examination may be the time when a health care professional discusses with an adolescent such critical issues as the use of tobacco, alcohol, drugs, and steroids. Teachers and parents should reinforce the hazards associated with the use of these substances.

• **Physical Conditioning.** Most sports require muscle strength and a degree of flexibility. Children need to train, just as adults do. While it was once thought that resistance training with weights was harmful to young people, current research points to benefits and no risk when correctly used. Children should first learn the exercises without weights. Progressively greater levels of resistance (weights) should be introduced so as to gradually develop muscular strength throughout the body. Equipment should be appropriate in size for the young athlete. A qualified instructor should ensure that movements are correctly made.[31]

• **Pre-Activity Warm-up and Stretching; Post-Activity Cooldown.** Just as warming up, stretching, and cooling down are important for adults, they similarly help to prevent injuries in children. In fact, warm-ups and cooldowns may be even more necessary for children since they are less metabolically efficient and perspire less than adults. Unfortunately, these simple techniques are often overlooked when children go out to play ball. They are more often routinely incorporated in dance and gymnastics training. (See Chapter 4, Focus on Fitness, and Chapter 5, Routines: The Stars Are the Limit, for more information on this topic.)

• **Cross-Training.** Overtraining is a major cause of many injuries.[32] Ted Quedenfeld, Director of the Temple University Sports Medicine Centers, estimates that 60 percent of children's athletic injuries are related to overuse.[33] What constitutes overtraining is not entirely clear, but experts suggest erring on the side of caution. One study noted an increase in back injury for gymnasts who trained more than 16 hours per week.[34] Other studies note overuse arm and shoulder injuries associated with intensive programs of swimming and baseball. This is especially a problem for young pitchers.[35]

Children, like adults, need a balance in their athletic pursuits and their lives. Tennis and other specialty camps should be evaluated so that youngsters are not spending too many hours in repetitive movements. Dance programs should be similarly evaluated; care should also be taken to see that children are not expected to progress too rapidly. (See Chapter 5 for more information on cross-training. Chapter 16 describes the hazards of overtraining.)

• **Safety Equipment.** In most states, children are required to wear helmets while bicycling; however, only 15 percent of children do. It has been estimated that helmets, if worn by every biker between the ages of 4 and 14, could prevent 45,000 injuries and 155 deaths each year.[36] Helmets should also be used in hockey, football, skateboarding, and horseback riding, and they must fit properly.[37]

Other safety equipment—such as knee braces, mouth guards, and eye protectors—is not as well known or encouraged. Knee injuries occur frequently in young female soccer, basketball, and lacrosse players. Dr. Micheli, of Harvard Medical School, suggests that appropriate use of knee braces may prevent some of these injuries, although the prophylactic use of braces is currently controversial and awaits further investigation.[38]

In ice hockey, skating, and football, mouth guards can prevent dental injuries. Eye protectors with polycarbonate lenses are valuable in many sports, such as soccer and tennis.[39]

Dr. Clay Miller notes the importance of appropriate floors for ballet students. If your child is to study dance, make sure that the studio flooring is of wood, and preferably that a suspended floor construction was used. Basements with linoleum over concrete are not resilient, and jumps on these floors are more likely to lead to foot and ankle injuries.

Floors should be kept clean and should not be slippery.[40] All exercise should take place in a well-ventilated space to prevent respiratory problems.[41]

- **Proper Grouping.** Children are often grouped by age. This may be appropriate for young children, but in early adolescence, differences in pubertal growth account for significant variations in size and strength in children of both sexes—but especially in boys. Professors Roemmich and Rogol of the University of Virginia Health Sciences Center suggest that "maturity-based categorization, especially in contact and collision sports, would heighten the competition and lessen rates of injury."[42] Appropriately matched late maturers might experience greater sports success and thereby improve their self-image during these often psychologically stressful years.

Bountiful Benefits. While organized sports and athletics present certain risks, these can be minimized, as we saw in the sections above. And taken all together, the benefits far outweigh the risks.

Physical Fitness. Regular exercise has the potential for improving all the dimensions of physical fitness. Children who play sports or engage in other regular physical activities tend to be better coordinated, have greater balance, physical strength, and endurance than their peers.[43] Even children with chronic illnesses may benefit from being active. Dr. Barry Goldberg, writing in *The Physician and Sportsmedicine*, observed that while "a chronic disease can burden a child, it doesn't have to deprive him or her of sports participation. In fact, exercise can ameliorate the disease and enhance quality of life."[44]

Aerobic Fitness. If continued over the long term, regular aerobic exercise improves VO_2max, and by extension cardiac fitness. Drs. T. W. Rowland and A. Boyajian, of the Department of Pediatrics at Baystate Medical Center in Springfield, Massachusetts, studied 24 girls and 13 boys between the ages of 10 and 13. These children were in a physical education class that provided three 30-minute sessions of aerobic activity each week for 12 weeks at an average intensity level of 166 beats per minute heart rate. At the end of this period, VO_2max improved significantly.[45]

Enjoyment and Self-esteem. When children are involved in appropriate physical programs, they have fun. They enjoy the social nature of their sport or activity, and they develop positive attitudes about themselves.[46] Several studies confirm that teens who engage in athletic activities have higher self-esteem and are more popular with their peers.[47]

As an elementary-school teacher, I have observed a big difference between girls who participate in sports and those who do not. Part of the athletic process is to push yourself to be the best you can be. That in itself is rewarding for young women. Playing sports affords girls the opportunity to be part of a group with common goals, something that is rare in other areas of the curriculum. —Vivian[48]

What We Know

About 10 percent of American youngsters underexercise and are overweight. Many others participate in sports or other physical activities on a regular basis. While competition may pose certain health hazards, these can be minimized through judicious planning. The benefits of physical activity far outweigh any potential risks.

What to Do

Provide your child with the opportunity to participate in regular physical activity that is enjoyable to her or him and that is well organized and monitored. Encourage schools to incorporate 30 minutes or more of well-taught physical education into the curriculum for all children. Be a model and a guide for a healthful lifestyle.

Caution: If your child is not mature or coordinated enough to play a certain sport, having her or him on a team could be a set-up for failure and ridicule. For this reason, it is imperative to let children individually find the physical activity that is best for them.

Reducing Risks of Poor Health. Although cardiovascular disease is rare in children, coronary heart disease risk factors can be identified at young ages. Risk factors include obesity, lack of aerobic fitness, elevated blood pressure, and poor blood lipid profiles (cholesterol, HDL, LDL). All of these adverse features are significantly more prevalent in children who are not physically active.[49]

Developing Lifetime Attitudes. The joy of exercise learned at an early age can lead to a lifetime of physical fitness and improved quality of life.[50] This is an investment in our children that is well worth making.

I played soccer and basketball all through high school and am playing again in college. I swim and do aerobics, too. These activities have made such a difference in my life. They help me unwind from studying and give me extra energy. If I don't work out or play, I really miss it. I've also made great friends. My teammates have always been terrific. We support each other and have a lot of fun together. I want to be on a team and stay active my whole life if possible. —Heidi Melinda, age 21

1. Shelkun, P. H. Exercise and breast-feeding mothers. *The Physician and Sportsmedicine*, April 1991, 19 (4), 109.

2. Press, G. Baby carrier basics. *Parents*, August 1996, 71 (8), 23–28.

3. Scott, J. Where Johnny can come in to play. *New York Times*, November 15, 1995, c1, c8.

4. U.S. Department of Health and Human Services. *Physical Activity and Health: A Report of the Surgeon General*. Atlanta, GA: U.S. Department of Health and Human Services, Centers for Disease Control and Prevention, National Center for Chronic Disease Prevention and Health Promotion, 1996.

5. Allenson, Y. Professor Emeritus of Health & Physical Education, personal communication, November 1996.

6. Blank, J. H. Is your playground safe? *Sesame Street Parents' Guide*, May 1993, 26–29.

7. Truscott, J. A nation of little butterballs. *Vibrant Life*, November 1993, 9 (6), 18.

8. Maillet, J. O. Weight: Too heavy. Fortune: bleak. *New York Times*, November 5, 1995.

9. Brody, J. E. Personal health: A Michigan program shows the unhealthy trend among school-children is reversible. *New York Times*, October 24, 1984.

10. Steinhauer, J. Girls don't want to have gym. *New York Times*, January 4, 1995, c1, c6.

11. Frydenberg, E., & Lewis, R. Boys play sport and girls turn to others: age, gender and ethnicity as determinants of coping. *Journal of Adolescence*, 1993, 16, 253–266.

12. Steinhauer, J. Girls don't want to have gym. *New York Times*, January 4, 1995, c1, c6.

13. Kutner, L. Learning to swim. The first step is helping your child have fun in the water. *Parents*, June 1996, 88–90.

14. Castiglia, P. T. Sports injuries in children. *Journal of Pediatric Health Care*, January–February 1995, 9 (1), 32–33.

15. Treasure, D. C., & Roberts, G. C. Perception of success questionnaire: preliminary validation in an adolescent population. *Perceptual and Motor Skills*, 1994, 79, 607–610.

16. Cook, P. C., & Leit, M. E. Issues in the pediatric athlete. *Orthopedic Clinics of North America*, July 1995, 26 (3), 453–464.

17. Ryan, J. *Little girls in pretty boxes: The making and breaking of elite gymnasts and figure skaters*. New York: Doubleday, 1995.

18. Glassman, M. The first line of defense. *New York State Dental Journal*, August–September 1996, 61 (7), 48–50.

19. Ryan, J. *Little girls in pretty boxes: The making and breaking of elite gymnasts and figure skaters*. New York: Doubleday, 1995.

20. Castiglia, P. T. Sports injuries in children. *Journal of Pediatric Health Care*, January–February 1995, 9 (1), 32–33.

21. Bijur, P. E., Trumble, A., Harel, Y., et al. Sports and recreation injuries in U.S. children and adolescents. *Archives of Pediatric and Adolescent Medicine*, September 1995, 149 (9), 1009–1016.

22. Castiglia, P. T. Sports injuries in children. *Journal of Pediatric Health Care*, January–February 1995, 9 (1), 32–33.

23. Overbaugh, K. A., & Allen, J. G. The adolescent athlete. Part I: preseason preparation and examination. *Journal of Pediatric Health Care*, July–August 1994, 8 (4), p. 209.

24. Kishton, J. M., & Dixon, A. C. Self-perception changes among sports camp participants. *Journal of Social Psychology*, April 1995, 135 (2), 135–141.

25. Putukian, M. The female triad. Eating disorders, amenorrhea, and osteoporosis. *Medical Clinics of North America*, March 1994, 78 (2), 345–355.

26. Micheli, L. J. Sports injuries in children and adolescents. *Clinics in Sports Medicine*, July 1995, 14 (3), 727–745.

27. Cook, P. C., & Leit, M. E. Issues in the pediatric athlete. *Orthopedic Clinics of North America*, July 1995, 26 (3), 453–464.

28. Overbaugh, K. A., & Allen, J. G. The adolescent athlete. Part I: preseason preparation and examination. *Journal of Pediatric Health Care*, July–August 1994, 8 (4), 146–151.

29. Bratton, R. L., & Agerter, D. C. Preparticipation sports examinations. Efficient risk assessment in children and adolescents. *Postgraduate Medicine*, August 1995, 98 (2), 123–126, 129–132.

30. Overbaugh, K. A., & Allen, J. G. The adolescent athlete. Part I: preseason preparation and examination. *Journal of Pediatric Health Care*, July–August 1994, 8 (4), 146–151.

31. Castiglia, P. T. Sports injuries in children. *Journal of Pediatric Health Care*, January–February 1995, 9 (1), 32–33.

32. Micheli, L. J. Sports injuries in

children and adolescents. *Clinics in Sports Medicine*, July 1995, 14 (3), 727–745.

33. Castiglia, P. T. Sports injuries in children. *Journal of Pediatric Health Care*, January–February 1995, 9 (1), 32–33.

34. Goldstein, J. D., Berger, P. E., Windler, G. E., et al. Spine injuries in gymnasts and swimmers. An epidemiologic investigation. *American Journal of Sports Medicine*, 1991, 19, 463–468.

35. Micheli, L. J. Sports injuries in children and adolescents. *Clinics in Sports Medicine*, July 1995, 14 (3), 727–745.

36. Vander Schaaf, R. Safe cycling: Kids' health and safety. *Parents*, August 1996, 71 (8), 35–37.

37. Castiglia, P. T. Sports injuries in children. *Journal of Pediatric Health Care*, January–February 1995, 9 (1), 32–33.

38. Micheli, L. J. Sports injuries in children and adolescents. *Clinics in Sports Medicine*, July 1995, 14 (3), 727–745.

39. Castiglia, P. T. Sports injuries in children. *Journal of Pediatric Health Care*, January–February 1995, 9 (1), 32–33.

40. Miller, C. Safe footing for young dancers. *The Physician and Sportsmedicine*, July 1996, 24 (7), 22.

41. Cook, P. C., & Leit, M. E. Issues in the pediatric athlete. *Orthopedic Clinics of North America*, July 1995, 26 (3), 453–464.

42. Roemmich, J. N., & Rogol, A. D. Physiology of growth and development. Its relationship to performance in the young athlete. *Clinics in Sports Medicine*, July 1995, 14 (3), 483–502.

43. Ignico, A. A., & Mahon, A. D. The effects of a physical fitness program on low-fit children. *Research Quarterly for Exercise and Sport*, 1995, 66 (1), 85–90.

44. Goldberg, B. Children, sports, and chronic disease. *The Physician and Sportsmedicine*. October 1990, 18 (10), 44.

45. Rowland, T. W., & Boyajian, A. Aerobic response to endurance training in children. *Pediatrics*, October 1995, 96 (4 Pt 1), 654–658.

46. Overbaugh, K. A., & Allen, J. G. The adolescent athlete. Part I: preseason preparation and examination. *Journal of Pediatric Health Care*, July–August 1994, 8 (4), p. 209.

47. Browne, B. A., & Francis, S. K. Participants in school-sponsored and independent sports: perceptions of self and family. *Adolescence*, Summer 1993, 28 (110), 383–391.

48. Damelio-Sherman, V. Just buy it. (Letters). *The New York Times Magazine*, July 14, 1996, 7.

49. Brody, J. E. Personal health: A Michigan program shows the unhealthy trend among schoolchildren is reversible. *New York Times*, October 24, 1984.

Hager, R. L., Tucker, L. A., & Seljaas, G. T. Aerobic fitness, blood lipids, and body fat in children. *American Journal of Public Health*, December 1995, 85 (12), 1702–1706.

Maillet, J. O. Weight: Too heavy. Fortune: bleak. *New York Times*, November 5, 1995.

U.S. Department of Health and Human Services. *Physical Activity and Health: A Report of the Surgeon General*. Atlanta, GA: U.S. Department of Health and Human Services, Centers for Disease Control and Prevention, National Center for Chronic Disease Prevention and Health Promotion, 1996.

50. Shephard, R. J. Physical activity, health, and well-being at different life stages. *Research Quarterly for Exercise and Sport*, 1995, 66 (4), 298–302.

14 *Keeping it Going: The Older Athlete*

ADELAIDE HAAS, PH.D.

*I came in first in my age group, but if I had been five years **older**, I would not even have placed in the race. Three women in their sixties were much faster than I was. I wonder what it will be like when they are in their seventies and I'm a young 65?*
              —Dale, age 55, competes in local 5 & 10K running races

Most of us assume that as we get older, our athletic ability will diminish. We predict that our speed, strength, and endurance powers will slacken. We also may become afraid to push ourselves. More and more people our age seem to be injuring themselves and even dying. Is our exercise routine worth the risks? In this chapter some of the changes that occur with age will be explored. We consider limitations that may begin to show. More importantly, ways of maintaining healthy fitness throughout life will be examined. As Professors William Evans and Irwin Rosenberg, of the Center on Aging at Tufts University, point out, "chronology is not destiny."[1] Each of us ages differently; our objective should be to do it as well as we possibly can.

THE ACTIVE GENERATION

Bonnie Prudden, fitness guru to many young and old, describes those in the United States who were born before 1940 as "the last fit Americans." They had the advantage of growing up active. Most of them walked to school in all kinds of weather. They did not spend hours in front of the television or computer as young children, because neither had yet entered their homes. Much of their recreation consisted of physical activities such as running, jumping rope, or playing ball. This background laid a foundation for making them "naturally" fit.[2] Some of you older readers may have built on this and might continue to be energetic.

THE AGING PROCESS

Like it or not, no human function remains constant throughout life. As children, we could not compete with adults intellectually or physically; we were developing toward our full potential. And once we reach our peak, we find as older adults that we cannot stay there; we notice changes that we attribute to aging. While it may take firm resolve, we should not become discouraged with the physiological differences we encounter with advancing years.

> *On a recent ski weekend my 23-year-old granddaughter, Daniele, commented to me, "it must be great to be over 70 and ski free of charge." I retorted, "I'd rather be 23, and pay my own way." On the other hand, when I look around, I know that I can still ski faster and with better control than most of the younger people on the mountain.* —Sally, age 75

The Circulatory System

In order for your body to function, your blood stream must deliver oxygen to every cell, as we described in Chapter 3. The efficiency with which oxygen is transported is dependent on the work of your heart, lungs, and circulatory mechanism. This is known as **aerobic capacity** or **VO_2max.**

VO_2max is often considered the best single measure of overall fitness.[3] The more fit you are, the more able your body is to breathe in air and transport it to your muscles, permitting them to work at a high level. Put another way, a person with a high aerobic capacity or VO_2max can exercise longer and harder than an individual with a lower capacity.

As we age, our VO_2max declines. There are several reasons for this age-associated reduction in aerobic capacity:

- The heart muscle tends to decrease in size and responsiveness, so it pumps less oxygen-rich blood to the muscles.
- The muscles of the rib cage diminish in their ability to expand and contract. Since the lungs expand passively, and are dependent on the enlargement of the chest cavity to take in air, the effect is a lessened volume of air entering the body.
- Overall weakened muscle strength reduces the amount of oxygen that the muscles can use.[4]

While some decline is inevitable, regular exercise over time reduces the impact.

Target Heart Rates.   As we just noted, aerobic capacity diminishes in part due to a decline in heart efficiency. One measure of this is that our maximum number of heart beats per minute decreases with advancing age.

TABLE 14.1

....

Target Heart Rates Associated with Age

Age	Maximum Heart Rate Per Minute	Target Heart Rate Range* Per Minute	Per 10 Seconds
20	200	120–160	20–27
30	190	114–152	19–25
40	180	108–144	18–24
50	170	102–136	17–23
60	160	96–128	16–21
70	150	90–120	15–20
80	140	84–112*	14–19**

....

* 60% – 80% of maximum
** extrapolated

CAUTION: Individual factors, including the use of some medications for high blood pressure, affect heart rate. Your medical caregiver and your own common sense are your best guides.

Adapted from the following sources: Cooper, K.H. & Cooper, M. *The New Aerobics for Women.* New York: Bantam, 1988, pp. 33–34; Group Health Cooperative, on line at http://www.ghc.org/health_info/self/fitness/x2w_thr.html; and Mercy Hospital Medical Center, Des Moines, Iowa, on line at http://www.mercydesmoines.org/health/articles/hrt-rate.htm.

If you've ever taken an aerobics class, you have no doubt learned that target heart rates, as measured by your pulse, decline with each decade. You are simply not expected to make your heart beat as fast as you age. However, in general, the older woman may *feel* as though she is exerting herself to the same degree with a lower heart rate compared to the younger woman whose heart rate is higher during exercise. (See discussion of Perceived Rate of Exertion, later in this chapter and in Chapter 4, Focus on Fitness.) Table 14.1 provides target ranges for different ages based on studies at the Cooper Aerobics Activity Center in Dallas, Texas, and elsewhere.

Age is not the only factor in determining your target heart rate. The more fit you are, the higher you may allow your rate to go. For example, a 70-year-old woman who is in excellent shape may aim for a heart rate of 120 while engaging in aerobic exercise, while an unconditioned 20-year-old might also have the same target rate. The goals are based in part on your resting heart rate and on your recovery time. So if you have a low resting rate and your pulse bounces back quickly after a vigorous workout, due to either youth or fitness, you may train at relatively higher levels of intensity.

On the other hand, the more fit you are, the less your heart rate will increase for a given activity. In essence, if you lower your resting heart rate, your target heart rate can also be lowered and you will still achieve positive training effects. This is important, as many people erroneously believe they need to exhaust themselves in order to get any benefits. Furthermore, exercise physiologists point out that it is desirable to train at varying intensity levels.[5] (For specific guidelines on determining your target heart rate, refer back to Chapter 4, Focus on Fitness.)

Heart Health and Fitness. As we get older, we may be afraid that over-exertion will lead to heart attack. The origin of this fear of exercise may stem from ancient Greek times, when Phidippides died following his long hard run from Marathon to Athens.[6] Even today, we likely know someone who was running or shoveling snow and then collapsed of cardiac arrest. For example, Jim Fixx, the well-known runner and author of *The Complete Book of Running*, died of a heart attack at age 52 following a run.[7]

A careful investigation of the risks of cardiovascular problems associated with exercise was reported in the *Journal of the American Medical Association*. Researchers studied over 1,000 women, 17 to 73 years of age, as they engaged in a combined total of 110,037 hours of exercise over a five-year period. They reported *no* "cardiac events" for these women. The study also included almost 2,000 men, of whom two experienced acute, but not fatal, heart problems. One of the men, a 61-year-old businessman, who had not been training, collapsed in the middle of a 3.2 km race. The other man, age 35, ran a fast 4 km, although he had not been exercising regularly. He suffered a heart attack following the cold shower he took after running. (Showers after exercise are discussed later in this chapter.) Both men survived and resumed their exercise routines not long after these incidents. The researchers conclude that a very small risk of cardiovascular events exists for adults who exercise. The risk may be associated with lack of regular exercise, competition, smoking, and the presence of heart disease.[8]

Would we be better off just taking it easy? The answer is an emphatic "No." Ample evidence exists to demonstrate that people who are not physically fit more often have serious or fatal heart attacks than those who exercise regularly. It is generally agreed today that regular exercise helps to prevent heart and circulatory problems that can lead to a premature demise.[9]

Gauge Your Reactions to Exercise. As you exercise, your pulse rate will increase and you may sense your heart beating faster. You should expect to perspire and to breathe more deeply and rapidly. These are normal responses. However, if you experience any of the following exercise-related symptoms, *do not* continue exercising and *do* obtain medical advice.

Warning Signs

- Marked difficulty in breathing or catching your breath.
- Nausea, diarrhea, vomiting.
- Chest pain or tightness.
- Fainting, dizziness, headache, lightheadedness.
- Prolonged, marked exhaustion following exercise.
- Unrelenting muscle/joint pain, marked cramping.[10]

You should consult with your physician before beginning any exercise program. This is especially true as you get older and if you have high blood pressure, diabetes, or other medical conditions, or are taking medicine.

• **The One-Mile Timed Walk.** Chapter 4, Focus on Fitness, contains a description of the Rockport One-Mile Timed Walk test. If you do not have any known medical problems, this may be appropriate for you to use. However, be sure to stop should you exhibit any of the warning signs listed above. You will note that as you age, your aerobic capacity normally decreases. This is indicated by your need to take more time to walk a mile and a corresponding increase in heart rate associated with this exertion.

• **The Home Stress Test.** If weather or other limitations make the timed one-mile walk test difficult to accomplish, our adaptation of Bonnie Prudden's Step Test may provide a reasonable substitute. Ms. Prudden does not provide specific heart rate targets or aerobic capacity estimates. She states that this test is to determine your current level of fitness and chart personal improvement.[11]

In the procedures that follow, you'll note that in step 1, we suggest taking your pulse for a full 60 seconds. All other times we recommend that you take your pulse for 15 seconds and multiply by 4. The reason for this is that resting rate is best assessed by a full minute's count. On the other hand, since your rate drops rapidly following exercise, the 15-second count is used for all other measurements.

1. Lie down and relax for 10 minutes. Then take your pulse for 1 full minute. Record this under *Rest*.
2. Stand up. Take your pulse for 15 seconds and multiply by 4. Record this under *Standing*.

FIGURE 14.1

....

Bonnie Prudden's Heart Action Step Test

Date	Rest	Standing	Action	Steps	After 1 min.	After 5 min.

....

Adapted with permission from Bonnie Prudden.
Source: Bonnie Prudden's After Fifty Fitness Guide. New York: Ballantine Books, 1986, p. 79.

3. Step on and off a stair as many times as you can in one minute. Count "1" as you bring the first foot up; say "and" as you bring the second foot up. Count "2" as you bring the first foot down; say "and" as you bring the second foot down. Say "3" as the first foot goes up again, and so on. Take your pulse for 15 seconds immediately following this stepping activity. Record your pulse rate (using the 15 second times 4 method) as *Action*, and the number of steps as *Steps*.
4. Wait 1 minute after recording your action pulse and take your pulse again. Count the beats in 15 seconds and multiply by 4. Record this under *After One Minute*.
5. Sit down for 5 minutes. Take your pulse for 15 seconds, multiply by 4, and record this number under *After Five Minutes*.[12]

• **Estimate Your Level of Exertion.** In the 1980s, Gunnar Borg of the University of Stockholm, Sweden, devised a system for **rating perceived exertion** (RPE). The original Borg Scale was based on values from 6 to 20, with 6 equivalent to the estimate of a 60-beats-per-minute heart rate (resting rate), and 20 equivalent to 200 beats per minute (maximum exertion). This has been updated, so that 0 now indicates relaxation and 10 is the hardest effort possible. The reason for the modification is that age and condition influence the degree of intensity for an individual at any given heart rate. The ratings on the

TABLE 14.2

....

Gunnar Borg's Rating of Perceived Exertions (RPE) Scale

Rating Scale

Original RPE	New RPE	Description	Equivalent Intensity Level	Heart Rate*
6	0	Nothing		60 bpm**
9	1	Very Light		90 bpm
12	3	Fairly Light	60% MHR***	120 bpm
13	4	Somewhat Hard	70% MHR	130 bpm
15	5	Hard		150 bpm
16	6	Very Hard	80% MHR	160 bpm
19	10	Almost Max		190 bpm

....

Adapted from the following sources: Edwards, S. *The Heart Rate Monitor Book.* Port Washington, NY: Polar CIC Inc., 1993; and Howley, E. T., & Franks, B. D. *Health fitness: Instructor's handbook.* Champaign, IL 1992.

*Equivalent Heart Rates were the basis for the original scale; in fact they will vary considerably depending on the condition and age of the individual.

** bpm = beats per minute

*** MHR = maximum heart rate

original scale were quite accurate for younger and fitter individuals, but the new numbers should be applicable to the general population. Table 14.2 shows both original and new ratings of perceived exertion as they compare to *approximate* heart rate, percentage of maximum heart rate (MHR), and verbal descriptions.[13] The Borg Scale provides a rough measure of how hard your body is working. With practice, most of us can competently estimate the intensity of our exercise, especially when the effort is relatively hard. Dr. C. C. Dunbar and colleagues at the University of Pittsburgh compared individuals' judgments of exertion on a treadmill with clinical measures of oxygen used and heart (pulse) rate; they confirmed that most people are fairly accurate in estimating the intensity of their exercise simply by judging how they feel.[14]

• **Measure Your Heart Rate.** Instruments that monitor heart rate during exercise have become widely available to amateurs and professionals alike. These heart rate monitors are biofeedback devices that can be set at a predetermined target zone. The idea is to push yourself sufficiently to obtain a training effect but not so much that you collapse in exhaustion, although as we have just reported, the probability of the latter is exceedingly remote. (See Table 14.1, Target Heart Rates Associated with Age, and Chapter 4, Focus on Fitness.) When your activity level causes your heart rate to fall below or above the targeted area, most instruments will notify you with a beeping sound. It is then up to you to adjust your workout. This is especially important for those who have a tendency to over-exert, particularly during recovery from heart or other medical problems. It is interesting that optimal heart rate for distance training is much lower than many athletes realize. With a heart rate monitor, individuals are more aware of their level of exertion and can compare it to the recommended targets for serious competitors.

Heart rate monitors also offer the capacity for setting alternative training objectives on different workout days. This is desirable in developing a competitive edge—if only with yourself.

Take a Medically-Monitored Stress Test. If you have any of the warning signs noted earlier, or you have been diagnosed with a medical condition, you should consult your physician, who will likely recommend a stress test. While not infallible, medically-monitored stress tests may provide an indication of how safe aerobic exercise is for you. Treadmill tests can help determine your level of cardiovascular fitness and may indicate a need for further diagnostic testing.[15]

• **Routine Stress Test.** The simplest procedure measures your pulse, your blood pressure, and your heart's electrical activity through the use of an electrocardiogram (ECG) as you walk or run on a treadmill. If no abnormalities are found, you do not develop any warning symptoms, and your system returns to its resting condition relatively rapidly, you will probably be advised that you may exercise reasonably without fear.

• **Echocardiogram Stress Test.** Your heart's size, motion, and valve function can be visualized on a computer monitor through the use of high-frequency sound waves. A transducer—a small recording device—is placed against your chest. You then walk or run on a treadmill. The sound waves are recorded and studied by your physician. The findings will suggest the appropriateness of your exercise activities.

• **Nuclear Stress Test.** Heart function and blood flow may be studied by injecting a small amount of radioactive material into the bloodstream through an intravenous (IV) tube. Thallium or technetium-99m (Cardiolite) are the most commonly used radioactive tracers. A nuclear camera is used to capture an image of your heart. Typically, your heart will be studied during treadmill exercise; at a later time, the same measures will be obtained without exercise. The two profiles are then compared to evaluate the safety of an exercise program.

This procedure is not dangerous; you need not worry about the small amount of radioactive material used unless you are pregnant or nursing. The most common side-effect is a somewhat annoying metallic taste in your mouth. You probably will be advised to avoid any food, drink, and medications that may contain caffeine for the 4 to 6 hours before testing. Nuclear cardiology studies, although generally free of risk, are usually recommended only if there is a reason to suspect problems.

Improve Your Heart's Condition

I was inconsolable after Sam, my husband of 55 years, died. I wanted to die also. Knowing that I had 'a heart condition,' I decided to simply wear myself out. I took every opportunity to climb stairs, walk distances, and carry heavy groceries. I was convinced that I would use up my heart's allotment of beats and quickly follow my departed husband. But the opposite occurred. When I visited my physician about a year after Sam died, my doctor remarked on my excellent condition. He told me that my physical activity actually had strengthened my heart. Along with this physical improvement my attitude toward life also became better. I became a volunteer at a local hospital; I joined a walking club, and once again I feel good about myself.

—Molly, age 73

While Molly's approach clearly backfired and turned her life around in a positive way, women with known heart problems should seek medical advice before beginning a program of formal or informal exercise.

A team of physicians at the Veterans Administration Medical Center in Salt Lake City studied the effects of a four-month aerobic conditioning program on heart rate, blood pressure, maximal oxygen consumption, and physical work capacity of 55- to 70-year-old, previously sedentary women and men. Their subjects engaged in either fast walking or jogging at a prescribed target heart rate or stretching exercises for one hour, three days per week. The researchers found that all those who participated in any part of the program were able to stay on a treadmill longer, had lower resting and recovery heart rates, and lower resting systolic blood pressure at the end of the four months compared with the beginning. Four years after the study was completed, about two-thirds of the people who were in the program reported that they were still exercising because they enjoyed both the activity and the benefits.[16]

If you have reason to be concerned about your heart function, you should not exercise without medical guidance. A heart rate monitor might be especially helpful for you to stay within recommended target heart rates.

What to Do

If you do not have any medical contraindications and are free of warning signals when you exercise, regular aerobic exercise is valuable. You should not work at the same intensity level every time you train. Lower levels produce important benefits, and these targets should constitute a major part of your program.

I had a heart attack at age 50. My family and I were totally stunned when this occurred. I was not overweight, did not smoke, and appeared fit. I played tennis twice a week, coached girls' soccer, and was generally active. On the other hand, I had a hysterectomy at age 45, was not on hormone replacement therapy (HRT), and had borderline high (240) cholesterol. Since an angiogram and other tests revealed occluded arteries, I had heart by-pass surgery five days following the heart attack. Several weeks after the surgery, I was on a slow walking exercise regimen. Within a month I could walk for about an hour. Today, one year later, I am back to playing tennis and my previously active life. I have cut fat from my diet, and I take hormone replacement medication. I am truly grateful for the new lease on life.

—Barbara, age 51

Brittle Bones

We can often estimate a woman's age by watching her walk on ice and snow. Children and young people will run and slide, letting the falls come where they may. Middle-aged folks are typically deliberate but cautious. As we move into older age, we tend to watch every step. We don't want to risk falling. We have heard about hip fractures, long convalescences, and other tales of woe. In fact, the likelihood of breaking a hip doubles with every six or seven years after age 40.[17] Is it surprising that we watch our step?

Osteoporosis. The word osteoporosis comes from "osteo," which refers to bones, and "porosis," which means full of holes. If you have osteoporosis, the mineral content in your bones is insufficient. This results in fragile bones that tend to be thin around the edges and vulnerable to breakage. Loss of the mineral calcium in the bones is a corollary of aging. However, the degree to which our bones become osteoporotic is dependent on several factors in addition to aging. (See Table 14.3.)

Are You at Risk for Osteoporosis? Although we think of osteoporosis as an older women's disease, it strikes men too, and the consequences for them are just as serious. The difference is that it is more common among women, especially following natural or surgical menopause. Bone loss may begin in younger females, too, as a result of menstrual dysfunction. (See Chapter 11, Menstrual Matters.)

As you can see in Table 14.3, genetics, medical history, tobacco use, lifestyle, as well as estrogen depletion, all may play a role in whether or not you develop osteoporosis. If you are a black woman, you are considerably less likely to develop osteoporosis than a white or Asian woman.[18]

If, in the past, you had a substantial period of anorexia, engaged in considerable dieting and fasting, or exercised to excess, your body may have produced insufficient

TABLE 14.3

....

Factors Associated with Osteoporosis

Genetic or Medical Factors

Caucasian or Asian ancestry

Family history of osteoporosis

Early menopause (natural or surgical)

History of anorexia

History of amenorrhea

Diabetes

Kidney or liver diseases

Behavioral Factors

Smoking

High alcohol or caffeine use (more than 2 drinks / 4 cups a day)

Too little or too much weight-bearing exercise

Being confined indoors

Low dietary intake of calcium and vitamin D

....

Source: Haas, A., & Puretz, S. L. *The Woman's Guide to Hysterectomy: Expectations & Options.* Berkeley, CA: Celestial Arts, 1995.

Doress-Worters, P. B. & Siegal, D. L. *The New Ourselves, Growing Older.* New York: Simon & Schuster, 1994.

estrogen. A history of estrogen deficiency may make you more vulnerable to osteoporosis. On the other hand, too little exercise may decrease bone density, also placing you at risk. So weight-bearing exercise in moderation seems the best option.

Smoking, consuming more than two alcoholic drinks per day, or drinking more than four cups of caffeinated coffee, tea, or cola, all make you a more likely candidate for osteoporosis. However, ample amounts of calcium, vitamin D, and sunshine may offer some protection. (See Chapter 10, Food for Fitness.)

Determine Your Bones' Health. If you are in a high-risk group, it might be worthwhile to be evaluated for osteoporosis. The simplest means is to check your height every six months. If you are getting shorter, this may be a signal for concern, and you should check with your doctor about further testing. Before panicking, however, recognize that small differences in height are often hard to detect because hair style and posture contribute to inaccurate readings.

Bone densitometers provide a more reliable way for physicians to evaluate women who are symptom-free. These devices accurately detect the mineral content of bone using a method called **dual photon absorptiometry.**[19] The most-used machine is the **dual energy X-ray absorptiometer** (**DEXA**). It gives very little radiation exposure, takes less than half an hour, and the procedure may cost between $100 and $500. This is covered by many insurance plans, but as of this writing, Medicare only pays the cost if a problem is detected. Measures of the spine and hip generally are considered most useful. Test results are compared to a set of normal values of healthy young women as well as to age-matched women who do not have osteoporosis or other bone disease.

Protect Yourself Against Brittle Bones. While you cannot do anything about the genetic correlates associated with osteoporosis, you should be able to modify some of the other risk factors. Table 14.4 summarizes some things you can do to combat osteoporosis. The sooner you start, the better.

• **Hormone Replacement Therapy.** Physicians Cauley, Seeley, and Ensrud, reporting in the *Annals of Internal Medicine*, studied almost 10,000 women over age 65 at four clinical centers. They found that women who started estrogen therapy within five years of menopause and continued its use had 50 percent fewer nonspinal fractures than those not taking estrogen. Estrogen was especially helpful in preventing hip fractures in women older than 75, with an 80 percent reduction in incidence.[20] (For women with an intact uterus, estrogen is given in combination with progesterone.)

• **Non-hormonal medications.** Supplementing your diet with 1,200 to 1,500 mg of elemental calcium a day can help slow bone loss. Calcium carbonate is the most concentrated form available, and it can be purchased inexpensively as a drugstore or supermarket brand supplement or as an antacid tablet. These products are as effective as more costly "natural" health food preparations. If you take calcium supplements, be aware that the recommended daily allowance (RDA) of 1,200 to 1,500 mg for women over age 50 is based on the active calcium amount. Some compounds, such as calcium lactate, contain relatively small amounts of elemental (active) calcium. For example, a 1,200-mg tablet of lactate may mean only about 180 mg of available calcium. Be sure to carefully read the label of any product you use. You will not need to supplement by the full RDA amount since the foods you eat also contain calcium.[21] The level of supplementation you choose will depend on your diet. (See Chapter 10, Food for Fitness.)

Alendronate sodium tablets (5 mg/day for prevention and 10 mg/day for treatment of osteoporosis) are approved by the Food and Drug Administration as a means of increasing bone density and reducing the risk of vertebral fractures. Studies of post-menopausal women have shown that this chemical cuts the risk of bone fracture in half and significantly reduces height loss associated with osteoporosis. Alendronate, marketed under the brand name *Fosamax*, is available by doctor's prescription.[22]

A combination of low-dose (25 mg) **slow-release sodium fluoride** together with a regimen of calcium citrate also has been found to reduce the incidence of vertebral fractures in postmenopausal women. However, slow-release sodium fluoride has not yet been approved by the Food and Drug Administration. Excessive amounts of fluoride can cause internal bleeding and encourage abnormal bone growth. Once appropriate dosages are determined, slow-release sodium fluoride may prove helpful in the future for some individuals.[23]

• **Exercise.** If you have been exercising most of your life, you may have been "investing" in hip fracture protection. In a study in Rancho Bernardo, California, 1,014 women and 689 men with an average age of 73 years were asked to recall their level of exercise during their teens, 30s, and 50s. Those who were both currently active and had a history of physical exercise had greater bone mineral density in their hips than those who were more sedentary.[24]

But even if you just started to exercise, and you are past menopause, you may still preserve your bone integrity and reduce your risk of fractures. Tufts University scientists studied postmenopausal women between 50 and 70 years of age who were not receiving estrogen replacement and were formerly sedentary. Engaging in a high-intensity strength training program twice a week improved their muscle mass, strength, and balance and prevented bone density loss. Also, they were less likely to fall and less likely to break a bone if they did tumble.[25]

Bone mineral density can be improved by some types of exercise. Postmenopausal women who exercised on stationary bicycles regularly for a period of eight months were found to have greater bone density than women of similar age who didn't exercise. In fact, the bikers gained bone density while the sedentary women lost it. This is particularly interesting since it shows a reversal in bone loss.[26] (Other research cast doubt on the ability to build bone once it has been lost.[27])

Even walking at least one mile three times a week may protect against bone fractures, according to a study of over 3,000 residents of a Florida retirement community who averaged about 73 years of age. Walkers were significantly less likely than matched non-walkers to break any bones during the following year.[28]

Some researchers have emphasized that only those bones that have been the direct

What We Know

As we get older, our bones become more brittle, although our genetic makeup, estrogen levels, and exercise history influence the likelihood of osteoporosis. Bone mineral density can be reliably measured by the dual energy x-ray absorptiometer (DEXA). Whatever the outcome, we can take specific measures to reduce the probability of broken bones.

What to Do

If you are past menopause and fall into a high-risk group (See Table 14.3), talk to your physician about using hormone replacement therapy or alendronate sodium (Fosamax). At any age, weight-bearing exercise and sufficient calcium, in the diet and through supplements, may prevent and even reverse bone loss.

recipient of weight-bearing exercise improve in bone density. They point out that a specific site needs to be "overloaded" or stressed in order to be made stronger. This has been termed **site specificity**. In other words, tennis players have stronger bones in their forearms, and runners have stronger leg bones. These investigators note that if you wish to preserve bone integrity throughout your body you must embark on a strength training program that will involve all your bones.[29]

Flexibility

It's been said that decreased flexibility is the surest sign of aging. From having trouble touching your toes to being unwilling to change mealtimes, becoming rigid is often associated with advancing years. Physical therapists talk about your body's flexibility in terms of "range of motion" (ROM), and they recommend gentle stretching exercises to keep limber. Lack of flexibility limits what we can do, but over-stretching also is not recommended as that may result in pain and injury.

How Loose Are You?   Flexibility involves all parts of the body, and you would be wise to systematically assess your own limberness. Just because you can run a marathon does not assure that your body is loose enough to serve all potential needs. In fact, when you exercise vigorously, you tax your muscles, causing them to shorten. For this reason, the more you exercise, the more important it is to stay limber.[30] A number of measures of flexibility exist. In addition to the tests described in Chapter 4, Focus on Fitness, we've compiled a package from various sources,[31] so that you can test yourself from head to toe.

Test Yourself

Head and Neck Flexibility. While sitting tall in a straight-backed chair or stool, turn your head from side to side, then up and down, looking first at the ceiling and then at the floor. Now try looking forward while dropping your right ear toward your right shoulder; do the same thing on the other side. If you are of average flexibility, you should be able to do all these movements easily, with no discomfort.

Shoulder Flexibility. Test 1. Hold your right arm straight up against your right ear. Bend the elbow and move your right hand down your back as far as it will go. Try to meet your right hand with your left hand coming up your back. Switch hands. You should be able to get your fingertips to touch. You may find this easier on one side than the other. **Test 2.** Raise and lower your arm out to the side and try to make a 90 degree angle with your body. Try the same thing to the front. Repeat with the other arm.

Elbows. Let your arms hang down at your sides. Bend each elbow so that each arm forms a 45-degree angle. The lower part of your arm should be in front of you and your finger tips should be 8 to 12 inches from your shoulder.

Legs and Knees. Test 1. From a standing position, lift one leg out to the side. Can your legs form about a 40-degree angle? Do the other side. You may hold on to a wall or chair for support. **Test 2.** From a standing position, bend your knee and lift your thigh straight in front of you with your foot hanging down toward the floor. Your thigh should form a 45-degree angle with the rest of your body. Do the same on the other side.

Back and Hamstrings. Sit on the floor, legs straight out in front of you. Bend at the waist. You should be able to touch your toes with your fingertips.

Feet. In the same position as above, point your toes toward the floor. You should be able to move them about 40 degrees down from the flexed, straight-up position.

Getting and Staying Limber.   Several guidelines are helpful for achieving and maintaining optimum flexibility. While these were described in detail in Chapter 4, Focus on Fitness, a short review follows.

Easy Does It. Static stretching is considered best and safest. These stretches let the force of gravity assist your muscles in stretching beyond their normal length. The idea is to take a position and slowly and gently relax into your stretch. You should try to hold the stretch for about 15 seconds to permit your muscles to relax fully. It helps to take full breaths in and out as you hold your stretch. While years ago you may have been advised to bounce and push to the limit in a "ballistic" movement, research has demonstrated that easy, gravity-guided stretches are safer and more beneficial.[32]

Stretch after Warming Up and Cooling Down. Never begin your exercise or sport full force without a warm-up period. This consists of getting your heart rate up slightly by moving your body around and also stretching gently to limber those muscles that will be used. When you have finished your workout you should similarly slowly decrease your activity. Never stop moving abruptly. Always give yourself time to cool down and go through transition safely. Stretching is especially helpful following a workout. At this time your muscles are warm and your blood circulation is good. (Refer back to Chapter 4, Focus on Fitness, for a more complete discussion.)

Routines. The sequence for your entire routine should be: warm-up, stretch, workout, cooldown, stretch. In Chapter 4, Focus on Fitness, we discussed this in further detail. When you stretch you should consider your sport and make sure that appropriate muscles have been limbered. Secondly, include basic stretches in your routine, such as arm circles, body twists, leg stretches, sitting toe touches, squats, and an Achilles tendon stretch. You might consider Hatha Yoga or T'ai Chi, two Eastern disciplines that offer valuable methods for improving flexibility. See Chapter 4 for pictures of stretches that might be included in your fitness program.

Stretches to Avoid. As we get older, some stretches may cause more problems than they solve. Mary Ann Uznis, a physical therapist, advises that we especially protect the neck and knees.[33] For example, the yoga position known as the "plow," where you are on your back with legs and feet up and over your shoulders, may overly strain your back and neck. Often you are the best judge of what is and is not appropriate. Your stretches should make you feel good and limber. You should not feel pain; if you do, back off and try modified, gentler versions of the exercise.

Strength

When once a jar of jelly may have been easy to open by simply turning the cap, now many of us use more brain than brawn. We may heat the cover, puncture it, or tap it on the side. Some of us may still prefer to hand it over to an individual deemed stronger (a man?). It is not only that we are getting smarter, we are actually—sadly—also getting weaker.

We're Not As Strong As We Were. Physical strength declines with age. The culprits appear to be primarily muscle atrophy, decrease in number of fast-twitch muscle fibers, and loss of some motor nerves.

Muscles that are not used tend to decrease in size; they atrophy. Most people lose about 30 percent of their total number of muscle cells between the ages of 20 and 70. In

What We Know

We all tend to become less flexible as we get older, but regular gentle stretching helps to keep us limber.

What to Do

You should engage in static stretching following your warm-up and, if possible, after the cooldown portion of your exercise routine. Avoid stretches that hurt and those that may strain your back and neck.

addition, remaining muscle cells tend to get smaller. Taken together, less bulk translates into less strength.

As we described in Chapter 3, Body Works, muscles are composed of both fast-twitch and slow-twitch fibers. Slow-twitch are called into play to maintain posture and to engage in low-intensity movement. Fast-twitch fibers are required in high-exertion activities like sprinting. Researchers have shown that after about age 60, most of us have relatively fewer fast-twitch fibers contributing to our loss of muscle power. In addition, the number of motor neurons that stimulate our muscle fibers also decreases, further reducing our strength.[34]

Keeping and Building Strength.   Fortunately, if we continue to use our muscles, we may minimize the loss in strength, at least for a while. The muscles we use regularly tend to remain relatively strong. This was demonstrated by an investigation of grip strength of machine workers. Those who had been on the job for years and were now in their fifties had just as much isometric strength as workers 10, 20, and 30 years their junior.[35] It may be, however, that loss in strength occurs after age 50 or 60.[36] But there is some good news! Vigorous strength training at any age can actually *reverse* the decline and cause muscle cells to get larger and strength to increase.[37]

Speed and Endurance

Much as Dale, quoted at the beginning of this chapter, hopes to run faster as she gets older, the odds are not in her favor. As we age, most of us are not able to move as quickly as we did when we were younger, and our endurance may diminish.

World class masters runners exhibit a slow but steady decline in running speed. Table 14.5 shows running times for women World Class Record holders at various ages. Although it varies depending on the event, it may be reassuring to some readers that, in general, the biggest reduction in speed usually does not occur until after about age 70!

Why Do We Slow Down?   Speed is most accurately considered in two parts. One is reaction time, and the other is speed of movement. The former concerns how long it takes to get moving; the latter deals with the movement itself. While changes in the central nervous system as we age cause us to respond more slowly, the reduction in number of fast-twitch muscle fibers we talked about earlier is primarily responsible for reducing the speed of our movements. Age-associated rapid reaction time and speed of movement account for the fact that most world-class sprinters are in their late teens or early twenties, although in recent years some have continued training into their thirties.[38]

TABLE 14.5

....

Women's World Records for Running at Selected Ages

Time in Minutes & Seconds

Age	100 Yards	1-Mile	5-Kilometer	10-Kilometer
35	0:10.80	4:17.33	15:15.20	31:35.52
40	0:12.50	4:54.69	16:44.28	35:20.59
45	0:11.70	5:28.90	16:17.60	32:41.98
50	0:12.47	5:29.83	17:46.20	37:35.00
55	0:14.80	5:50.60	18:49.00	38:38.60
60	0:15.50	6:46.30	19:16.80	45:09.74
65	0:15.50	6:41.64	22:24.61	46:54.87
70	0:16.20	7:26.00	24:52.83	50:28.33
75	0:27.50	13:12.00	28:12.90	53:20.50
80			30:21.85	60:47.20
85			41:56.20	

....

Source: Masters Age Records 1990, Pasadena, CA: National Masters News, 1990.

Later in life, especially after menopause, women often gain weight, and our body-mass index increases. The amount of body fat we carry around often increases as our muscle weight decreases. Excess body mass may serve to slow us down![39]

Why Do We Poop Out?

When I was in my twenties and thirties a day of skiing meant just that. I was sure to get onto the slopes when they opened. I downed a quick sandwich and cup of hot chocolate for lunch, and then returned to ski until the lifts closed. Today, at age 57, I am relaxed about starting my skiing day. I enjoy a leisurely lunch, and I'm usually content to leave the slopes by 3 P.M. —Kitty, age 57

Many research physiologists attribute part of our age-related decline to a quicker buildup of lactic acid in our muscles during exercise. The influence of lactic acid may be felt in several ways. It takes us longer to get our heart rate and respiration back to normal after a

TABLE 14.6

....

Aerobic capacity of women at different ages and fitness levels

Fitness Level

Age	Poor	Average	Excellent
20–39	<26*	26–39	>39
40–49	<24	24–34	>34
50–59	<22	22–31	>31
60–69	<20	20–28	>28

....

* Numbers refer to VO_2max (milliliters × kilograms of body weight per minute). See Chapter 4, Focus on Fitness, for further information.

Adapted from Costa, D. M., & Guthrie, S. R. (Eds.). *Women and Sport: Interdisciplinary Perspectives.* Champaign, IL: Human Kinetics, 1994, p. 171.

vigorous workout. This means that whereas once we could coast for a while and then return with full vigor, with advancing years this becomes more difficult. Lactic acid may also contribute to the aches and pains that we feel long after the exercise is over. Is it any wonder that we need to quit early?[40] The role of lactic acid was discussed more fully in Chapter 3, Body Works.

To further exhaust us, our maximum oxygen consumption (VO_2max) decreases with age, as we discussed earlier in this chapter. Dr. Susan L. Evans and her colleagues at the Department of Kinesiology at the University of Colorado studied 31 highly trained female runners aged 23 to 56 who participated in a 10K race. They took numerous physiological measures of these runners who had placed first, second, or third in their age and sex class in either 1993 or 1994. They confirmed that both running velocity and aerobic capacity decrease with advancing age, resulting in more time required to run a given distance.[41]

The American Heart Association has compiled normative data for VO_2max for women of different ages and fitness levels. (See Table 14.6.) No matter how fit you are, you can expect your VO_2max to decrease with age.

Is There an Up Side?   With advancing age, we may not be as fast or last as long as when we were younger, but those who continue to exercise throughout life have far greater speed and endurance than their non-exercising sisters. If you stop to look at the accomplishments of the masters athletes (Table 14.5), you'll agree that their times for *all* events are formidable. And as we noted earlier, the most marked declines do not occur until after age 70. But even here, studies have shown that elderly nursing home patients can improve their speed and endurance in treadmill and stationary bicycle exercises when they engage in a conditioning program.[42]

PUTTING IT ALL TOGETHER

As we age, we are not as strong, fast, or coordinated as we once were. In addition, our stamina declines. To further compound the matter, advancing age often brings illnesses that may limit our athletic prowess. We'll first review some common physical problems, then take a more cheerful look at the brighter side of our advancing years.

Working Out with Injuries and Medical Problems

Later years often bring considerable health problems. Table 14.7 shows the percentage of women over age 65 with various chronic conditions. So if you are in that age bracket and experience medical complaints, you will note that you have plenty of company.

Musculoskeletal Problems. In his provocative book, *The Exercise Myth*, Henry A. Solomon, M.D. cites studies reporting the incidence of injuries in various sports. He concludes from the data that about two-thirds of runners are forced to cut back or stop entirely due to injury at least once during their running career, and almost half of all squash players are hurt while playing their sport.[43]

In our own survey of 497 women, we found that 42 percent of those who were over age 50 had injured themselves sufficiently during exercise at one time in their lives to alter their activity; however, almost all (99 percent) resumed their active lives after a period of rest and recuperation.

> *Mother's position on her own injuries, reiterated every time the subject came up, was that you couldn't do anything athletic for twenty, thirty, forty years without suffering damage of some sort, could you?*[44]
> —Jane Smiley in *Barn Blind*. NY: Fawcett, 1980, p. 138.

Until fairly recently, medical researchers believed that women were more vulnerable to orthopedic injury compared to men. This likely contributed to the rationale for limiting women's physical activity.[45]

Today, however, activity and training rather than gender have been found to influ-

TABLE 14.7

....

Some chronic health conditions in women over age 65

Condition	% of Women
Arthritis	55
Hypertension	41
Ischemic heart disease	12
Other heart disease	19
Orthopedic impairment	19
Chronic sinusitis	17
Diabetes	10
Varicose veins in legs	10
Chronic bronchitis	7
Frequent constipation	7
Abdominal hernia	6
Cerebrovascular disease	6

....

Data from: Cohen, R. A., & Van Nostrand, J. F. Trends in the health of older Americans: United States, 1994. National Center for Health Statistics. *Vital Health Statistics*, 3 (30) 1995.

ence the likelihood of injury. For example, while exercise experts Mona Shangold, M.D. and Gabe Mirkin, M.D. observe that women are more likely than men to get hurt while exercising, they suggest that this is because, in general, women do not know how to condition themselves as well as men do. Shangold and Mirkin maintain that "Men were taught to get in shape *before* exercising; women were taught to get in shape *by* exercising."[46] This may hold true especially for older women.

> *Before I started exercising I was fine . . . no sprains, no aches and pains. But now, my knees often hurt and my back feels stiff. Sometimes I need to modify the routine that the aerobics instructor is teaching so that it doesn't hurt me. If I didn't love it and feel that it was still good for me, I'd quit. I'm thinking about taking aspirin before class, but I was told that's dangerous since it might tempt me to push myself too hard.* —Maxine, age 46

As we age, we are more likely to accumulate injuries. Fortunately, this can be minimized, as we pointed out before, by warming up, stretching, and cooling down. In addition, proper equipment, thoughtful planning, finding an alternative activity, and cross-training can make exercise safer. See Chapter 5, Routines: The Stars Are the Limit.

Circulatory Problems. Researchers are generally in agreement that exercise is beneficial for individuals with adult-onset diabetes, high cholesterol, high triglyceride levels, and depression. What kind of exercise is appropriate for people with high blood pressure remains a matter of medical discussion.[47]

High Blood Pressure. Almost half of women over age 65 have hypertension. Endurance exercise is often recommended as a way of preventing high blood pressure, but those who are already hypertensive may be the recipients of mixed information. Individuals with high blood pressure are at greater risk for cardiovascular disease than others. Because of this, it is argued that there is an increased danger of a fatal heart attack or incapacitating stroke as a result of vigorous exercise. Recent research suggests that this concern is largely unwarranted. Nevertheless, certain guidelines should be followed.

• **Use Medications Appropriately.** If your blood pressure is over 140/90 mm Hg (hypertension), you should be under a doctor's care. If your readings are above 180/105 mm Hg, this is considered moderate to severe high blood pressure and you will probably be advised to stop *heavy* exercise until your pressure has been satisfactorily reduced. Medication will likely be prescribed.

Diuretics and ACE-inhibitors are generally preferred. Beta-blockers are also effective in lowering blood pressure, but they may interfere with exercise by reducing your maximal aerobic capacity and also give you an exaggerated perception of your exertion level. Calcium channel blockers are sometimes prescribed for hypertension, but their efficacy in reducing heart attacks has been questioned. Since all of these drugs are sold under a variety of brand names, you should be sure to ask your doctor or pharmacist about the medication prescribed for you. New medications are continually being developed and some of these may prove to be particularly valuable.[48]

• **Drink Plenty of Fluids.** Anyone engaged in athletics should make sure to avoid dehydration. This is particularly true for any individual who is taking hypertensive medication, particularly diuretics. (See Chapter 10, Food For Fitness, for more information about fluid intake.)

• **Adjust Your Workout.** In the past, individuals with high blood pressure may have been advised that while aerobic exercise was fine and even helpful, weight training should be avoided. Recent studies have shown that eliminating strength training from your routine is usually not necessary.[49]

The keys to safe weight training are: do not lift more than about 50 percent of your maximum one-repetition weight, and avoid holding your breath. By keeping your weights under 50 percent of maximum and engaging in about 12 to 15 repetitions per set, you will build muscle tone without forcing an abnormally high blood pressure response. Breath holding (the **Valsalva maneuver**), sometimes associated with trying to lift maximum weights, is never recommended, but should be avoided even more carefully if you have high blood pressure.[50]

Caution! If your high blood pressure is associated with a heart abnormality, such as enlargement of the left ventricle, vigorous exercise may pose a serious risk. In such a case, your physician may encourage you to engage in moderate activity, but caution you against heavy strength training and some competitive events.

Anyone with *severe* high blood pressure should avoid straining and lifting unduly heavy weights. Similarly, sports such as rock climbing, competitive rowing, and gymnastics may not be appropriate for you. These activities may cause the systolic pressure to rise to seriously dangerous levels.[51]

• **Shower Wisely**. Beware of cold showers. When you take a cold shower, the blood vessels in the skin constrict so as to keep your vital organs warm. Narrowing of the blood vessels tends to increase blood pressure because the same quantity of blood is trying to force its way through a more narrow passageway. For this reason, if your blood pressure is normally elevated, cold showers may raise it to potentially dangerous levels.[51]

On the other hand, you don't want to jump into a steaming shower, sauna, or hot tub immediately after exercising either. It takes about 45 minutes for your body to fully return to its non-exercising condition. Excessive heat interferes with the cooldown process and delays your heart's return to normal function. A shower with lukewarm water should cause no problems. Some women just towel off, powder, and put on dry clothes after a workout, saving the complete washup for later.[52]

Adult Onset Diabetes. Individuals with diabetes are generally advised to engage in regular vigorous physical activity.[53] The usual reminders to warm up and cool down apply. If you have diabetes, you should continue to exercise and follow the guidelines we described in Chapter 4, Focus on Fitness.

• **Weight Training**. Simply put, for non-diabetic people, control of sugar levels (glucose) in the bloodstream occurs naturally. The hormone insulin stimulates the body's muscles to take in and use the sugar they've ingested. With diabetes, the body becomes less tolerant of sugar and less able to utilize it. Developing your muscle mass will increase your muscles' need for glucose, thereby reducing the excess in the bloodstream. For this reason, a combination of weight training and aerobics is of special value for those with diabetes.[53]

What We Know

The older we get, the more likely it is we have experienced musculoskeletal injuries and have illnesses that may limit our exercise.

What to Do

Consult with a sports-minded physician before beginning or resuming workouts. Be sure to follow the guidelines for adequate fluid intake, warm-ups, and cooldowns. Be willing to switch or modify your activities in keeping with your physical condition. Something is better than nothing!

• **Fluid Intake.** As we noted earlier, all athletes should be sure to stay well hydrated; this is especially true if you have diabetes. Drink frequently before, during, and after working out. Remember that even if you don't feel thirsty, you should take in water. Cold-weather exercise requires water replenishment, just as warm-weather exercise does. Do not let yourself get dehydrated.

• **Injuries.** With diabetes, blood circulation is typically impaired, making injuries slower to heal. For this reason, you may want to be extra careful to avoid hurting yourself. In addition, the sensation of pain, especially in the extremities, is often decreased. This may make you less aware of simple problems such as cuts or sores. A podiatrist may recommend special footwear to prevent injuries to your feet. You should select a physical activity with these limitations in mind—and then go out and do it![54]

Keep On Moving

Do the Differences Make a Difference?   As we age, we slow down. We are not as physically strong, and we have less endurance. Some of us may have given up team sports like softball or soccer because we felt that we were no longer doing our bit. We may have switched from tennis singles to doubles or from tennis to golf because that rhythm now suits us better. If we live long enough, we will all experience a decline in athletic ability. However, regular exercise will keep us fit longer and make our later years more pleasurable.

Working Out Smarter. We are wise to modify our exercise routines as we age and should not be disappointed if we can't do what we once did. If you've been physically active all of your life, you are at a definite advantage. It's easier to continue doing something you know rather than starting from scratch. Remember the old saw about teaching an old dog. . . . However, that isn't always the case. One gutsy 60-year-old woman who responded to our questionnaire noted that after years as an avid skier, she recently tried snowboarding for the first time and loved it! But that's *not* for everyone.

• **The Advantages of Practice.** The more you do anything, in general, the better you'll be at it. Years of a sport or other physical activity may provide you with skills that younger folks do not possess. What they may have in energy, strength, and reaction time, you may match in know-how and trained muscles. While this is not always an even trade, it is a motivator to continue with an activity with which you have experience.

• **Listen to Your Body.** For many of us, nothing beats an exercise high! We get that endorphin rush, and we want to work out forever. Sometimes our friends encourage us to keep pushing, go faster, work harder. But our inner voice is wiser. If you feel pain, discomfort, serious fatigue, or breathlessness, these are signs that something is wrong. Slow down; walk easily until your body stabilizes. This is true at any age, but especially so during our later years. There is wisdom in our bodies, and we would be fools not to listen.

- **Duration over Intensity.** When you engage in very strenuous exercise, your blood pressure rises, and when you stop it tends to drop rapidly. Sudden cessation may make you dizzy or cause you to faint. For this reason, especially if you have circulatory problems, you'd be advised to switch from activities calling for spurts of energy to those that are gentler but last longer. An extended cooling-down period is also helpful.[55]

> *I joined the "silver sneakers" branch of the Appalachian Mountain Club about six months ago. This group of older people meets for long hikes most weekends of the year. To my delight I found that many of the hikers were formerly runners who decided to stretch out the pleasures of their exercise.* —Delores, age 64

- **Low or High Impact?** Because our bones may be more susceptible to breakage and heal more slowly as we age, we would be prudent to select activities that are relatively gentle to our skeletal structure. Low-impact aerobics, such as those provided in "step" classes, may be preferable to jumping around, especially on a hard surface. Many runners find that a cushioned track, grass, or a dirt trail is easier on their systems than road work. Swimming provides a wonderful total body workout without taxing our bones. Yoga and t'ai chi are other ways of getting solid exercise with almost no risk of injury.
- **The All Important Warm-up and Cooldown.** With advancing years, transitions require more time. Taking a good ten minutes to build up from your non-exercise state to workout level will help prevent damage to all parts of your body. Unwarmed, you are more likely to tear a muscle or tendon. Similarly, allow yourself time to come down from your exercise peak slowly, giving your body a chance to readjust. Remember, stopping suddenly will rapidly and perhaps dangerously lower your blood pressure, causing dizziness, fainting, and/or falling.[56]

Here's to Long Life and Good Health.   As the classic toast suggests, everyone wants a long life and good health. But does exercise play a role?

Longevity. While it would be nice to say that exercise guarantees a long life, the evidence is mixed. You don't have to look far to find older people who feel fine and have never exercised or younger ones who worked out faithfully and died prematurely. But what are the odds?

Dr. John W. Rowe, director of the MacArthur Foundation Consortium on Successful Aging, concludes that, "Only about 30 percent of the characteristics of aging are genetically based: the rest—70 percent—is not."[57]

Recent evidence suggests that regular exercise throughout life contributes to a longer lifespan. For example, Dr. S. N. Blair and colleagues at the Institute for Aerobics Research in Texas compared longevity of women and men who were in five different fitness categories. Those who were sedentary were placed in category one; individuals who ran 30 or more miles a week were in category five. Following more than 13,000 subjects for eight years, the investigators found that women who were in the least fit category died at a rate more than four times greater than those who were most fit. They attributed this largely to higher rates of cardiovascular disease and cancer among their unfit subjects. They found that even a little exercise will contribute to longer life. The researchers suggest that "an unfit woman might reduce her risk of dying by almost 50 percent if she became fit."[58] Dr. Lawrence Kushi and associates at the University of Minnesota School of Public Health studied more than 40,000 post-menopausal women and concur that even moderate activity as infrequently as once a week reduces the risk of death, and vigorous physical activity at least four times a week confers even greater longevity benefits.[59]

Quality of Life. The relationship between good health and exercise is well documented. Even previously sedentary women appear to gain from physical activity. For example, Dr. Patricia Gillett studied women between the ages of 60 and 72 who had not exercised in the past. After an 11-week program that included one hour of aerobic dance three times a week, the dancers reported improved energy, sleep, flexibility, strength, mobility, feelings of self-esteem, and general well-being compared with the non-dancers.[60] Regular exercise is effective in providing protection against osteoporosis, heart disease, and excess weight.[61] It can often contribute to relief of the bodily aches and pains, constipation, diarrhea, and more serious physical problems that may plague us as we age.[62] Working out, especially in the company of others, has also been documented to counter the depression that is common among the elderly.[63] Regular exercise has been so successful in making life better as we age that it has been recommended as a "preventative prescription" instead of drug therapy.[64]

Superstars. In 1955, Emma (Grandma) Gatewood was the first woman to "thru-hike" the Appalachian Trail, a 2,000-mile wilderness path stretching from Maine to Georgia. She was 68 years old and completed this trip in 146 days, pitching her plastic shower curtain for shelter and eating only cold food (such as cheese, raisins, and nuts) that she bought in local groceries along the way.[65] She repeated this accomplishment several times prior to her death in 1973 at age 85.

Record-holding female competitive athletes reveal some impressive accomplishments. Ruth Rothfarb and Ida Mintz, both over 80 years of age, ran marathons (26 miles) in slightly over five hours. Those are roughly 11.5-minute miles. Many younger people cannot do even one mile at that rate.

Helen Zechmeister holds the world dead lift record for women between the ages of 75 and 79. She lifted 220.5 pounds. Other women of all ages continue to compete as runners, bicyclists, swimmers, oarswomen, and in track and field events. While the records for those who are older do not match those of younger competitors, they remain impressive and far exceed what most ordinary people hope to do at any age.[66]

For those who are interested in competition, master's events for older athletes are available at local, national, and international levels.

Join the Fun. With advancing years, we may have more time to enjoy ourselves. Perhaps we've retired from our jobs, and our children are grown. Many organizations are geared to active "seniors." The Over the Hill Gang, International, which has its home base in Colorado, offers discount skiing, river rafting, bicycling, and even "heli-skiing" for the most adventurous. Other groups, such as North Wind Tours and Mountain Travel, provide hikes of varying levels of difficulty and duration—with food, lodging, and baggage delivery—for older outdoor lovers. Some of these opportunities are for men and women, and others are geared to women alone. You can select your preference.

The 2,000-mile Appalachian Trail has been attracting more and more groups of older women who band together to hike sections at a time or to even become "thru-hikers" and do the whole thing. One group, The Happy Hikers, has members ranging in age from 60 to 80. They hike once a week and always celebrate each other's birthdays on the trail with cakes they pack in.[67] Can you think of a better way to mark advancing years?

Whether you choose to exercise alone or with others, the benefits are great. It does not matter whether you are already well-conditioned or just starting out: The only way to reap the health and happiness rewards is to keep on moving.

ENDNOTES

1. Evans, W., Rosenberg, I. H., & Thompson, J. *Biomarkers: The 10 keys to prolonging vitality*. New York: Fireside, 1991.
2. Prudden, B. *Bonnie Prudden's after fifty fitness guide*. New York: Ballantine Books, 1986.
3. Cooper, K. H., & Cooper, M. *The new aerobics for women*. New York: Bantam Books, 1988.
    Evans, W., Rosenberg, I. H., & Thompson, J. *Biomarkers: The 10 keys to prolonging vitality*. New York: Fireside, 1991.
4. DiGiovanna, A. G. *Human aging: biological perspectives*. New York: McGraw-Hill, 1994.
5. Edwards, S. *The heart rate monitor book*. Port Washington, NY: Polar CIC Inc., 1992.
6. Hayflick, L. *How and why we age*. New York: Ballantine Books, 1994.
7. Henderson, J. Joe Henderson's journal: He's on the list. *Runner's World*, 1995, 30 (1), 14.
8. Gibbons, L. W., Cooper, K. H., Meyer, B. M., et al. The acute cardiac risk of strenuous exercise. *Journal of the American Medical Association*, October 17, 1980, 244 (16), 1799–1801.
9. Spirduso, W. W. *Physical dimensions of aging*. Champaign, IL: Human Kinetics, 1995.
10. Doress-Worter, P. B., & Siegal, D. L. *The new ourselves, growing older: Women aging with knowledge and power*. New York: Simon & Schuster, 1994.
11. Personal communication with Bonnie Prudden, May 1, 1997.
12. Prudden, B. *Bonnie Prudden's after fifty fitness guide*. New York: Ballantine Books, 1986.
13. Edwards, S. *The heart rate monitor book*. Port Washington, NY: Polar CIC Inc., 1992.
    Evans, W., Rosenberg, I. H., & Thompson, J. *Biomarkers: The 10 keys to prolonging vitality*. New York: Fireside, 1991.
    Howley, E. T., & Franks, B. D. *Health fitness: Instructor's handbook*. Champaign, IL: Human Kinetics, 1992
14. Dunbar, C. C., Robertson, R. J., Baun, R., et al. The validity of regulating exercise intensity by ratings of perceived exertion. *Medical Science Sports Exercise*, January 1992, 24 (1), 94–99.
15. Cooper, K. H., & Cooper, M. *The new aerobics for women*. New York: Bantam Books, 1988.
16. Steinhaus, L. A., Dustman, R. E., Ruhlin, R. O., et al. Aerobic capacity of older adults: a training study. *Journal of Sports Medicine Physical Fitness*, June 1990, 30 (2), 163–172.
17. Doress-Worter, P. B., & Siegal, D. L. *The new ourselves, growing older: Women aging with knowledge and power*. New York: Simon & Schuster, 1994.
18. Cummings, S. R., Nevitt, M. C, Browner, W. S., et al. Risk factors for hip fracture in white women. *New England Journal of Medicine*, 1995, 332 (12), 767–773.
19. Kritz-Silverstein, D. & Barrett-Conner, E. Early menopause, number of reproductive years, and bone mineral density in postmenopausal women. *American Journal of Public Health*, 1993, 83 (7), 983–988.
20. Cauley, J. A., Seeley, D. G., Ensrud, K., et al. Estrogen replacement therapy and fractures in older women. *Annals of Internal Medicine*, 1995, 122 (1), 9–16.
21. Consumer Reports. Calcium: How to get enough. *Consumer Reports*, August 1995, 60 (8), 510–513.
    Prince, R. The calcium controversy revisited: Implications of new data. *Medical Journal of Australia*, September 1993, 159 (6), 404–407.
    The Nation's Health. Institute of Medicine recasts dietary requirements for calcium. *The Nation's Health*. September 1997, 6.
22. Liberman, U. A., Weiss, S. R., Broll, J., et al. Effect of oral alendronate on bone mineral density and the incidence of fractures in postmenopausal osteoporosis. *New England Journal of Medicine*, 1995, 333 (22), 1437–1443.
23. Pak, C. Y., Sakhaee, K., Adams-Huet, B., et al. Treatment of postmenopausal osteoporosis with slow-release sodium fluoride. Final report of a randomized controlled trial. *Annals of Internal Medicine*, September 15, 1995, 123 (6), 401–408.
24. Greendale, G. A., Barrett-Connor, E., Edelstein, S., et al. Lifetime leisure exercise and osteoporosis. The Rancho Bernardo study. *American Journal of Epidemiology*, May 15, 1995, 141 (10), 951–959.
25. Nelson, M. E., Fiatarone, M. A., Morganti, C. M. et al. Effects of high-intensity strength training on multiple risk factors for osteoporotic fractures. A randomized controlled trial. *Journal of the American Medical Association*, December 28, 1994, 272 (24), 1909–1914.

26. Bloomfield, S. A., Williams, N. I., Lamb, D. R., et al. Non-weightbearing exercise may increase lumbar spine bone mineral density in healthy postmenopausal women. *American Journal of Medical Rehabilitation*. August 1993, 72 (4), 204–209.

27. Allen, S. H. Exercise considerations for postmenopausal women with osteoporosis. *Arthritis Care Research*, December 1994, 7 (4), 205–214.

    Drinkwater, B. L. 1994 C. H. McCloy Research Lecture: Does physical activity play a role in preventing osteoporosis? *Research Quarterly for Exercise & Sport*, September 1994, 65 (3), 197–206.

28. Sorock, G. S., Bush, T. L., Golden, A. L., et al. Physical activity and fracture risk in a free-living elderly cohort. *Journal of Gerontology*, September 1988, 43 (5), 134–139.

29. Drinkwater, B. L. 1994 C. H. McCloy Research Lecture: Does physical activity play a role in preventing osteoporosis? *Research Quarterly for Exercise & Sport*, September 1994, 65 (3), 197–206.

30. Shangold, M., & Mirkin, G. *The complete sports medicine book for women*, revised. New York: Simon & Schuster, 1992.

31. Kusinitz, I., & Fine, M. *Your guide to getting fit*, 3rd ed. Mountain View, CA: Mayfield Publishing Co., 1995.

    Prudden, B. *Bonnie Prudden's after fifty fitness guide*. New York: Ballantine Books, 1986.

32. Shangold, M., & Mirkin, G. *The complete sports medicine book for women*, revised. New York: Simon & Schuster, 1992.

33. Uznis, M. A. Forum: more exercise alternatives. *The Physician and Sportsmedicine*. August 1995, 23 (8), 7.

34. DiGiovanna, A. G. *Human aging: biological perspectives*. New York: McGraw-Hill, 1994.

35. Petrofsky, J. S., & Lind, A. R. Aging, isometric strength and endurance, and cardiovascular responses to static effort. *Journal of Applied Physiology*, 1975, 38, 91–95.

36. Spirduso, W. W. *Physical dimensions of aging*. Champaign, IL: Human Kinetics, 1995.

37. Evans, W., Rosenberg, I. H., & Thompson, J. *Biomarkers: the 10 keys to prolonging vitality*. New York: Fireside, 1991.

    Spirduso, W. W. *Physical dimensions of aging*. Champaign, IL: Human Kinetics, 1995.

38. DiGiovanna, A. G. *Human aging: biological perspectives*. New York: McGraw-Hill, 1994.

    Evans, W., Rosenberg, I. H., & Thompson, J. *Biomarkers: the 10 keys to prolonging vitality*. New York: Fireside, 1991.

39. Spirduso, W. W. *Physical dimensions of aging*. Champaign, IL: Human Kinetics, 1995.

40. DiGiovanna, A. G. *Human aging: biological perspectives*. New York: McGraw-Hill, 1994.

41. Evans, S. L., Davy, K. P., Stevenson, E. T., et al. Physiological determinants of 10-km performance in highly trained female runners of different ages. *Journal of Applied Physiology*, May 1995, 78 (5), 1931–1941.

42. Naso, F., Carner, E., Blankfort-Doyle, W., et al. Endurance training in the elderly nursing home patient. *Archives of Physical Medicine and Rehabilitation*, March 1990, 71 (3), 241–243.

43. Solomon, H. A. *The exercise myth*. San Diego, CA: Harcourt Brace Jovanovich, 1984.

44. Smiley, Jane. *Barn Blind*. New York: Fawcett Columbine, 1980.

45. Solomon, H. A. *The exercise myth*. San Diego, CA: Harcourt Brace Jovanovich, 1984.

46. Shangold, M., & Mirkin, G. *The complete sports medicine book for women*, revised. New York: Simon & Schuster, 1992.

47. Jacober, S. J., & Sowers, J. R. Exercise and hypertension. *Journal of the American Medical Association*, June 28, 1995, 273 (24), 1965.

48. Jacober, S. J., & Sowers, J. R. Exercise and hypertension. *Journal of the American Medical Association*, June 28, 1995, 273 (24), 1965.

    Psaty, B. M., Heckbert, S. R., Koepsell, T. D., et al. The risk of myocardial infarction associated with antihypertensive drug therapies. *Journal of the American Medical Association*, August 23/30 1995, 274 (8), 620–625.

    Tanji, J. L. Exercise & the hypertensive athlete. *Clinics in Sports Medicine*, April 1992, 11 (2), 291–302.

    Tanji, J. L. & Batt, M. E. Management of hypertension: adapting new guidelines for active patients. *The Physician and Sportsmedicine*, February 1995, 23 (2), 47–55.

49. Jacober, S. J., & Sowers, J. R. Exercise and hypertension. *Journal of the American Medical Association*, June 28, 1995, 273 (24), 1965.

50. Tanji, J. L. Exercise & the hyper-

tensive athlete. *Clinics in Sports Medicine*, April 1992, 11 (2), 291–302.

51. Jacober, S. J., & Sowers, J. R. Exercise and hypertension. *Journal of the American Medical Association*, June 28, 1995, 273 (24), 1965.

    Tanji, J. L. & Batt, M. E. Management of hypertension: adapting new guidelines for active patients. *The Physician and Sportsmedicine*, February 1995, 23 (2), 47–55.

52. Shangold, M., & Mirkin, G. *The complete sports medicine book for women*, revised. New York: Simon & Schuster, 1992.

53. Evans, W., Rosenberg, I. H., & Thompson, J. *Biomarkers: the 10 keys to prolonging vitality*. New York: Fireside, 1991.

54. Canabal Torres, M. Y. Exercise, physical activity, and diabetes mellitus. *Boletin Associacion Medica de Puerto Rico* (San Juan), Feb 1992, 84 (2), 78–81.

    Sims, L., Stamm, D., & Parajon, R. Proper footcare is important for everyone, especially diabetics. *Poughkeepsie Journal*, January 23, 1996, Family Health, 7.

55. DiGiovanna, A. G. *Human aging: biological perspectives*. New York: McGraw-Hill, 1994.

56. Prudden, B. *Bonnie Prudden's after fifty fitness guide*. New York: Ballantine Books, 1986.

57. Brody, J. E. Good habits outweigh genes as key to a healthy old age. *New York Times*, February 28, 1996, c9.

58. Blair, S. N., Kohl III, H. W. Paffenbarger, Jr., R. S., et al. Physical fitness and all-cause mortality: A prospective study of healthy men and women. *Journal of the American Medical Association*, November 3, 1989, 262 (17), 2395–2401.

59. Kushi, L. H., Free, R. M., Folsom, A. R., et al. Physical activity and mortality in post-menopausal women. *Journal of the American Medical Association*, April 23/30, 1997, 277 (16), 1287–1292.

60. Gillett, P. A. Senior women's fitness project: A pilot study. *Journal of Women & Aging*, 1993, 5 (2), 49–66.

61. Hazzard, W. R. Weight control and exercise: Cardinal features of successful preventive gerontology. *Journal of the American Medical Association*, December 27, 1995, 274 (24), 1964–1965.

62. Pahor, M., Guralnik, J. M., Salive, M. E. et al. Physical activity and risk of severe gastrointestinal hemorrhage in older persons. *Journal of the American Medical Association*, 1994, 272 (8), 595–599.

63. Butler, R. N., Collins, K. S., Meier, D. S., et al. Older women's health: Clinical care in the postmenopausal years. A roundtable discussion part 2 (clinical conference). *Geriatrics*, June 1995, 50 (6. 33–6, 39–41.

    Chavez, V. Z., Lopez, Y. O., Martin, M. J., et al. Benefits of physical exercise in the elderly. *Revista Cubana de Enfermeria* (RNM), July–December 1993, 9 (2), 87–89.

64. Fujita, Y. Avoidance of drug therapy in the elderly: Exercise as a preventative prescription. *Drugs and Aging*, January 1995, 6 (1), 1–8.

65. Dale, F. T. Mighty and mischievous Grandma Gatewood. *Appalachian Trailway News*, July/August 1995, 9–14.

66. Spirduso, W. W. *Physical dimensions of aging*. Champaign, IL: Human Kinetics, 1995.

67. Tyner, G. From menopause to Medicare—and beyond. *Appalachian Trailway News*. July/August 1995, 15–17.

15 *Getting Personal*

ADELAIDE HAAS, PH.D.

If a sprain caused by tennis prompts the use of an elastic bandage around your wrist, chances are you'll wear it proudly and eagerly explain how your injury came to pass. But not all problems associated with exercise are talked about openly. In this chapter, we get "personal." Our discussion will include bathroom functions and sexual concerns.

THE PROCESS OF ELIMINATION

Bladder Matters

While they may not openly discuss it, about one-third of all women (twice as many women as men) experience some degree of involuntary urinary leakage, whether they exercise or not. Some consider this serious enough to give up the exercise that they associate with the problem. Many others treat the leakage as a mild inconvenience that can be tolerated or managed in one way or another.[1]

Types of Urinary Incontinence. While certain exercises tend to bring on urinary leakage, "exercise incontinence" is not considered a "type" since the problem is rarely confined just to working out. Leakage during exercise is most likely **urinary stress incontinence.**

   Stress Incontinence. Loss of urine associated with exercise, coughing, sneezing, and so on is usually considered stress incontinence. It is the result of increased abdominal pressure and can often be controlled by quickly sitting down.[2] We will discuss stress incontinence in more detail a little later.

   Urge Incontinence. An unexplainable, uncontrollable need to urinate is most likely urge incontinence. This type is not related to exercise or activity. Urinary infections, tumors, and side-effects of certain drugs may cause this problem.[2]

Neurogenic Incontinence. Some disorders involving the nervous system, such as Parkinson's disease and diabetes mellitus, may affect the nerves that control the muscles necessary for normal bladder function. Again, this problem is not generally related to activity.[2]

Continuous Incontinence. A steady leak of urine is probably due to a fistula (an abnormal body passage or opening) caused by trauma from surgery or extremely difficult vaginal delivery.[2]

Causes of Urinary Stress Incontinence. **Urinary stress incontinence** is the medical term for involuntary loss of urine resulting from increased abdominal pressure. Coughing, straining, laughing, hitting a tennis ball, running, and jumping up and down can all result in loss of support to the bladder, thereby leading to leakage of urine. A study by University of Michigan physician/researchers examined the characteristics of women who reported involuntary expulsion of urine during exercise. They found that stress incontinence is *not* related to race, occupation, educational level, height, weight, menopausal status, use of diuretics, high blood pressure medication, estrogen replacement therapy, or birth control pills. Urinary stress incontinence *is* most closely influenced by childbirth.[3]

A Hidden Cost of Childbirth. The best single predictor of stress incontinence is the number of babies a woman has had by vaginal delivery. Table 15.1 shows the relationship between the number of vaginal childbirths and urinary stress incontinence.

As you can see in Table 15.1, while not having children is no guarantee that incontinence will never be a problem, the likelihood of experiencing stress incontinence increases dramatically with the number of children a woman has had. Almost 75 percent of women who have given birth vaginally to three or more children are unable to control urine leakage at least some of the time.[3]

Sally Inch, author of *Birthrights*, persuasively demonstrates that childbirth itself should not cause incontinence. Rather, the manner of birth may be more to blame. For example, the use of forceps for delivery or a poorly performed episiotomy (incision that enlarges the vaginal opening) may weaken muscles associated with urine control. In addition, delivering a baby in a lying-down position and "pushing uphill," sometimes with a bladder that is not completely empty, may contribute to later continence problems.[4]

Today about one-fourth of all births are by cesarean section. While it is unlikely that any women choose this surgery in order to avoid urinary problems later in life, C-sections are associated with a reduced incidence of incontinence.

TABLE 15.1

Urinary Stress Incontinence and Number of Vaginal Childbirths

Number of Vaginal Childbirths	Percent Reporting Incontinence
0	22
1	38
2	57
3	73

Data from Nygaard, I., DeLancey, J. O. L., Arnsdorf, L., et al. Exercise and incontinence. *Obstetrics and Gynecology*, 1990, 75 (5), 848–851.

The Bounce Effect. The more you jump around when you exercise, the more likely you are to get that uncontrollable urge to release urine. More than a third of women who run or engage in high-impact aerobics experience some incontinence. On the other hand, few women have urinary problems while lifting weights. Table 15.2 shows the relationship between various exercises and urinary stress incontinence.

Don't Jump to Conclusions. Urinary stress incontinence should not be a reason to stop exercising. The Michigan researchers found similar problems with urinary control among women who were not regular exercisers. In addition, only one woman in their study of 326 women indicated that she lost urine only during exercise and at no other time. All the other women experienced some incontinence at different times of their day as well. Such commonplace (and often hard-to-avoid) activities as laughing, coughing, sneezing, lifting furniture, vacuuming, and lawn mowing were reported to bring about wetness. In fact, incontinence was found to occur more often during routine daily activities than during exercise.[5]

A Problem of Aging? The Michigan research team found that urinary stress incontinence was related to aging among women who had never given birth by vaginal delivery. In this group, leakage was reported by 9 percent of those 30 or younger, 41 percent of those between 30 and 49 years of age, and 50 percent of those between 50 and 65. Among women who had given birth, age was apparently not a factor, although other studies[6] report that all forms of urinary incontinence (see Types of Urinary Incontinence above) are more common among older women.

TABLE 15.2

··

The Relationship between Various Activities and
Urinary Stress Incontinence

Exercise	Number Participating	% Incontinent during activity
Running	99	38
High-impact aerobics	94	36
Tennis	37	27
Low-impact aerobics	134	22
Walking	164	21
Golf	38	18
Bicycling	81	16
Racquetball	31	13
Swimming	87	12
Weight lifting	54	7

··

Table adapted from Nygaard, I., DeLancey, J. O. L., Arnsdorf, L., et al. Exercise and incontinence. *Obstetrics and Gynecology*, 1990, 75 (5), 848–851.

However, advancing age, by itself, should not be considered the leakage culprit. Weakened muscles, often from too much sitting and too little exercise, may impair bladder control. Certain medications, such as some tranquilizers, antidepressants, and antihistamines, taken by many older women, may also interfere with bladder control.[7]

Reduced estrogen around the time of menopause causes thinning of the vaginal walls and may similarly affect the urethra with resultant incontinence. Also, surgical complications associated with hysterectomy and repair of uterine prolapse or cystocele (protrusion of the bladder through the vaginal wall) may affect urinary and related structures and/or neural mechanisms.[8]

Managing Stress Incontinence.   Although stress incontinence is quite common among women, we are often reluctant to talk about it. This is unfortunate, because other women can sometimes suggest solutions and let us benefit from their experience. The following suggestions are things you can do on your own. If the problem persists, you should see your physician for a full diagnosis. Medical and surgical approaches are discussed later in this section.

Watch Your Fluid Intake. While it is important to drink about eight glasses of water a day (more in warm weather and if you exercise a great deal), some of us who are inclined toward variety may substitute other fluids such as coffee, tea, soda, or even alcoholic beverages. Caffeinated and alcoholic drinks do *not* count in the minimum recommendations. These drinks are diuretics and cause a frequent urge to urinate, thus dehydrating rather than hydrating your system.

You may be tempted to cut down altogether on your fluids, reasoning that if you don't drink much, you'll need to urinate less. While this appears to be logical, too little water may result in dehydration, with resultant complications such as exhaustion and fainting. This is not the route to take!

• **Tank Up.** The two days before a major race or other athletic competition is the time to fully hydrate your body. Mary, a 55-year-old grandmother who has successfully completed 16 marathons and one ultra (50-mile race) in the past 15 years, uses the following routine:

> *I drink as much water as I can tolerate for several days before a marathon. My urine becomes clear. I continue to drink heavily immediately prior to and during the race. Most of this liquid is absorbed and used by my body during the competition. Should I need to urinate during the event, I let it happen! Especially during warm weather, this is not a problem. I assure you that I am not alone! —Mary, age 55*

Other runners try to drink as much water as they can the previous day, but avoid all liquids for one to two hours before the event. If they feel thirsty immediately before a competition, they simply rinse their mouth with water and spit it out. Water taken during a competition generally is used by the body and urinary urgency does not occur.

Try to modify these regimes for your daily or regular workout. Plan your day so you take lots of fluids two hours or more before you exercise; then consider stopping. You will prevent both dehydration and urgency. You should drink large amounts of water, or water and sport liquid (see Chapter 10, Food for Fitness) *after* the session or event. *Remember: It is most important to avoid dehydration!*

Improve Your Toilet Habits. As an adult, you may spurn advice about toileting, but if you are experiencing stress incontinence the following hints may be helpful.

• **Empty Your Bladder Fully.** Do you ever notice a need to urinate immediately after urinating? Don't hesitate to return to the toilet to continue to empty your bladder. Several suggestions may be helpful. (1) After urinating, stand up, walk around the bathroom for a minute or so (brush your teeth; comb your hair), then sit down again on the toilet. (2) Let water run lightly while you are urinating; this may encourage your own flow. (3) Press gently on your lower abdomen and lean forward while sitting on the toilet to push more urine from your bladder.

• **Clean Yourself Thoroughly After Using the Toilet**. Remember to always wipe from front to back to avoid infecting your vagina and urinary tract with fecal matter. Europeans are accustomed to a bidet where they can wash their genital area carefully after a bowel movement or sexual activity. Since most of us don't have this piece of equipment, we can substitute a quick jump in the shower. Just remove your bottom garments, including shoes, and either squat under the bathtub faucet, or use a removable shower head to carefully cleanse yourself. As another alternative, a moist towelette, found in the baby section of most supermarkets, may be more effective than toilet paper after moving your bowels.

Do the Kegel. In the 1940s, Dr. Arnold Kegel, a gynecologist, devised a set of pelvic floor exercises to help women who suffered from urinary incontinence following child delivery. **Kegel exercises** improve vaginal tone and help to prevent the release of urine during coughing, laughing, sneezing, or exercise. Kegel-type training also can enhance sexual satisfaction.

Kegel exercises strengthen the **pubococcygeal** (PC) muscles that encircle and support the vagina. Many variations of these pelvic floor exercises now exist. The basic movements are described below. Be sure not to tighten your abdomen or buttocks or hold your breath while doing these exercises. The point is to isolate and gain control over the PC muscles.

1. Lie on your back with knees bent. Contract by tightening your vaginal muscles as if you were squeezing or holding a tampon in place. Maintain this position for three or four seconds; relax for ten seconds. Do this five times in a row, three times a day. Increase the length of time you hold the vaginal contraction to eight seconds and the number of sets to ten. Remember to relax the full ten seconds between contractions and to keep breathing throughout.
2. When you are able to hold the tense position for eight seconds, top each long contraction with three quick short contractions.
3. When you are comfortable with exercise 2, you are ready to do these contractions in a variety of positions, such as standing and sitting.
4. After some practice, if you have successfully mastered steps 1 through 3, you are ready for step 4. Concentrate on moving an *imaginary* object from the outside of your vagina to a place deep inside. You should have a drawing in sensation.

5. The last exercise is the opposite of the previous one. In step 5, you bear down, focusing on pushing an imaginary object out of your vagina. Visualizing a large tampon may be helpful.

When you have gone through all five steps, continue to do all of the exercises several times a day. An advantage to Kegel exercises is that by stage 3, you can do them anywhere, anytime. Whether you are waiting on line at the grocery, watching television, driving a car, or reading, no one need know that you are working on urine control.[9]

Lose Some Weight. Extra flesh in the abdominal area may contribute to pressure on the bladder. If this is true in your case, losing weight may be helpful. Obviously, this is easier said than done. You may feel that you are already doing all that you can to control your weight. However, some careful examination of your eating habits and exercise routines (See Chapters 5 and 10) may help tighten up those abs.

Consider Panty Shields. Most supermarkets and drugstores carry an array of protective devices. Don't hesitate to use these if necessary. First of all, it is important not to restrict your activities because of incontinence. Secondly, panty shields are not visible under your clothing; you can keep them a private matter.

Keep Exercising. The overall value of exercise cannot be denied: you feel better physically and psychologically, you look better, and you are likely healthier than your non-exercising sisters. Remember that exercise itself is not a *cause* of urinary incontinence. While jogging and jumping around may prompt some leakage, you can generally keep this from becoming a real problem by planning and sometimes utilizing professional assistance.

Professional Assistance with Urinary Incontinence. In the past, most women were reluctant to discuss lack of urinary control with their medical caregiver. And sadly, many health care professionals were not trained to provide adequate guidance.[10] Fortunately, today we are more open and better informed. If the suggestions given above do not solve your problems, you should consult your primary physician. Careful evaluation of your particular situation may lead to a referral to a urologist, gynecologist, physical therapist, or other specialist.

Estrogen Replacement Therapy. The functions of estrogen in the female body are multiple. In addition to its role in reproduction, estrogen lowers the risk of osteoporosis and heart attack. Estrogen also contributes to vaginal moisture and urethral tone. Some researchers have found that replacing estrogen in women who are not producing it adequately may assist in improving urinary control.[11]

Body fat of less than 10 percent of your total weight, caused by exercise and/or diet, may interfere with estrogen production. (Normal body fat for a fit post-pubescent female is between 16 and 25 percent; over 30 percent is considered obese, although the number is slightly higher for women over age 50. Desirable body-fat percentages for males are considerably lower.)[12] If you are premenopause, increasing your weight usually prompts a normal return of estrogen. Occasionally a physician may prescribe birth control pills, which contain estrogen, to further assist you. (See Chapter 11, Menstrual Matters.)

Decreased amounts of estrogen are also associated with menopause. Hormone replacement therapy (HRT), including both estrogen and progesterone, is frequently recommended at this time. In addition to reducing hot flashes, mood swings, and vaginal dryness, it may help reverse urinary incontinence.[13]

Note: The determination as to whether to take HRT should be made after balancing the benefits with the potential drawbacks, for example the possible increased risk of breast cancer.

Drug Therapy. Various medications, such as alpha-adrenergic drugs (ephedrine), beta blockers, and imipramine may help in improving urinary control. Dr. Rene Genadry, an Associate Professor of Gynecology and Obstetrics at The Johns Hopkins Medical Institutions, reviewed numerous studies of pharmacological treatment and concluded that a combination of some of the above substances, including estrogen, is more effective than any single drug.[14]

Help with Kegel Exercises. Many women master the Kegel exercises, described earlier in this chapter, by carefully following these or similar instructions; however, about 40 percent of women require professional help. Although pelvic floor exercises seem quite straightforward, expert guidance to make sure that you are doing them correctly is generally advocated.[15]

• **What's Your Grade?** Physical therapists and other medical professionals often use a system of muscle grading to assess function. While the concept of grading is more generally applied to muscles of the arms and legs, it is also useful in describing the muscles of the pelvic floor. *Normal* muscle ability occurs when a test position is held against gravity and maximum pressure. This describes the ability to hold urine even with a very full bladder or to stop the flow of urine in mid-stream. A *fair* grade is when the flow of urine can be stopped with the help of gravity (for example: sitting down), but a cough, laugh, or jump will force some leakage. A *poor* or *zero* grade is the inability to alter the flow of urine.

Caution! Do not stop and start the flow of urine as an exercise; it should only be done as a test procedure. Repeatedly stopping your flow may cause the urine to back up and result in upper urinary tract infection.[16]

Once the strength of the muscles of your pelvic floor has been evaluated or graded, the effectiveness of any training program can be measured against this baseline information.

• **Biofeedback.** Monitoring your ability to stop your urinary flow provides an easily observable indication of how well you are developing your muscles. This form of feedback, however, is *not* recommended as a training procedure since it may result in bladder infection, as noted above. Safer biofeedback mechanisms include the use of a **vaginal perineometer, vaginal cones,** or, more simply, your finger.

The perineometer is an instrument that typically consists of a balloon-type probe placed into the vaginal cavity. This is hooked up to a recording device, such as a computer. As you contract your PC muscles, numerical values are shown on a screen. You are then able to visualize how effective your pelvic floor exercises are.

Vaginal cones come in different weights, normally from 20 to 70 grams (about one to three ounces). They are shaped like tampons and consist of a metal weight covered by smooth plastic. As PC muscles strengthen, you should be able to retain successively heavier cones by voluntary contraction.

A finger or tampon placed in the vagina can be held in place or forced out by muscle contraction. The success of this effort is easily observed.

Electrical stimulation has also been used to develop awareness of the muscles required for bladder control. An electrode is introduced into the vagina. Repeated brief spurts of electrical stimulation, a few seconds in duration, followed by rest, are provided during sessions that last 10 to 15 minutes. These stimulate a spontaneous PC muscle response, thereby helping the woman localize the contractions necessary for urinary control.[16]

Biofeedback techniques have been reported to significantly improve or cure urinary stress incontinence in about 80 percent of the women who use this approach.[17] Pelvic floor exercises without biofeedback, but with the assistance of a physical therapist or other skilled professional, are effective in more than half of women. Studies have shown that once the muscles have been adequately trained, their effectiveness in controlling incontinence is maintained for at least 5 years.[18]

Mechanical Support. A diaphragm used for contraceptive purposes may provide some support to the back wall of the urethra, thus helping to block the flow of urine. A **pessary** may be even more helpful. This rubber or silicone device is similar to a diaphragm but is a bit larger and firmer. Placed into the top of the vagina, a pessary helps support the bladder, resulting in a decrease in stress incontinence. A pessary is sometimes recommended in cases of a prolapsed uterus. You will need to see your medical provider to have one fitted.[19]

Surgery. If urinary incontinence persists and exercises and mechanical measures prove unsatisfactory, surgery may be appropriate. Surgery is used typically to reposition a "dropped" bladder. It cannot strengthen weakened pubococcygeal muscles. The surgical option has inherent risks and benefits, which need to be carefully explored before proceeding.[20]

When You Have to Go on the Go

Know Your Neighborhood.   If urinary urgency is a problem while you are running or working out, you need to plan your routine. Exercising in a gym or confined space has the advantage of bathroom facilities nearby. You can simply walk out of class or your activity and tend to business.

Location becomes an issue if your exercise of choice is running or outdoor bicycling. If you are on the streets of a city, scout out available restrooms *before* the situation becomes desperate. Restaurants, bars, supermarkets, gas stations, hotels, hospitals, police stations, and other municipal buildings frequently have toilets available to the public. Plan your route so that you will never be too far from one of these.

If you work out at a stadium with a running track or at a public park, you will often find that restrooms are available. Check their location before you have a pressing need.

I enjoy running on trails in a state park that is a few miles from my home. On one of my jogs, I felt an urgency and squatted behind some bushes several feet from the trail. At the moment of putting myself together, two other women runners came by. I was clearly embarrassed and tried to hide the fact that I had urinated in the woods, when one of the passersby called "Don't worry, I do that all the time." —Loni, age 36

Do It Like a Man.   Males urinate outdoors in public, often quite easily. They may simply step off a trail to relieve themselves. Of course, they have the advantage of being able to stand up. But you, too, can stand while peeing. A plastic funnel and tube, available in pharmacies and designed originally for women confined to bed, can also be used by the woodswoman or athlete. The funnel top of this "pee-shooter" is placed against the opening of your urethra. You then release and direct a stream of urine through the plastic tube, without needing to crouch. You will find that your pubic area remains dry, and no toilet paper is necessary.

If you are wearing shorts, you can avoid pulling your pants down and possibly remain standing, even without special equipment. Simply pull the crotch fabric firmly over to one side. With practice you should be able to urinate without getting yourself wet.

Avoid Paper Pollution. If you decide to squat in the woods and use toilet paper, place it in a plastic bag, carry it out, and then discard in an appropriate receptacle. If this is not possible, another alternative might be to dig a hole with a stick and bury the paper in some soil and leaves. Although paper will eventually decompose, in the weeks that it takes

What We Know

Urinary stress incontinence is very common, especially in women who have given birth to several children. Running and high-impact aerobics are most likely to bring about the urgency.

What to Do

Do not limit your water intake! Avoid caffeinated beverages. Try to time your drinking so that it does not interfere with your activity. Do urinate immediately before exercising and take steps to fully empty your bladder. Consider Kegel exercises or biofeedback training (with professional assistance). If the situation is severe and you cannot relieve it through simple methods, consult your health caregiver about the use of a pessary, medication, or as a last resort, surgery.

to happen, wads of used toilet paper near a hiking or running trail are both unhygienic and unsightly, so make every effort to either carry paper out or bury it well.

Incidentally, spreading your vaginal lips with your fingers will help you avoid wetting your pubic hair. In this case, no toilet paper is needed at all.

Runners' Runs

People who exercise regularly are rarely constipated. Aerobic workouts, in particular, increase the contractions of the colon.[21] Exercise, in moderation, can also relax the bowel.[22] But this can have a downside.

Nearly half of all women runners have experienced nausea, vomiting, and/or loose stools *after* a vigorous competition or workout.[23] About one in three women runners has had the urgent need to defecate *during* a run.[24] While "**runners' runs**" occur in people of both sexes, this condition is more common among women and probably among younger runners.[25]

Dr. Randall Swain of the Department of Family/Sports Medicine at West Virginia University in Charleston summarized the findings of several studies. This summary is presented in Table 15.3. Dr. Swain observes the wide range in reported problems, depending on the particular study, and concludes "all one can say is that these problems do occur and the frequency is at least one in ten runners."[26]

Prevention.   No definitive technique exists for avoiding runners' runs. The suggestions below are based on individual case reports as well as medical research.

Watch What You Drink and Eat. Certain foods, such as dairy products, coffee, tea, and colas, may contribute to bowel urgency. Try avoiding these. Also, check your intake of dietary fiber; you may be having too much of a good thing!

Eat lightly the night and morning before a major event. Foods high in potassium, like cantaloupe and bananas, are helpful. Be sure to drink enough, especially on warm days and during long workouts. Sometimes insufficient liquid (dehydration) is associated with gastrointestinal problems during exercise.

Some runners find it helpful to take anti-diarrheal medication such as *Pepto-Bismol* or over-the-counter loperamide before a major competition; however, this should not be a routine practice. Cathartics and laxatives to force a movement before a race are *not* recommended.[27]

"Gut Training". Dr. Frank M. Moses, of the gastroenterology service unit at Walter Reed Army Medical Center in Washington, D.C., reports that it may be possible to train one's gut. To do this, cut back your exercise duration and intensity to a point where you do not feel bowel pressure. Stay with this level of exercise for a week or so. If you

TABLE 15.3

....

Incidence of Gastrointestinal Problems during Exercise

Type of Problem	Percent Reporting *
Cramping	11–30
Urge to Defecate	12–54
Defecating during Exercise	16–44
Diarrhea during Exercise	8–30

....

* Since these data are compiled from several studies, the number of subjects on which these percentages are based varies.

Composite data based on Swain, R. A. Exercise-induced diarrhea: when to wonder. *Medicine and Science in Sports and Exercise*, 1994, 26 (5), p. 524.

gradually increase your routine, your digestive system should be able to tolerate more vigorous exercise.[27]

Regulate Your Timing. Regular habits are helpful to physical well-being. Routines can provide comfort to both mind and body. Try to eat meals and do exercise at regular times. While it is wise to allow several hours for your body to digest food prior to exercise, you might be amazed at the accommodations your system can make.

I joined the army at age 18. Every morning about 30 minutes after breakfast, my troop was expected to run ten miles. I had prided myself on my physical fitness before joining, and thought this should not be a problem. However, for the first two weeks, I suffered from nausea and often diarrhea during and after the run. My drill sergeant, more empathic than those pictured in most movies, advised me to give it time. My body would adjust. In fact, after those initial weeks, I ran the ten miles with no ill effects. —Rosemary, age 44

When preparing for a major competition, try to have a bowel movement before the event. Get up several hours earlier than you might think necessary. Drink a large glass of juice and a glass of warm water; eat a piece of fruit and a muffin. Then jog lightly. This may move things along, prompt a movement, and spare you gastrointestinal pressure later.

FIGURE 15.2

···

Hints for Avoiding Runners' Runs

1. Try to be regular in your habits: a usual time for bowel movements and a set time for exercise.
2. Do no exercise sooner than three hours after eating.
3. Keep well hydrated; drink lots of fluids.
4. Do not drink coffee or other caffeinated beverages.
5. Avoid the use of laxatives.
6. Be careful not to have an excess amount of fiber in your diet.
7. Try to have a bowel movement *before* you exercise, and especially before a major event.
8. Consider taking over-the-counter loperamide or *Pepto-Bismol* 30 minutes before an event.
9. Try drinking lactose-reduced milk instead of regular milk, or limiting your intake of dairy products.
10. If the problem persists and/or is severe, see your physician.

···

Sources: Moses, F. M. The effect of exercise on the gastrointestinal tract. *Sports Medicine*. 1990, 9 (3), pp. 159–172.

Shangold, M., & Mirkin, G. *The Complete Sports Medicine Book for Women*. New York: Simon & Schuster, 1992.

Swain, R. A. Exercise-induced diarrhea: when to wonder. *Medicine and Science in Sports and Exercise*, 1994, 26 (5), p. 524.

In Case of Urgency.   As with urinary incontinence, knowing your neighborhood toilet facilities in advance can permit a quick retreat.

If you need to move your bowels in a wooded area, go well off trail, dig a hole several inches deep, then cover your excrement and toilet paper with dirt and leaves. Use a stick you found for the purpose beforehand, and stir. Top with additional leaves and dirt. For a full, environmentally sensitive discussion, the entertaining book by Kathleen Meyer, *How to Shit in the Woods* (Ten Speed Press), is strongly recommended.[28]

"A Stress Test for the Colon".   Dr. Randall Swain presents evidence to support his hypothesis that "running (may be) . . . 'a stress test for the colon.'" He proposes that vigorous exercise may bring out an underlying medical condition rather than being the primary cause of gastrointestinal (GI) distress. He reports that in one study of 109 runners, 91 (83 percent) might have had diarrhea or related difficulties for reasons other than running. These other factors include: irritable bowel syndrome (15 percent), lactose intolerance (15 to 20 percent), and high fiber diet (25 percent).[29] Although the incidence of underlying GI disturbances among athletes sounds high, if you suffer from persistent bowel problems associated with exercise you would be wise to consult a physician for appropriate medical consultation and tests.

Flatulence

Gas may contribute to stomach cramps and interfere with your routine. If you exercise with others, flatulence can also be an embarrassment. Trying to conceal gas is primarily a female concern. In some male groups, flatulence is openly joked about, and they do not attempt to keep this natural function hidden. Relieving the gas freely may help to avoid or reduce abdominal distress. (When it comes to urination and flatulence, men may have some advantages!)

As a woman, it might help to know that exercise flatulence is quite common, although some people are more prone to this than others. As you work out, the colon tends to contract, causing you to pass gas. While you might accept flatulence openly, as many men do, there are things you can do to minimize it. Prevention of flatulence is usually best accomplished through modification of your diet. In some individuals, foods such as milk, onions, beans, celery, carrots, brussel sprouts, cabbage, and pastries are likely to cause intestinal gas. Experiment with avoiding these foods.

Consult Your Health Care Provider.   If you are bothered by significant abdominal cramping, flatulence, diarrhea, or other gastrointestinal distress associated with exercise, you would be wise to consult your physician. As we indicated earlier, a continuing problem may signal bowel disease and warrants careful professional evaluation.

SEX AND EXERCISE

In the 1950s and '60s, athletes were often cautioned to avoid sexual activity prior to a major event. College football players were instructed to be in bed (*alone*) by 9:30 the night before the big game. Some coaches even warned them that masturbation would sap their strength. How valuable were these instructions? Surprisingly little research has been pub-

---

What We Know

At least one in ten runners has experienced the need to have a bowel movement either immediately after or during a workout or competition.

What to Do

If diarrhea is a frequent problem related to your exercise routine, consult a physician, because your distress may be symptomatic of an underlying problem such as lactose intolerance or irritable bowel syndrome. Avoid excess fiber, caffeine, laxatives, and possibly dairy products. Try to schedule a regular time for your bowel movements and a regular time for your exercise.

lished on the relationship between exercise and sexuality, and much that exists focuses on men. We'll share both the scientific and the anecdotal data on the next few pages.

The Energy Equation

Human energy is *not* like a tank of gas, where the more you use for one purpose the less you have for another. In fact, in some ways, it is quite to the contrary. To become strong, you need to expend energy or train. Several important questions remain to be considered: (1) How soon prior to a major athletic event can you afford to use sexual energy? (2) Does exercise affect sexual interest? (3) Does a commitment to fitness affect a relationship?

The Winning Advantage. Dr. Charles Garfield has studied factors associated with peak performance. He noted that sex before a major event does not impair performance. On the contrary, it may even help. The night before a major competition, athletes are likely to feel tense and unable to sleep. Orgasm and the "afterglow" are good relaxants.[30]

The medical editor of *Runner's World*, Dr. Gabe Mirkin, reported that he "interviewed a runner who broke a world record one hour after masturbating." Mirkin further observed that the energy expended during sex is remarkably little. "Sex takes about as much energy as walking up two flights of stairs."[30]

Confirming this observation, in a sample of 500 women runners responding to a *Runner's World* survey,[30] 57 percent reported that sex before running does not affect their training (27 percent said that it did, and 16 percent did not know). Responses from men were similar.

So, while the research is limited, most survey respondents and experts agree: You do not deplete your energy resources by having sex prior to an athletic event. You may, in fact, make yourself even more competitive.

Libido

How does exercise influence interest in sex? The simplest measure of desire is frequency of activity. However, how often people engage in sex is also influenced by many other factors such as partner availability, desirability, and interest; attitudes toward masturbation; health; living arrangements; privacy issues; and so on.

Frequency Studies. There is little scientific information on the relationship between exercise and frequency of *female* sexual activity. Dr. James R. White, and his associates at the University of California, San Diego, studied the frequency of sexual activity and orgasm among 95 previously sedentary, middle-aged men. Most of the subjects were put on a program that consisted of an average of one hour of intense aerobic exercise three or four days a week for nine months. The others were placed on a walking schedule for comparable time periods.

All the men kept diaries. When month one and month nine were compared, those in the highly aerobic group reported increased sexual activity, including orgasms. In fact, the more aerobic gain an individual man made, the more likely his sexual capacity also increased. The walkers did not show an increase in sexual activity.[31]

Whether aerobic exercise contributes to sexual desire and activity in women remains to be confirmed. When the women in our study were asked, "What benefits have you experienced that you attribute to exercise?," almost all wrote that they "look and feel better," "have greater self esteem," "have more energy," and similar responses that might suggest a more positive outlook toward sex as well. Melanie Roffers, a health club director cited in *Runner's World*, more precisely noted, "Physical fitness increases energy for everything, including sex."[32]

The Fatigue Factor. Just as the coaches of yesterday were afraid that their players would tire themselves out with sex, and therefore would compete poorly, some people are afraid that physical exercise will leave them too tired for sex.

Moderate exercise or even intense exercise for moderate periods of time is likely to *increase* your physical energy and desire for sex. But overtraining, which leaves you exhausted, may in fact detract from your sexual interest and capacity. Overtraining, as we discussed in Chapter 4, has other adverse affects and should be avoided for many reasons.

Feeling Sexy.   All forms of exercise, from aerobic dance to yoga, contribute to women's increased feelings of sexiness. First of all, when you engage in a physical activity, you become more in touch with your body. Your focus becomes more physiological. When the body is aroused sexually, muscles throughout the body respond. The improved tone brought about by exercise may enhance these sexual feelings.

Secondly, when you are physically active, you look better. When you are more attractive, your spirits are higher, and you feel good about yourself. These positive feelings are often reflected in a feeling of sexiness.

Finally, for many women, being desired is a powerful aphrodisiac. As your body blossoms with the good health and tone provided by exercise, its appeal to others will also increase. A positive cycle may develop: The better you look and feel, the more desired you will become, the greater your libido and sexual satisfaction will be, the more you will be motivated to keep exercising so as to look and feel great, etc.

In its 1985 survey, *Runner's World* attempted to determine what effect running has on sex life. They found that 70 percent of the women who responded reported that running influenced their sex drive. Of these, 79 percent said they are now more sexually responsive and 83 percent said that running enhanced their sex life. Male responses were similar.[32]

Orgasm

Orgasm, also called sexual climax, has been defined as "the intensely pleasurable feelings resulting from stimulation of the genital organs."[33] While men generally almost always climax as a result of sexual intercourse, women report more variability.[33] In the next few sections we will see how orgasm may become more predictable and satisfying as a result of exercise.

Physiology.   According to Masters and Johnson, two biological processes are active during the sexual response cycle. One is **vasocongestion**, the increased blood flow to and enlargement of the genitals, breasts, and other body tissues. The second is **myotonia**, which is the buildup of tension and energy in nerves and muscles.[34]

    Trained Muscles. A body that is generally well trained may more easily permit the processes of vasocongestion and myotonia to occur. Regular physical exercise increases the efficiency of the blood flow to all parts of the body, including the genitals. The result may be more reliable, pleasurable orgasm.

    The Kegel exercises described earlier in this chapter have been found to not only help alleviate urinary incontinence, but also to train the muscles of the pelvic floor to facilitate sexual arousal and orgasm. These exercises are often taught to women who are seeking help with sexual response.[35]

    Hormones. During and after menopause, the normal production of the female hormone estrogen is diminished. Similarly, overtraining and/or extreme weight loss that brings body fat to less than about 10 percent can reduce estrogen production, thereby interfering with normal menstrual periods. Estrogen also facilitates lubrication of the vaginal area during sexual arousal. With limited lubrication, you may feel less aroused as well as less responsive to sexual activity. Normalizing your weight and easing up on your exercise routine should permit the return of normal estrogen. (See Chapter 11, Menstrual Matters, for a more complete discussion.)

    Although a connection between estrogen and sexuality can easily be made, as we just did above, Dr. Jay Shinfield, professor of obstetrics and gynecology at Thomas Jefferson University in Philadelphia, believes that hormonal changes in exercising women probably do not greatly affect sexuality. He notes "there is not a very good correlation between hormone levels and female sexuality."[36] Low levels of vaginal lubrication can be compensated

What We Know

Physical exercise is likely to enhance your sexual interest and responsiveness. Severe overtraining, however, may result in extreme weight loss, loss of menstrual periods, estrogen depletion, and fatigue. Therefore, exercising to excess for a long period of time may impair your sexuality.

What to Do

Enjoy your workouts for themselves and for the health, fitness, and appearance benefits they yield. Don't overtrain!

for by the application of gels (such as *K-Y*) during intercourse or slow-release products such as *Replens*. Nevertheless, if you believe your estrogen levels are low, you should consider modifying your exercise schedule and consult your medical caregiver.

Partner Politics

Good sex involves far more than hormones and muscles. The relationship of the people involved is paramount. Exercise can have both positive and negative effects on partner politics. Since fit people tend to look better and be more sexually responsive, this can enhance your relationship, as we discussed earlier. On the other hand, if you work out, but your partner does not, problems may ensue.

Jealousy. If you are in a relationship and your exercise routine involves working out in a gym, running, playing tennis, or any number of activities with attractive people, and it almost surely will, your significant other may feel jealous. Your partner may comment about your hanging out with (fill in the name) and make derogatory remarks about your exercise friends.

Time. Your exercise will likely require a significant amount of time. These are hours that perhaps could have been spent with your partner.

> *I recently entered a new relationship. My past two ended because I could not give the amount of time these men seemed to want from me. In addition to my elementary school teaching job, I love to dance. Four evenings a week and every Saturday morning are taken by jazz, African, and modern dance classes. This is my passion, and I do not want to give it up. My new boyfriend exercises regularly; this consists of half-hour runs every other morning and weight training of less than an hour on alternate days. But, his evenings and Saturdays are free, and he wants to spend them with me. I've cut back on my dance classes. This feels like the right thing to do. At the same time, John understands my need to dance. . . . but just a little less. I really want to make this new relationship work. —Erin, age 35*

Women who are training for marathons need to put in many hours of road work each week. Partners left alone during these times may feel neglected. They may complain directly or express hostility in unrelated ways. In cases where the relationship is shaky, the partner may even look for and find a new relationship.

Self-Esteem. The partner we select usually reflects our self-perception. We tend to seek a partner who we believe is comparable in intelligence, appearance, social status, and so on. Sometimes through the years, changes occur which affect an individual's sense of self. If you have begun and maintained an exercise routine and your partner has not, you are likely to have improved your self-esteem while that of your partner may have deteriorated. This difference may cause resentment. Women and men are equally vulnerable to feeling excluded or irritated by a partner who exercises.

> *I do not have the luxury of exercising. Sometimes I become annoyed just seeing my husband's weights lying in the corner of the living room. I've asked him to keep them somewhere else. I know I shouldn't do this, but sometimes when I come home from work and find him exercising, I ask him if he doesn't have anything better to do. Frankly, I'm jealous. I've gained a few pounds since we were first married, and with my job, running after the children, and taking care of the house, I can't fit in exercise. He's encouraged me to start, but at this point, I don't know how. —Sally, age 33*

Working Out Conflict. The problems described above may appear formidable. Yet adjustments can be made to keep your relationship strong and your sex passionate even with partner differences in exercise habits.

1. Recognize and discuss any frustrations that may occur as a result of your individual exercise patterns.
2. Re-evaluate your exercise program—is it extreme? Be ready to make adjustments in length of time and/or time of day devoted to exercise.
3. Focus on compatibilities, the things that initially brought the two of you together.
4. Consider engaging in some activities which interest your partner. Perhaps your partner can similarly be brought into your exercise world. However, you may need to accept the fact that your significant other does not want to share or take part in an exercise regime.
5. Plan to spend time together doing things that you both enjoy. Make these hours a priority.
6. Don't stop exercising! With accommodations and sensitivity you should be able to maintain intimacy and affection while sustaining your commitment to physical fitness.

ENDNOTES

1. Doress-Worters, P. B. & Siegal, D. L. *The new ourselves, growing older.* New York: Simon & Schuster, 1994.
   Genadry, R. R. Evaluation and conservative management of women with stress urinary incontinence. *Maryland Medical Journal*, 1995, 44 (1), 31–35.
   Nygaard, I., DeLancey, J. O. L., Arnsdorf, L., et al. Exercise and incontinence. *Obstetrics and Gynecology*, 1990, 75 (5), 848–851.
2. Benson, R. C. & Pernoll, M. L. *Benson & Pernoll's Handbook of Obstetrics & Gynecology*, 9th ed. New York: McGraw Hill, 1993.
3. Nygaard, I., DeLancey, J. O. L., Arnsdorf, L., et al. Exercise and incontinence. *Obstetrics and Gynecology*, 1990, 75 (5), 848–851.
4. Inch, S. *Birthrights.* London: Merlin Press, 1989.
5. Nygaard, I., DeLancey, J. O. L., Arnsdorf, L., et al. Exercise and incontinence. *Obstetrics and Gynecology*, 1990, 75 (5), 848–851.
6. Doress-Worters, P. B., & Siegal, D. L. *The new ourselves, growing older.* New York: Simon & Schuster, 1994.
   Henderson, J. S., & Taylor, K. H. Age as a variable in an exercise program for the treatment of simple urinary stress incontinence. *Journal of Obstetrical, Gynecological and Neonatal Nursing*, July–August 1987, 16 (4), 266–172.
7. Margolis, S. (Ed.). *The Johns Hopkins Medical Handbook.* New York: Random House, 1995
8. Doress-Worters, P. B., & Siegal, D. L. *The new ourselves, growing older.* New York: Simon & Schuster, 1994.
   Margolis, S. (Ed.). *The Johns Hopkins Medical Handbook.* New York: Random House, 1995
9. Cammu, H., & Van Nylen, M. Pelvic floor muscle exercises: 5 years later. *Urology*, 1995, 45 (1), 113–118.
   Haas, A., & Puretz, S. L. *The Women's Guide to Hysterectomy: Expectations & Options.* Berkeley, CA: Celestial Arts, 1995.
10. Doress-Worters, P. B., & Siegal, D. L. *The new ourselves, growing older.* New York: Simon & Schuster, 1994.
    Turner, T. Continence. Muscle control. *Nursing Times*, March 9–15, 1994, 90 (10), 64–69.
11. Benson, R. C., & Pernoll, M. L. *Benson & Pernoll's Handbook of Obstetrics & Gynecology*, 9th ed. New York: McGraw Hill, 1993.
    Hilton, P., Tweddell, A. L., & Mayne, C. Oral and intravaginal estrogens alone and in combination with alpha-adrenergic stimulation in genuine stress incontinence. *International Urogynecology Journal*, 1990, 1, 80–86.
    Sultana, C. J., & Walters, M. D. Estrogen and urinary incontinence in women. *Maturitas*, 1994, 20 (part 2–3), 129–138.
12. Howley, E. T., & Franks, B. D. *Health fitness instructor's handbook*, 2nd Ed. Champaign, IL: Human Kinetics: 1992.
13. Benson, R. C., & Pernoll, M. L. *Benson & Pernoll's handbook of obstetrics & gynecology*, 9th ed. New York: McGraw Hill, 1993.
14. Genadry, R. R. Evaluation and conservative management of women with stress urinary incontinence. *Maryland Medical Journal*, 1995, 44 (1), 31–35.
15. Brubaker, L., & Kotarinos, R. Kegel or cut? Variations on his theme. *The Journal of Reproductive Medicine*, 1993, 38 (9), 672–678.
16. Wallace, K. Female pelvic floor functions, dysfunctions and behavioral approaches to treatment. *Clinics in Sports Medicine*, 1994, 13 (2), 459–481.
    Unsworth, J. Stress incontinence: treatment using pelvic floor re-education. *British Journal of Nursing*, 1995, 4 (6), 323–4, 326–7.
17. Genadry, R. R. Evaluation and conservative management of women with stress urinary incontinence. *Maryland Medical Journal*, 1995, 44 (1), 31–35.
18. Cammu, H., & Van Nylen, M. Pelvic floor muscle exercises: 5 years later. *Urology*. 1995, 45 (1), 113–118.
    Dougherty, M., Bishop, K., Mooney, R., et al. Graded pelvic muscle exercise: Effect on stress urinary incontinence. *Journal of Reproductive Medicine*, 1993, 38 (9), 684–691.
19. Nygaard, I. Prevention of exercise incontinence with mechanical devices. *Journal of Reproductive Medicine*, 1995, 40 (2), 89–94.
20. Benson, R. C. & Pernoll, M. L. *Benson & Pernoll's Handbook of Obstetrics & Gynecology*, 9th ed. New York: McGraw Hill, 1993.
21. Cooper, K. H., & Cooper, M. *The New Aerobics For Women.* Toronto: Bantam Books, 1988.
22. Janowitz, H. D. *Your gut feelings: a complete guide to living better with intestinal problems.* Yonkers, NY: Consumer Reports Books, 1994.
23. Moses, F. M. The effect of exercise

on the gastrointestinal tract. *Sports Medicine*, 1990, 9 (3), 159–172.

24. Shangold, M., & Mirkin, G. *The Complete Sports Medicine Book for Women*. New York: Simon & Schuster, 1992.

25. Moses, F. M. The effect of exercise on the gastrointestinal tract. *Sports Medicine*, 1990, 9 (3), 159–172.

26. Swain, R. A. Exercise-induced diarrhea: when to wonder. *Medicine and Science in Sports and Exercise*, 1994, 26 (5), 524.

27. Moses, F. M. The effect of exercise on the gastrointestinal tract. *Sports Medicine*, 1990, 9 (3), 159–172.

28. Meyer, K. *How to shit in the woods*, 2nd ed. Berkeley, CA: Ten Speed Press, 1994.

29. Swain, R. A. Exercise-induced diarrhea: when to wonder. *Medicine and Science in Sports and Exercise*, 1994, 26 (5), 523–526.

30. Castleman, M. Can running improve your sex life? *Runner's World*, April 1985, 20 (4), 50–58.

31. White, J. R., Case, D. A., McWhirter, D., et al. Enhanced sexual behavior in exercising men. *Archives of Sexual Behavior*, 1990, 19 (3), 193–209.

32. Castleman, M. Can running improve your sex life? *Runner's World*, April 1985, 20 (4), 50–58.

33. Haas, K., & Haas, A. *Understanding sexuality*, 3rd edition. St. Louis, MO: Mosby Yearbook, 1993.

34. Masters, W. H., Johnson, V. E., & Kolodny, R. C. *Human sexuality*, 3rd edition. Glenview, IL: Scott, Foresman, 1988.

35. Haas, K., & Haas, A. *Understanding sexuality*, 3rd edition. St. Louis, MO: Mosby Yearbook, 1993.

36. Schinfield, J. S. Effects of athletics on male reproduction and sexuality. *Medical Aspects of Human Sexuality*, 1989, 23 (2), 119–126.

Understanding Aches and Pains

DONNA I. MELTZER, M.D.

CHAPTER 16

True or False?

1. Women are the weaker sex and therefore should not participate in certain sports.
2. Women are always more likely to get injured than men while playing sports.
3. The risks of injury outweigh any benefits a woman would derive from exercise.
4. Women should not play in any contact or collision sports for fear of injuring their reproductive organs.
5. Strains and sprains are more common among women athletes.
6. "Runner's knee" affects women and men at an equal rate.
7. Only women who engage in hard-core exercise suffer injuries.
8. Women are more prone to "shin splints" because of an inborn weakness.
9. Serious breast injuries are frequently reported among female athletes.
10. Athletic injuries tend to be more gender-specific than sports-specific.

If you believe in any of the above statements, this chapter should interest you, because none of them are true! Over the years, lots of articles and books have been written about sports injuries and treatment, but very few have focused on the female athlete. It is apparent to us now that some musculoskeletal conditions are unique to women. Let's see if we can begin to understand some of these aches and pains better.

The passage of Title IX legislation in 1972, which prohibited discrimination on the basis of gender, opened up new opportunities for females to participate in sports. With more and more women taking part in recreational, competitive, and elite athletic events, we have witnessed the expected and the unexpected from an injury standpoint. That is, with increased participation, the number of injuries sustained by women has naturally increased, yet not for the gender-based reasons that might be expected.

Sports injuries are a fact of life. We now know that most injuries are sports-specific and not gender-specific. In other words, when a woman and a man play the same sport, they are both more or less hypothetically prone to the same type of injury. However, there are some important exceptions. Keep in mind that this is not an exhaustive guide that will teach athletes to diagnose and treat injuries for each body part. (That would be a book by itself.) As we discuss each area, we will highlight some of the musculoskeletal aches and pains that may be specific to you, the exercising female.

STARTING AT THE TOP

Fortunately, serious head injury occurs less frequently than minor head trauma in athletic activities. Minor head trauma or concussions—with or without a loss of consciousness—are usually associated with contact sports such as football and lacrosse. Blows to the head are also encountered in other athletic activities not normally thought of as contact sports: cycling, gymnastics, and horseback riding. In fact, head or neck injuries can occur in virtually any sport where there is a risk of collision or falling.

Warning Signs

While concussions are one of the more common types of head injury, they are also sometimes difficult to recognize. A mild concussion is characterized by confusion without any loss of consciousness. The hallmark of a moderate concussion is the added finding of amnesia. A severe concussion is associated with a loss of consciousness. The medical treatment for concussions will depend on the severity of the injury.

No athlete should continue to play when concussion symptoms are present—whether the symptoms occur at rest or with exertion. By symptoms, we mean headache, confusion, memory problems, or dizziness. Sometimes, these symptoms may persist for days to months after a head injury. In addition, the affected person may also seem irritable, experience difficulty with concentration, and tire easily. This may be a sign of post-concussion syndrome. If you have suffered a blow to the head and have these symptoms, you should discuss this with your physician.

Preventing Head Injury

Head, neck, and facial injuries can be prevented with the use of appropriate protective headgear. Helmets should feel comfortable and fit properly and, most importantly, must be worn. We all know that a helmet sitting on a shelf at home provides little protection to the active athlete.

PAIN IN THE NECK

In earlier chapters, it was pointed out that women are generally not as tall as men, and we usually also have shorter extremities. It is therefore not unusual for women cyclists to complain of back and neck strain—especially if they ride a bicycle that has a less-than-ideal fit. Adjusting the seat and handlebars may remedy neck strain. (Moving the seat forward, raising the handlebars, decreasing the drop of the handlebars, and shortening the stem size of the handlebars are all tricks that may work for you.) See Chapter 9 for more information on choosing a bicycle.

Also, make sure that your helmet fits properly. A helmet that rides too low on your forehead will force you to keep your head up in order to see, thereby creating neck strain. If correcting these problems does not help, you should see your physician. Treatment may consist of massage therapy to help relieve back and neck spasms, medications, stretching exercises, or injection of trigger points.[1]

Otherwise, women and men are prone to many of the same neck aches and injuries. Since the neck is much less stable compared to other parts of the spine, it is also more prone to injury. Our neck muscles are also not as strong as all the other muscles supporting the spine. All athletes should try to improve neck strength and range of motion.

BREASTS AND CHEST

Blows to the chest wall, although temporarily stunning, usually are not considered serious provided the athlete recovers quickly. More critical injuries occasionally occur after major trauma to the chest wall and may result in rib fracture or lung damage. These injuries are usually accompanied by significant pain and shortness of breath.

Blunt trauma to the breasts is always a possibility in collision and contact sports, but serious injuries are rare. Female athletes can wear well-padded bras or other protective gear to prevent injury. More information on sports bras is presented in Chapter 8, Dressing for the Job.

Breast soreness and injuries associated with exercise have been described by some athletes, but are probably underreported due to a paucity of studies and because little attention has been paid to this area.[2] In one survey, 85 intercollegiate athletes at the University of Washington were asked about breast pain and bra use. Only 20 percent of these varsity athletes (participating in track and field, basketball, crew, volleyball, and tennis) reported occasional breast pain. Their breast discomfort was usually premenstrual or associated with cold weather exposure. Only one injury was reported: a blow to the breast of a basketball player.[3] Surprisingly, just 10 percent of the athletes in this survey wore sports bras, while the rest wore other types of bras. While no research has yet documented this, it is plausible that large-breasted females may suffer more exercise-related breast discomfort because of inadequate support.

Chafing was the only breast problem reported in an informal poll of 27 female marathon runners.[4] In two other surveys, 31 percent and 72 percent of female athletes reported breast problems or soreness associated with exercise at one time or another.[4] This chafing problem ("jogger's nipples" or "bicyclist's nipples") was briefly discussed in Chapter 8.

A LOAD ON ONE'S SHOULDERS

The shoulder joint is one of the most complex joints in the human body. Unlike many of the other joints, the shoulder is a very shallow ball and socket joint, which implies a certain amount of instability. Unfortunately, shoulder pain and instability trouble many athletes, females and males alike. Athletes involved in throwing and racket sports, gymnastics, and swimming are particularly prone to shoulder injuries. Shoulder injuries are difficult to diagnose, primarily due to the complex arrangement of muscles and ligaments around the joint and their wide range of intricate movements.

Injuries to the shoulder can be divided into those problems which arise suddenly, often after trauma, and those that are the result of repetitive overuse. Some shoulder problems may be unique to women because our shoulders are narrower and our upper arms are shorter and less powerful. Our attention will be directed toward the overuse injuries.

Impingement Syndrome

The most common shoulder overuse injury is "impingement syndrome," which occurs when the space in the joint is narrowed so that the rotator cuff muscles and their surrounding tissues become irritated and inflamed. (The rotator cuff muscles are a set of four muscles that hold the shoulder joint together and allow it to rotate.) Pain is usually felt in the front and side of the shoulder. Treatment normally consists of relieving pain and inflammation with ice and NSAIDs (non-steroidal anti-inflammatory drugs) and reducing the activities that aggravate the injury. (For more information on NSAIDs, see Appendix.) This should be followed by physical therapy to restore normal motion and strengthen the rotator cuff muscles.[5]

You may wonder whether some shoulder problems are more common in certain athletic activities and whether these conditions plague women more often than their male counterparts. For example, in swimming, the crawl and butterfly are strokes that have been associated with impingement syndrome more often among women.[6] A gender difference may be the cause: Women, with our shorter arm lengths, must take more strokes to cover the same distance as a taller male swimmer. Also, since we have less upper body musculature, we must work harder to swim the same distance.[7]

Steps to Recovery.   The first step toward recovery is to evaluate your training techniques; next, you should strengthen your rotator cuff muscles through specific exercises. Proper warm-ups are fundamental in preventing further injury. It's also important to identify mechanical errors that occur during training or rehabilitation that actually worsen the problem. Who would ever think that a rehab program for the shoulders could actually aggravate a shoulder injury? Make sure that any upper body exercise equipment you use does not place your hands in a starting position behind your ears, as this can literally force the arm out of the socket.[8] Weight machines should be used with caution by those who have impingement and probably should not be used repeatedly by people with shoulder instability.[9]

Loose Ligaments

Up to this point, we have not addressed the topic of loose or lax ligaments. The wonderful flexibility of female gymnasts certainly lends credence to the impression that women may have looser ligaments compared to men. There is a reason for skirting this issue— primarily because medical studies have been inconclusive as to whether women actually have "looser" ligaments and joints compared to men.

Notwithstanding, laxity in shoulder ligaments has been blamed for an increased number of shoulder complaints in female athletes.[10] This may lead to instability of the shoulder joint or to subluxation, a condition in which the shoulder seems somewhat "disjointed" or "dislocated." Subluxation appears as a spectrum of symptoms ranging from "silent" impingement (which causes no symptoms), to significant pain with overhead arm movement, to actual dislocation.

MY ACHING BACK

Low back pain can strike anyone—young and old, males and females, sedentary and active individuals, and players of all types of sports. In fact, 80 percent of the adult population experiences back pain at some time.[11] The causes are varied, as are the diagnoses. The often-used term "lumbar strain" is a diagnosis by default. Sometimes an initiating insult cannot be identified—in fact, the actual cause of low back pain may be determined in only 12 to 15 percent of patients.

A movement as innocent as bending over and tying one's shoes has been implicated in serious back disorders, yet lifting weights over a hundred pounds may not cause a problem. Fortunately, most low back pain is self-limited and will resolve itself in a few weeks with a little TLC.

Not all sufferers of low back pain need extensive medical work-ups and intervention. Some patients seek medical attention for back pain and are surprised, if not angry, when their physician does not order X-rays, CAT scans, or MRIs. It is up to your family doctor to try to differentiate the serious from the not-so-serious back pain. Taking a good history and performing a focused physical exam will enable your physician to determine the extent to which further medical tests are mandated.

Red Flags

Red flags that your back pain is potentially serious include the following symptoms: muscle weakness, bladder or bowel problems, changes in sensation in the legs, pain only at night, and soreness in association with weight loss, fever, or undue fatigue. Further investigation may be indicated in these cases, and also in cases of severe unrelenting back pain or major trauma resulting in any of the above symptoms.

Possible Causes.   As with some of the other injuries discussed earlier, back problems can cause acute or chronic pain. Factors that may predispose an athlete to low back pain include leg length discrepancy, improper techniques, and sudden increases in the intensity or duration of training. On the other hand, excessive lifting and twisting motions, weak back and abdominal muscles, and poor flexibility of the hip, thigh, and back muscles can increase the risk of chronic low back pain. (See Chapter 4 for more information.)

Other causes of back pain include fractures, arthritis, infections, and some anatomical conditions. Poor posture has also been implicated as a cause of lower back and neck pain.

Back Pain and the Young Athlete

When a young athlete complains of back pain, the approach and workup should be a bit more aggressive. A recent study at Children's Hospital in Boston compared the diagnoses of low-back complaints in 100 adults with 100 athletic adolescents. More serious diagnoses—such as stress fractures—were found in the adolescent group. Early diagnosis and treatment of youngsters with back pain can lead to complete healing without surgery.[12]

Slipped Disks

Not all backs that hurt are due to "slipped" or herniated discs. (In fact, many people who have these protruding disks have no symptoms whatsoever.) More common causes of pain are lumbar (lower back) strains and sprains. (Strains involve damage to a muscle or tendon, while sprains involve injury to ligaments.) Lower back strains are often precipitated by a trivial lifting or twisting maneuver. Although sprains and strains can be accompanied by severe muscle spasms, usually there is no pain traveling down the legs. Pain can often be relieved by lying down and a short period of rest.

On the other hand, people with symptomatic herniated disks may complain of low back or buttock pain that radiates down the legs. They may also have a "pins and needles" sensation, or numbness and weakness in the legs. A herniated disk can be caused by a simple lifting or twisting motion. When the above symptoms are accompanied by bladder or bowel problems, further diagnostic tests are indicated, as this may be a medical emergency requiring immediate surgery.

Leg Lengths

It's debatable whether having legs of different lengths could contribute to back pain. Some studies have shown that a leg length discrepancy of less than or equal to half an inch may be within normal errors of measurement. Other studies have shown that 4 percent to 8 percent of the general population has up to a half-inch difference in leg length. If you have chronic back pain and a physical exam shows more than a half-inch difference in your leg lengths, you may want to consider having your footwear fitted with shoe lifts.[13]

"Athletic Backs"

What about back problems unique to women athletes? Many female cyclists, recreational and elite, have complained of back pain after long rides. The complaint is often magnified in cyclists who ride ill-fitting bike frames. A common scenario is the female with a short torso who is forced to lean forward to reach the handlebars on her "man's" bike because of its long top tube and stem.[14] Adjusting the seat height and position may prevent many low back problems.[15] Refer to Chapter 9, Gearing Up, for more information.

In gymnasts, back problems may be due to trauma (for example, a bad fall) or to minor repetitive insults to the back. Young female gymnasts have been shown to have a higher incidence of spondylolysis.[16] **Spondylolysis** is a mouthful of a word that describes a fracture of the pars interarticularis, part of the lumbar spine. It probably occurs more frequently in female gymnasts because their routines often involve more hyperextension of the back, especially when they land after a dismount.[17] Volleyball players are also susceptible to this problem because they tend to arch their backs as they spike balls.

Runners, joggers, dancers, swimmers, and divers may also suffer from back pain and injuries. Much of the time it is an overuse phenomenon. Occasionally back pain may be due to improper technique.

Even golfers are not immune to injury. Studies have shown that female pro golfers are more likely to suffer injury to the left wrist than to the lower back. On the other hand, among male professional golfers, injuries to the back are more common, followed by those of the left wrist. (The left hand is affected more because most people are right hand dominant and it is the nondominant hand that undergoes more twist.) In the amateur arena, the findings are a bit different. Female amateur golfers list the elbow as being more commonly injured than the back. Male amateurs have more lower back injuries, followed by the elbow, hand, and wrist.[18]

Low Back Pain Rehabilitation

Rehabilitation of low back pain starts with identifying treatable causative factors (such as poor posture) and improper lifting techniques or athletic maneuvers. Pain control is also important and usually NSAIDs (nonsteroidal anti-inflammatory drugs) are the mainstay, rather than narcotic pain-killers.

For acute back pain due to muscle strains or ligament sprains, a short rest period of two or three days may be advised. A rest period does not generally mean strict bed rest, which should probably be avoided. Instead, it usually means refraining from the activity that may have precipitated the back injury in the first place. For others, it may involve cross-training or enrolling in an exercise program to strengthen weakened muscles.

We now know that exercise is central to the successful management of back pain. Your family doctor or trainer may be able to guide you toward the most suitable rehab program for you.

Tips for Getting Back in Shape

- Bed rest is out; exercise is in.
- Start maintaining or building general endurance by walking, swimming, or riding a stationary bicycle.
- If you tend toward exercise addiction, start slowly and don't overdo it.
- If you lean toward a sedentary lifestyle, stop procrastinating—exercising two minutes a day is better than doing nothing at all.
- Don't expect a miracle cure overnight. Healing takes time.

ELBOW AILMENTS

Tennis Elbow

Aside from your garden variety strains, sprains, and fractures, most injuries to the elbow are of the overuse type. **Lateral epicondylitis** is the medical term for "tennis elbow," which is the most common overuse injury of the elbow.[19] Tennis elbow is caused by repetitive stress to the forearm muscle, and this stress is transmitted up to where the muscle tendon inserts into the outer elbow knob. Not surprisingly, you do not have to be a tennis player to suffer from this ailment. Because many carpenters and factory workers who constantly extend their wrists against a load also suffer from this ailment, the term "industrial athlete" was coined.[20] Individuals who play any racket sports or who participate in throwing activities—novices and professionals alike—may be at risk.

Tennis elbow usually results in tenderness on the outside (lateral) part of the elbow. Pain is generally made worse with motions like handshaking.

Treatment and rehabilitation will depend on the severity of the pain. If you are a tennis player, inspect your racket and analyze your form. Is the racket the correct size and grip for you? Is it strung too tightly? Are you hitting most balls on the "sweet spot" of the racket? Some players may need to rest the elbow if they have suddenly increased their training or playing time. Others may find that icing the elbow, taking NSAIDs to reduce inflammation, or using an arm brace can be helpful in reducing pain during play.

Golfer's Elbow

Pain on the inside of the elbow is called **medial epicondylitis**, also known as "golfer's elbow." Like tennis elbow, it is an overuse injury that in this case is not restricted to golfers. Usually the pain of golfer's elbow is made worse with certain movements, such as throwing a ball or serving in tennis. As with tennis elbow, treatment involves relative rest, medications to reduce inflammation, and therapy to increase strength and flexibility.

PRIVATE PARTS

Unlike men, who have their testicles to protect, women's reproductive organs are very well sheltered inside the body—hence ovarian or uterine injury is rarely encountered. However, women *can* suffer painful bruising and abrasions to the vulva caused by straddle injuries, such as falling onto the crossbar of a bicycle or falling and straddling the balance beam.

In some cases, women have incurred vaginal injuries while waterskiing and jetskiing at high speeds.[21] Waterskiers should wear padded bottoms or other protective clothing to avoid suffering a traumatic "water douche." If a waterskier falls into a sitting position or is pulled through the water at high speeds while trying to stand from a crouching position, the tremendous water pressure can cause a vaginal laceration.

On the other hand, women rarely suffer traumatic sports-related injuries to the urethra, because of built-in protective properties. For example, in contrast to the male urethra, the female urethra is shorter and not rigidly attached to the pubic bone.[22]

Although the link between urinary tract infection (UTI) and bicycling has not been extensively studied, Barry Weiss, M.D. has described several cases of UTI in women who engaged in long bicycle rides. He surmises that incomplete emptying of the bladder combined with the pressure of the bicycle seat on the urethra causes inflammation and then infection.[23] A similar mechanism has been used to explain why both young and older male cyclists develop prostatitis, inflammation and infection of the prostate gland. Long-distance cyclists take note!

Female cyclists also frequently complain of saddle problems, which result from women's comparatively shallower pubic arch. A bike outfitted with a man's long-nosed seat aggravates the situation.[24] This discomfort can be remedied with better padding and the use of a seat specifically designed for females, that is, with a short nose and wide rear.[25] (See Chapter 9, Gearing Up: Making Informed Equipment Decisions, for more information.) But saddle-related problems aren't unique to women—numbness of the male sex organs and impotence have been reported and probably are underreported due to the sensitive and private nature of the subject.

WEAK KNEES

The knee is one of the most frequently injured joints. Whether women suffer more knee injuries than men has been subject to much debate and is still unresolved.

One study comparing all athletic injuries over a seven-year period at the University of Rochester Section of Sports Medicine provides us with some interesting data including differences between sexes, sports, and age groups.[26] The population studied included professional, intercollegiate, high school, and intramural athletes from the university and the surrounding community. The knees were the most frequently injured joints in both male and female athletes, and sprains and strains were the most commonly diagnosed injuries. Patellofemoral pain syndrome was the second most common knee diagnosis for females, while it ranked number five for males. Dislocation of the kneecap was also seen more frequently in females than males.

Our discussion of knee injuries will be limited to: sprains and strains, patellofemoral syndrome, meniscal (cartilage) problems, iliotibial band syndrome, and dislocation of the kneecap. These problems are common to all athletes and some additional ones are perhaps unique to women. Read on, as this will make more sense after a short anatomy review.

Getting to Know Your Knee

The knee is essentially a complex hinge joint made up of the large thigh bone (**femur**) and the shin bone (**tibia**) and stabilized by several important ligaments that enable you to bend, straighten out, and twist your leg. These two bones are cushioned by **menisci**, crescents of cartilage that sit on top of the tibia and help to stabilize the knee joint. Each knee has two shock absorbers: the medial and lateral menisci. Two ligaments, the **anterior**

(ACL) and **posterior** (PCL) **cruciate ligaments**, cross in the middle of the knee and provide front-to-back stability. Side-to-side stability is provided by the **medial** and **lateral collateral ligaments**. (See Diagram 16.1.) The kneecap (**patella**) sits in a groove between the two knobs that form the lower part of the thighbone. When the knee joint is subject to overuse, or when the athlete's foot is fixed and the knee is twisted or forced in another direction, injury and pain may result.

Figure 16.1
Front view of right knee

femur

iliotibial band

posterior cruciate ligament

anterior cruciate ligament

medial meniscus

lateral collateral ligament

medial collateral ligament

fibula

tibia

Sprains

When ligaments are stressed, sprains may result. Sprains can range from mild to severe. For example, in mild sprains the damage might only involve a few fibers; at the other extreme, it may be a complete rupture of the ligament, which is a severe injury that would render the joint unstable. New data suggest that women may experience more injuries to the anterior cruciate ligament (ACL) than men, but the cause is not known.[27]

Injuring the ACL. In one study of knee ligament injuries in volleyball players, the ACL was the most frequently damaged, although it is well known that ACL injuries can occur in any sport.[28] In fact, a common scenario is that the athlete lands on her foot and hears a loud pop in the knee, with subsequent pain and swelling.[29] When this occurs, the three most common diagnoses are ligament damage, a dislocated kneecap, or injury to the meniscus. A physical exam demonstrating joint instability often helps to confirm the diagnosis of damage to the ACL. Of course, damage can also occur to the other ligaments holding the knee in place. Injury to the MCL is seen when force is applied to the lateral (outside) part of the knee. Less common is a posterior cruciate ligament sprain. The PCL gets damaged when the top of the shin bone (tibia) suffers a blow. This can occur when an athlete falls and lands on the top part of the tibia. Usually there is less swelling with injuries to the PCL compared to the ACL.

Meniscal Injuries

When one foot is anchored to the ground and the rest of the body undergoes a twisting motion, damage to the meniscus (cartilage) can occur. Sometimes, meniscal injuries occur at the same time that the ACL is sprained, which may account for the pronounced pop heard or felt by the athlete. Minor damage to the meniscus may cause few or no symptoms. More severe injury results in swelling and pain and the sensation that the knee "locks" or gives way. While treatment often depends on the severity of the problem, initial management consists of icing the joint, taking NSAIDs, and doing quadriceps strengthening exercises.[30]

Patellofemoral Syndrome

Patellofemoral syndrome is reportedly twice as common in women as in men. This syndrome is now used to describe knee pain (around the kneecap) that, in the past, had several different names, including: runner's knee, chondromalacia (a misnomer meaning softening of the cartilage), or anterior knee pain.

In Chapter 2 we noted that women have a wider pelvis than men, which is one of the anatomical properties that contribute to their larger Q angle. Remember that the Q angle describes how the upper and lower leg bones meet at the knee joint. (Women who are knock-kneed tend to have larger Q angles.) Having a wider pelvis is probably partly responsible for the greater incidence of patellofemoral syndrome in women.[31] Patellofemoral pain syndrome is more of an overuse injury, rather than the result of major trauma.

Individuals suffering from patellofemoral syndrome typically describe dull pain and aching around the kneecap. Squatting or climbing stairs or hills may worsen the discomfort and cause sharper pain.[32] Some sufferers of this syndrome have noted that prolonged sitting can produce knee discomfort—the so-called "theater sign."[33] Although it's not specific to this syndrome, a snapping or popping sound associated with bending of the knees may be observed.

Treatment for patellofemoral syndrome includes the use of NSAIDs, applying ice, and modifying activity. Strengthening the quadriceps muscles is crucial to rehabilitation. Although stair climbing has been advocated for men, it is not advisable for the female athlete because the repetitive forces associated with climbing may also aggravate the problem.[34] (Women have wider pelvises, and thus tend to have larger Q angles, which increases patellofemoral forces and can actually worsen the pain. Stair climbing does strengthen the quadriceps muscles, but the added stress on the patella may aggravate the problem.) Remember, we noted that this syndrome is caused by overuse, so it is easy to see why stair climbing may worsen things. A better exercise for women is to put a rolled towel under the knee so it is slightly bent, then straighten out the leg.[35] (See Figures 4A, 4b in Chapter 17.) Start with one set of ten repetitions and build up to five sets. A brace may also be used to help stabilize the kneecap. In some cases, arch supports may solve the problem, especially for those whose knees tend to bend inward.[36]

Patellar Dislocation

Normally the patella (kneecap) slides along a groove in the femur. When it shifts out of this groove, it dislocates. A similar problem, where the patella slides slightly to one side, is called subluxation. Both dislocation and subluxation of the kneecap can occur after a twisting or jumping injury and result in the sensation that the knee has given way. As with ACL sprains, a popping sensation may be felt at the time of injury. Frequently, significant swelling of the knee joint occurs after the injury. Sometimes the kneecap falls back in place when the leg is straightened out.

Conservative treatment consists of immobilizing the joint so that the leg is kept straight for several weeks, followed by a quadriceps strengthening program. Some specialists advise surgery in individuals who have **genu valgum** (knock-knees), an increased Q angle, **patella alta** (a high-riding kneecap), and increased laxity of the ligaments.[37] These are all traits that are seen more frequently in women than men.

Iliotibial Band Syndrome

Pain on the outside of the knee may be due to iliotibial band syndrome. This overuse problem occurs when the band tightens and constantly rubs along the outside part of the thigh bone. Typically, it is a runner's injury, with pain that begins several minutes after exercise commences. It is not uncommon for the pain to intensify after several minutes of running.[38] Running downhill or on an uneven surface may cause or worsen this syndrome. Uneven leg lengths can further contribute to this problem. Treatment is aimed at stretching the iliotibial band. NSAIDs may be used for pain relief. Decreasing running mileage and using arch supports may also help.[39]

Recap on the Kneecap

It's a good sign if your physician spends a substantial amount of time examining your knee and listening to you talk about the details of your pain or injury, because more than 90 percent of all knee injuries can be diagnosed by a detailed history and careful physical exam.[40]

Certainly, there are times when X-rays, CT scans, and MRIs are needed to make or confirm a diagnosis. **Arthrograms** are X-rays taken after a dye is injected into the joint. Sometimes, when an individual does not improve with time and treatment, radiographic studies are performed. Another procedure performed by orthopedic surgeons is arthroscopy, in which small incisions are made in the joint to be studied. The surgeon will insert an **arthroscope**, a fiber optic device that has a light enabling the viewer to examine the inside of the joint. This is often done under anesthesia as a hospital outpatient procedure, which allows treatment to take place at the same time. Arthrograms are 90 percent accurate in diagnosing meniscal tears and 75 percent accurate in diagnosing torn ACLs and PCLs.[41] In the last few years, tremendous technological advances have prompted increased use of MRIs to assist in diagnoses of joint injuries. Whatever your situation, you should know why tests are or are not being ordered by your physician, and you should feel comfortable asking questions. It's equally important to understand the answers to your queries—if you don't, ask for clarification.

What We Know

Most knee pain can be diagnosed by a complete history and careful physical exam. Expensive X-rays, CT scans, and MRIs are often unnecessary.

THE LOWER LEG

As we travel down toward the foot, the next stop is the lower leg. The two long bones in the lower leg are the tibia (shin bone) and the narrower fibula. Several muscle groups surround these bones. The tibia, which supports most of your weight, tends to be more prone to injury than the fibula, which, although smaller, is protected by layers of muscle. Two lower-leg problems commonly encountered by athletes are shin splints and stress fractures.

Shin Splints

"Shin splints" is a catch-all term to describe pain on the anterior (front) or medial (inner) aspect of the lower leg. Researchers have recently proposed that shin splints be diagnosed more specifically to describe the cause of the problem.[42] Although athletes still use the term, physicians try to avoid its use because it is too vague. Identifying the cause of the pain can help with its treatment.

Female athletes may be prone to shin splints or exercise-related lower leg pain due to a variety of factors: faulty training techniques, inadequate conditioning, improper footwear, exercising on hard surfaces that lack good shock absorption, excessive foot pronation (foot rolling inward), or any combination of these conditions.[43] The discomfort of shin splints may range from a generalized soreness occurring as much as 12 hours after exercise to pain that commences immediately upon exercise.

Treatment consists of relative rest, ice, wrapping of the lower leg with elastic bandages, and NSAIDs. Absolute rest or cross-training may be indicated for shin pain that begins immediately or early in exercise.[44]

Stress Fractures

When you repeatedly overstress a bone, it can become fatigued and develop a hairline crack or stress fracture. Stress fractures can sometimes be confused with shin splints because the symptoms are similar. They are encountered more commonly in sports that involve running or jumping. Stress fractures are also more likely to occur in the tibia than the fibula.[45] As with shin splints, training errors, improper footwear, and running surfaces that stress the leg can lead to the development of a stress fracture. The diagnosis of a stress fracture can be confirmed by X-rays or a bone scan. It is not uncommon for X-rays to be normal early on and only show the fracture after healing has set in. Conversely, bone scans, which involve an injection of a small amount of radioactive material, can identify a fracture after only a few days of symptoms.

As with shin splints, treatment of stress fractures involves rest, modifying activities, and correcting problematic footwear or training techniques. Ice and NSAIDs may also provide relief.[46]

UNDERSTANDING ACHES AND PAINS   405

ANKLE AND FOOT PROBLEMS

The ankle has a unique structure that allows you to move your foot in many directions. The foot is the most complex bony structure in the lower body. It supports your body weight and is a major shock absorber. The following medical problems of the ankle and feet may interest the woman striving for fitness.

Ankle Sprains

Ankle sprains are not selective—they strike athletes and nonathletes, females and males. As with sprains of the knee, the ligaments of the ankle are subject to stress when twisted. Sprains can be subdivided into mild, moderate, or severe or classified as grades (one, two, or three) depending on the amount of damage to the ligaments. The most common mechanism causing an ankle sprain is inversion or turning inward of the foot as the heel of the foot strikes the ground.[47]

Examples of Treatment Approaches. Treatment is relatively straightforward and depends to a certain extent on the severity of the sprain: rest, icing, compression, and elevation. Simple grade one ankle sprains often can be wrapped in an ace bandage, whereas grade three sprains often require casting. Your physician will probably encourage you to perform range-of-motion exercises and then have you bear weight on your injured ankle as early as possible.

Plantar Fasciitis

The **plantar fascia** is a band of connective tissue that runs from your heel toward the toes. When it is too tight or gets inflamed, pain ensues. Typically, the pain of plantar fasciitis is worse in the morning upon arising and improves as the day goes on.

Since the symptoms of plantar fasciitis are annoying, often painful, and sometimes disruptive to activities of daily living, many people seek medical attention. Usually a diagnosis can be reached simply by taking a history and performing a physical exam. Occasionally X-rays are ordered to investigate other causes of heel or foot pain.

Heel spurs (little hooks of bone on the heel) are often found on X-rays, but they are probably not the source of the pain of plantar fasciitis.[48] Heel spurs are found in 15 percent of adults without foot pain, yet nearly 50 percent of individuals with foot pain will have heel spurs.[49] It may be that the heel spurs are a consequence, but not a cause, of foot inflammation.

Footwear Recommendations. Proper footwear for routine and athletic activities may help to lessen the inflammation of plantar fasciitis. Shoes that have a straight last and good hindfoot control (preventing pronation) are preferable. Running shoes should also be flexible at the ball of the foot but not in the middle of the arch.[50]

Care.   Treatment of plantar fasciitis may involve use of an arch support or heel cup, stretching exercises, and NSAIDs for pain relief. Splints worn at night (called tension night splints) have recently been shown to reduce early morning pain.[50] If conservative treatment fails, your physician may try injecting the area with a small amount of steroid.[51]

Pump Bump

Some women suffer from pump bump—so named because it was noted that an area on the back of the heel becomes enlarged in women who wear pumps. Basically, the shoe rubs against the heel and causes irritation resulting in a bump. Although it is not caused by athletic activity, pump bump may aggravate heel pain in some athletes. Treatment attempts to reduce the inflammation by modifying footwear or alleviating the irritation with felt padding or a heel cup.

WRAPPING UP

We have traveled a long road of injuries from head to foot. Most are common athletic injuries, including many that are unique to women. While some early studies indicated that women athletes were injured more often than men, many questions remain unanswered.

Was the higher incidence of injuries these studies showed due to lack of adequate conditioning and training, a physiological predisposition to injury, or because women could be the weaker sex? Or was this higher injury rate due to differences in socialization, lack of exposure to athletic activities, or inappropriate athletic equipment and apparel?

Many recent studies do not support a higher injury rate in females. However, as more women play mixed sex or contact sports, and develop more aggressive playing styles, we might see an increase in the number and severity of injuries. For now, the bottom line is that sports injuries are generally sports-specific and not gender-specific. In other words, it depends on the sport, not who is playing it.

1. Mellion, M. B. Neck and back pain in bicycling. *Clinics in Sports Medicine*, January 1994, 13 (1), 137–164.

2. Gehlsen, G., & Albohm, M. Evaluation of sports bras. *Physician and Sportsmedicine*, October 1980, 8 (10), 89–96.

   Haycock, C. E., & Gillette, J. V. Susceptibility of women athletes to injury. *JAMA*, July 12, 1976, 236 (2), 163–165.

3. Hunter, L. Y., & Torgan, C. The bra controversy: Are sports bras a necessity? *The Physician and Sportsmedicine*, November 1982, 10 (11), 75–76.

4. Gehlsen, G., & Albohm, M. Evaluation of sports bras. *The Physician and Sportsmedicine*, October 1980, 8 (10), 89–96.

   Schuster, K. Equipment update: Jogging bras hit the streets. *The Physician and Sportsmedicine*, April 1979, 7 (4), 125–126, 128.

5. Tearse, D. S. Shoulder problems in athletes: Hastening the return to full function. *Postgraduate Medicine*, February 1995, 97 (2), 67–81, 85.

6. Hunter, L. Y. Women's athletics: The orthopedic surgeon's viewpoint. *Clinics in Sports Medicine*, October, 1984, 3 (4), 809–827.

7. Arendt, E. A. Orthopaedic issues for active and athletic women. *Clinics in Sports Medicine*, April 1994, 13 (2), 483–503.

   Hunter, L. Y. Women's athletics: The orthopedic surgeon's viewpoint. *Clinics in Sports Medicine*, October, 1984, 3 (4), 809–827.

8. Lillegard, W. A., & Terrio, J. D. Appropriate strength training. *Medical Clinics of North America*, March 1994, 78 (2), 457–477.

   Hunter, L. Y. Women's athletics: The orthopedic surgeon's viewpoint. *Clinics in Sports Medicine*, October, 1984, 3 (4), 809–827.

   Arendt, E. A. Common musculoskeletal injuries in women. *The Physician and Sportsmedicine*, July 1996, 24 (7), 39–48.

9. Arendt, E. A. Orthopaedic issues for active and athletic women. *Clinics in Sports Medicine*, April 1994, 13 (2), 483–503.

   Hunter, L. Y. Women's athletics: The orthopedic surgeon's viewpoint. *Clinics in Sports Medicine*, October, 1984, 3 (4), 809–827.

10. Hunter, L. Y. Women's athletics: The orthopedic surgeon's viewpoint. *Clinics in Sports Medicine*, October, 1984, 3 (4), 809–827.

11. Bueff, H. U., & Van Der Reis, W. Low back pain. *Primary Care: Orthopedics*, June 1996, 23 (2), 345–364.

    Liang, M. H. Acute low back pain: Diagnosis and management of mechanical back pain. *Primary Care: Musculoskeletal Pain Syndromes*, December 1988, 15 (4), 827–847.

12. Micheli, L. J., Wood, R. Back pain in young athletes: Significant differences from adults in causes and patterns. *Archives of Pediatric Adolescent Medicine*, 1995, 149, 15–18.

13. Liang, M. H. Acute low back pain: Diagnosis and management of mechanical back pain. *Primary Care: Musculoskeletal Pain Syndromes*, December 1988, 15 (4), 827–847.

14. Cohen, G. C. Cycling injuries. *Canadian Family Physician*, March 1993, 39, 628–632.

15. Mellion, M. B. Neck and back pain in bicycling. *Clinics in Sports Medicine*, January 1994, 13 (1), 137–164.

16. Arendt, E. A. Orthopaedic issues for active and athletic women. *Clinics in Sports Medicine*, April 1994, 13 (2), 483–503.

17. Rubin, C. J. Sports injuries in the female athlete. *New Jersey Medicine*, September 1991, 88 (9), 643–645.

18. McCarroll, J. R. The frequency of golf injuries. In G. N. Guten (Ed.) *Clinics in Sports Medicine*, January, 1996, 15 (1) 1–26. Philadelphia: W. B. Saunders.

19. Fox, G. M., Jebson, P. J., & Orwin, J. F. Overuse injuries of the elbow. *The Physician and Sportsmedicine*, August 1995, 23 (8), 58–66.

20. Jones, J. W., Davidson, C. J., & Sevier, T. L. Managing sports-related overuse injuries. *Patient Care*, April 15, 1996, 55–71.

21. Wein, P., & Thompson, D. J. Vaginal perforation due to jet ski accident. *Australia New Zealand Journal of Obstetrics and Gynaecology*, 1990, 30 (4), 384–385.

22. Diekmann-Guiroy, B., & Young, D. H. Female urethral injury secondary to blunt pelvic trauma. *Annals of Emergency Medicine*, December 1991, 20, 1376–1377.

23. Weiss, B. D. Clinical syndromes associated with bicycle seats. *Clinics in Sports Medicine*, January 1994, 13 (1), 175–186.

24. Cohen, G. C. Cycling injuries. *Canadian Family Physician*, March 1993, 39, 628–632.

25. Dickson, T. B. Jr. Preventing overuse cycling injuries. *The Physician and Sportsmedicine*, October 1985, 13 (10), 116–123.

26. DeHaven, K. E., & Lintner, D. M. Athletic injuries: Comparison by age, sport, and gender. *The American Journal of Sports Medicine*, 1986, 14 (3), 218–224.

27. Arendt, E. A. Orthopaedic issues for active and athletic women. *Clinics in Sports Medicine*, April 1994, 13 (2), 483–503.

28. Sebastianelli, W. J., & Black, K. P. Knee ligament injuries: A guide to "Hands on" diagnosis of anterior cruciate problems. *Consultant*, February 1995, 35 (2), 163–174.

29. Ferretti, A., Papanderea, P., Conteduca, F., & Mariani, P. P. Knee ligament injuries in volleyball players. *The American Journal of Sports Medicine*, 1992, 20 (2), 203–207.

30. Stuart, M. J. with Couzens, G. S. Painful knees: When damaged menisci are the cause. *The Physician and Sportsmedicine*, March 1994, 22 (3), 96–106.

31. Buckley, R. L. Preventing and treating medical problems among women athletes. *Family Practice Recertification*, June 1989, 11 (6), 56–72.

    Davidson, K. Patellofemoral pain syndrome. *American Family Physician*, November 15, 1993, 48 (7), 1254–1262.

    Potera, C. Women in sports: The price of participation. *The Physician and Sportsmedicine*, June 1986, 14 (6), 149–150, 153.

32. Davidson, K. Patellofemoral pain syndrome. *American Family Physician*, November 15, 1993, 48 (7), 1254–1262.

    Ruffin, M. T. IV, & Kiningham, R. B. Anterior knee pain: The challenge of patellofemoral syndrome. *American Family Physician*, January 1993, 47 (1), 185–194.

33. Davidson, K. Patellofemoral pain syndrome. *American Family Physician*, November 15, 1993, 48 (7), 1254–1262.

    Ruffin, M. T. IV, & Kiningham, R. B. Anterior knee pain: The challenge of patellofemoral syndrome. *American Family Physician*, January 1993, 47 (1), 185–194.

    Wexler, R. K. Lower extremity injuries in runners: Helping athletic patients return to form. *Postgraduate Medicine*, October 1995, 98 (4), 185–193.

34. Hunter, L. Y. Women's athletics: The orthopedic surgeon's viewpoint. *Clinics in Sports Medicine*, October, 1984, 3 (4), 809–827.

35. Potera, C. Women in sports: The price of participation. *The Physician and Sportsmedicine*, June 1986, 14 (6), 149–150, 153.

36. Rubin, C. J. Sports injuries in the female athlete. *New Jersey Medicine*, September 1991, 88 (9), 643–645.

    Davidson, K. Patellofemoral pain syndrome. *American Family Physician*, November 15, 1993, 48 (7), 1254–1262.

37. Hutchinson, M. R., & Ireland, M. L. Patella dislocation: Recognizing the injury and its complication. *The*

Physician and Sportsmedicine, October 1995, 23 (10), 53–60.

38. Aronen, J. G., Chronister, R., Regan, K., & Hensien, M. A. Practical, conservative management of iliotibial band syndrome. *The Physician and Sportsmedicine*, June 1993, 21 (6), 59–69.

39. Wexler, R. K. Lower extremity injuries in runners: Helping athletic patients return to form. *Postgraduate Medicine*, October 1995, 98 (4), 185–193.

40. Mendelsohn, C. L., & Paiement, G. D. Physical examination of the knee. *Primary Care: Orthopedics*, June 1996, 23 (2), 321–328.

41. McCune, W. J., Matteson, E. L., & MacGuire, A. Evaluation of knee pain. *Primary Care: Musculoskeletal Pain Syndromes*, December 1988, 15 (4), 795–808.

42. Wexler, R. K. Lower extremity injuries in runners: Helping athletic patients return to form. *Postgraduate Medicine*, October 1995, 98 (4), 185–193.

43. Rubin, C. J. Sports injuries in the female athlete. *New Jersey Medicine*, September 1991, 88 (9), 643–645.

    Knortz, K. A., & Reinhart, R .S. Women's athletics: The athletic trainer's viewpoint. *Clinics in Sports Medicine*, October 1984, 3 (4), 851–868.

44. Bowyer, B. L., McKeag, D. B., & McNerney, J. E. When a beginning runner overdoes it. *Patient Care*, April 15, 1994, 28 (7), 54–86.

45. Gellman, R., & Burns, S. Walking aches and running pains: Injuries of the foot and ankle. *Primary Care:*

Orthopedics, June 1996, 23 (2), 263–280.

46. Knortz, K. A., & Reinhart, R .S. Women's athletics: The athletic trainer's viewpoint. *Clinics in Sports Medicine*, October 1984, 3 (4), 851–868.

47. Connolly, J. F. Acute ankle sprains: Getting—and keeping—patients back up on their feet. *Consultant*, August 1996, 36 (8), 1631–1646.

48. Bowyer, B. L., McKeag, D. B., & McNerney, J. E. When a beginning runner overdoes it. *Patient Care*, April 15, 1994, 28 (7), 54–86.

49. Engebretsen, L., & Bahr, R. Foot injuries: Office management for the woes of weekend warriors. *Consultant*, February, 1996, 36 (2), 209–225.

50. Batt, M .E., & Tanji, J. L. Management options for plantar fasciitis. *The Physician and Sportsmedicine*, June 1995, 23 (6), 77–86.

51. Bowyer, B. L., McKeag, D. B., & McNerney, J. E. When a beginning runner overdoes it. *Patient Care*, April 15, 1994, 28 (7), 54–86.

17

Fixing Things: An Approach To Rehabilitation

DONNA I. MELTZER, M.D.

Most rehabilitation programs aim to safely return an athlete to activity and to prevent reinjury. To do so, one must restore range of motion, strength, power, flexibility, and endurance, without incurring pain or further injury. Some injuries result from wear and tear or overuse, while others are sudden or acute in nature.

We now know that repetitive "microtrauma" occurring during athletic activities is the cause of most overuse injuries.[1] Muscle weakness, imbalance, and inflexibility are three of the many biomechanical factors that contribute to this tissue damage, which eventually has a cumulative effect resulting in an overuse injury.

With acute injuries, such as bad sprains or a suspected broken bone, it is usually easy to determine whether medical attention is needed. This is not always the case with overuse injuries. Overuse injuries tend to occur gradually: hence, some athletes might opt for self-treatment before seeing a physician because their pain does not seem too bad. We cannot emphasize enough that common sense should prevail. The information in this chapter is not designed to substitute for proper medical diagnosis and care.

RICE PRINCIPLES

Last summer while on vacation, I tripped and ended up going to a walk-in medical center because I was far away from home. An X-ray was taken and the doctor told me it was probably just a bad sprain. He prescribed "RICE" therapy. I had heard about this before and didn't think to ask too many questions. When I got home, I realized how little I knew about the specifics of RICE. —Joy, age 33

The RICE principles have been referred to many times in the previous chapter, and there is good reason—they are effective. In general, most acute injuries respond to RICE, which stands for rest, ice, compression, and elevation.

Resting

Resting an injury is one of the first steps toward healing. Continued movement of an injured part will result in increased bleeding and swelling and may worsen the damage. The amount of rest required will depend on the severity of the injury. An athlete with a minor injury is often managed with relative rest or partial sports participation. You and your health care provider can decide whether you need absolute or relative rest after an injury.

Icing

Application of cold packs to an injured body part constricts blood vessels and reduces bleeding, which then prevents excess inflammation and swelling. Cold treatments may also help to prevent painful muscle spasms.

There are a variety of methods available to ice an injury: ice cubes, gel packs, and chemical cold bags.[2] Ice cubes can be placed in a plastic food bag and then wrapped in a dish towel. Crushing the ice allows you to more easily mold the bag of ice. Alternatively, you may find that a bag of frozen vegetables (like peas) makes a great ice bag that you can re-use over and over again. Gel packs consist of a special material that remains pliable when frozen. They can be recycled, and they cool the skin faster than ice packs. Chemical cold bags are stored at room temperature until you activate them by squeezing them. They are great for traveling or for first aid use, but cannot be reused.

Whichever method you choose, try to ice the injured body part immediately. A general rule of thumb is to apply ice several times a day for the first 24 hours after an injury occurs. The frequency of application can then be tapered off gradually over the next 24 to 48 hours. The length of time you ice will depend on the size of the area injured and the depth of the injured structure. Some areas, like the knees and ankles, have little body fat and do not tolerate cold as well as better-padded areas like the thighs and buttocks. You can usually apply ice for 10 to 20 minutes per session. Do not be overzealous with the icing, as frostbite could occur should you continue cold applications after the injured part becomes numb.

Ice is also often used in the later stages of injury. Many physicians and trainers prescribe cold treatments for overuse injuries. After a workout, you may want to apply ice to an aching body part—whether you are recovering from an acute injury or suffering from an overuse problem.

What We Know

RICE principles are a practical and effective therapy for new and old injuries.

R<small>EST</small>

I<small>CE</small>

C<small>OMPRESSION</small>

E<small>LEVATION</small>

Compression

Compression is helpful in decreasing pain and swelling. Methods of compression include wrapping with an elastic bandage or splinting a limb with a brace. Putting on an elastic bandage takes more skill than you might think. Apply it firmly but not so tightly that it cuts off your circulation and acts like a tourniquet, which would cause more damage. The elastic bandage should be wrapped from the tip of the limb and directed inward toward the torso.

Elevation

Elevation of the injured part reduces blood flow to that site. This can be achieved by using a sling for the upper extremities. The lower limbs can be elevated with the use of chairs and pillows.

REHAB 101

Following an injury, strength and mobility can be restored with some of the routines described below. You do not always need a specially equipped gym or expensive gadgets to perform these exercises. What you need is willpower.

Our list of rehabilitative exercises is by no means inclusive. There are lots of different injuries and lots of different approaches to treatment. With this in mind, here are a few common exercise routines to help fix the body part that hurts and to keep it from hurting once it has been repaired.

ANKLE

Speed skater Bonnie Blair, who has won five gold medals, lists sprained ankles as her major sports medical problem. According to Blair, ". . . one of the most important parts of rehab is to make sure you're doing what you're supposed to. People have to realize that they're not going to get cured just at the doctor's office and the therapy office. A lot is going to come from you doing what you're told at home and trying to stay as regimented to that as possible."[3]

Following an acute injury, such as an ankle sprain, early motion promotes healing of tissues and limits formation of adhesions (which are like scars). Hence, many physicians recommend gentle movement of an injured part soon after injury.[4]

Rehab for a sprained ankle consists of exercises for range of motion, strength, and balance.[5] You can start by moving your injured ankle in clockwise and counterclockwise motions. The next step is to do the "alphabet exercise," which involves tracing the letters of the alphabet from A to Z in the air. Sit in a chair with the legs crossed, the injured leg

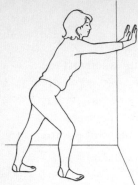

Figure 1
Ankle: Stretch

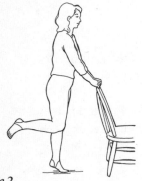

Figure 2
Ankle: Standing Heel-Raises

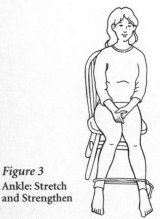

Figure 3
Ankle: Stretch
and Strengthen

on top. You can use your big toe as a pointer to trace the letters. Be sure to move the ankle and keep your hip and knee stationary.[6] (Remember, you want to restore motion to the ankle joint!) As your injury subsides, you will be able to outline bigger and bigger letters.

To stretch the muscles in the ankle (as well as in the back of the calf), stand at arm's length from a wall and, with the uninjured knee bent, lean against the wall. Hold this position with the abnormal foot on the ground for up to 30 seconds, doing five repetitions, three to five times daily.[7] Another approach is to hold for ten seconds with five to ten repetitions, two or three times a day.[8] See Figure 1.

Once your ankle range of motion has begun to normalize, standing heel raises can help to increase strength. While holding onto a table or sturdy chair for balance, lift your heel off the ground so the ball of your injured foot is bearing your body weight. You may want to start off by lifting both heels simultaneously and build up to doing one foot at a time. Gradually increase the number of repetitions and the amount of time you hold the position. While doing the one-leg version, you may want to keep your eyes closed so that you can concentrate on restoring your balance, an important part of ankle rehab. See Figure 2.

Next, you can further stretch and strengthen your ankle by placing an elastic cord around your feet and pulling your feet apart.[9] Try positioning your feet in different positions so that the different muscle groups are challenged. See Figure 3.

KNEE

Basketball star Dawn Staley is a five foot, six inch guard on the USA National Team and, in 1996, a first-time Olympian. She has had serious knee problems and has required surgery on both knees in the past. She reminds us that: "The rehab is all the same—it's pretty repetitive. It's a matter of disciplining yourself to do it. Some days you don't really feel like doing it. Those are the days you should work the hardest."[10]

Keep in mind that not all exercise routines are suitable for those with knee injuries. Since there are so many causes of knee pain, you should get clearance from your physician before proceeding with some of these rehab exercises. Many exercises are directed at strengthening the quadriceps so as to ease pressure on the knees.

While stair climbing has been advocated by some experts, it may actually worsen the overall situation for women with patellofemoral syndrome. Others feel that stair-climbing machines do not aggravate knee pain as much as actual stair climbing does, because the knee is not lifted as high.[11] Instead of stair climbing, women should do short arc extensions to strengthen the quadriceps.[12] To do this simple exercise, sit on the floor with legs extended in front of you. Place a rolled-up towel under the knee. Gently lift the foot

Figure 4a, 4b
Short Arc Extension

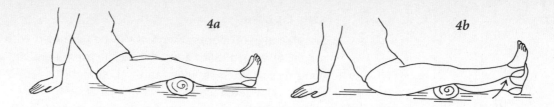

until leg is straight. Start with one set of ten, and built up to five sets per sitting. See Figures 4a and 4b.

Next, try straight leg raising in all four planes of hip motion. While flat on your back, lift the affected leg straight upwards (flexion). Then, roll to your side so that the problematic knee is on top. Gently raise the leg upwards (abduction). Next, lay face down and, while keeping the leg straight, lift it backwards (extension). Finally, roll to your side so the affected leg is on the ground and lift the leg upward (adduction). There is often minimal discomfort with these strengthening exercises because the knee is kept straight.[13]

Another approach to strengthen the quadriceps is to perform isotonic exercise with and without resistance or weights. Start by sitting in a chair, with a low stool nearby. Extend your injured leg and place your foot on the stool. Lift your leg to a horizontal position and hold for six to ten seconds.[14] Increase the number of repetitions as you improve. See Figures 5a and 5b.

Figure 5a, 5b
Knee: Quad Stregthening

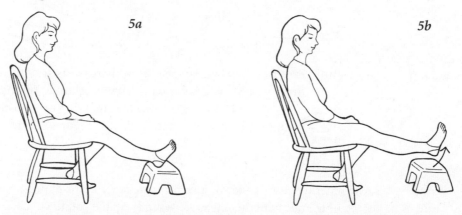

To better condition the inner thigh muscles and to help pull the kneecap into better alignment, try this routine: Lie on your back with knees bent and feet on the floor and place a pillow between your knees. Squeeze the pillow and hold for six to ten seconds. Aim for ten repetitions.[15]

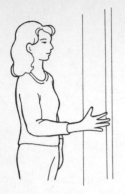

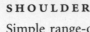

Figures 6a, 6b
Shoulder Isometrics

SHOULDER

Simple range-of-motion exercises can be perfomed with little pain, and are the best way to start a shoulder rehab program. Bend at the waist and hang your affected shoulder and arm straight down. Rotate the arm in small clockwise and counterclockwise circles.[15]

Once full, pain-free range of motion is achieved, exercise to strengthen the rotator cuff muscles can begin. One easy-to-perform isometric exercise involves standing in a doorway with the elbow bent to 90 degrees, as if you were about to shake hands. Push your palm against the doorway and hold for ten seconds. Repeat ten times. Next, push the back of your hand against the other side of the doorway, hold, and repeat the exercise.[16] See Figures 6a and 6b.

This exercise strengthens the external rotators of the shoulder. If desired, add two- to five-pound weights to increase resistance. Lie on your uninjured side and hold the affected arm against your side with the elbow bent 90 degrees. Slowly raise your forearm until it points upward. Add weight in small increments.[17] See Figures 7a and 7b.

Figure 7a, 7b
Shoulder: External Rotation

7a

7b

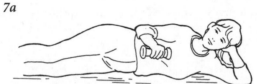

Figures 8a, 8b
Shoulder: Supraspinatus

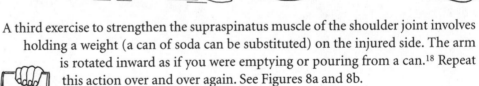

A third exercise to strengthen the supraspinatus muscle of the shoulder joint involves holding a weight (a can of soda can be substituted) on the injured side. The arm is rotated inward as if you were emptying or pouring from a can.[18] Repeat this action over and over again. See Figures 8a and 8b.

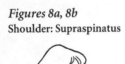

ELBOW

Any repetitive use of the wrist or forearm can set you up for tennis elbow. A routine of stretching and strengthening exercises may enable you to get back in the swing of things. To start, try this stretch: Straighten out your affected arm in front of you with the palm down and the elbow locked. Use the opposite hand to push the top of your hand and fingers toward the floor, resisting with the affected arm. Hold for about ten seconds and do five repetitions a few times a day.[19] You can also perform this stretch with your palm facing up.

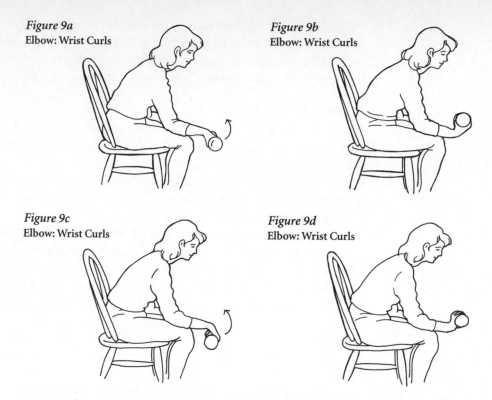

Figure 9a
Elbow: Wrist Curls

Figure 9b
Elbow: Wrist Curls

Figure 9c
Elbow: Wrist Curls

Figure 9d
Elbow: Wrist Curls

To strengthen the forearm, hold your arm straight out in front of you and make a fist. Cock up the wrist and, with the uninjured arm, try to push the wrist down. Gradually increase the number of repetitions.[19]

In addition to these strengthening exercises, you can also perform wrist curls with a small weight. If you do not have a dumbbell handy, you can improvise and find a household object that weighs about two pounds. Sit with your forearm resting on your lap. With your palm facing upward, bend the wrist up. Repeat the process with the palm facing down. See Figures 9a–9d. Gradually increase the weight and the number of repetitions.[20] This exercise can also be done in a standing position.

Roll-up exercises can also help to strengthen the forearm muscles. Tie a piece of rope about three feet long to a broomstick or cane, and attach a weight (about two pounds). Grasp the broomstick with your palms facing down and slowly lift the weight by bending your wrists up. Then *slowly* lower the weight back to the ground by bending your wrists down.[20] Gradually increase the number of reps and the amount of weight.

Two more exercises to strengthen the biceps and triceps utilize the dumbbell. Start-

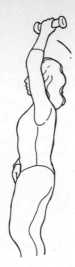

ing with your arm at your side and holding the weight, simply bend the elbow to lift the weight, with your palm facing forward.[20] To perform the triceps curl, lift the dumbbell over your head, keeping your arm straight. Slowly lower the weight behind your head, in the direction of the opposite shoulder, by bending your elbow. See Figures 10a and 10b.

BACK IN SHAPE

Connie Carpenter Phinney had an exciting Olympic career. At the age of 14, she competed in speed skating in the 1972 Olympics in Japan. In 1984, she brought home an Olympic gold medal in cycling. She also has a long history of chronic low back pain, dating back to her speed skating days. She now does yoga three days a week and is careful about not lifting up her five-year-old son. "As long as I maintain my flexibility and stomach strength, I'll be OK."[21]

A back program involves, first of all, the correction of poor posture and improper techniques that aggravate the spine. Exercises that stretch and strengthen the muscles that help flex and extend are also important. Many of these exercises can be done at home.

Figures 10a, 10b
Triceps Curl

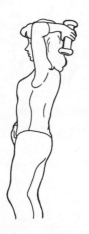

The pelvic tilt is a good back strengthener. Lie on your back with your knees bent and feet flat on the floor, then relax your back muscles. Simultaneously, use your belly muscles to press your back against the floor, forcing your hips to tip forward.[22]

The knee-hug stretch is another stretch performed while lying on your back. Bend one knee, bring it toward your chest, and hold for 30 seconds. Repeat with the other knee.[22]

The abdominal curl is performed while lying on your back with your knees bent and feet flat on the floor. Fold your arms across your chest and, while pressing your back against the floor, lift your head and shoulders off the floor and hold for about ten seconds.[22] (Proper form is illustrated in Chapter 4.) A more advanced step is to then clasp your hands behind your head and repeat the curl.

To strengthen the muscles that extend the back, get on all fours and arch your back upward like a cat or dog. You may also lie face down with a pillow supporting your hips and stretch out your arms and legs. Raise one arm while lifting the opposite leg off the ground, and hold for two seconds. Repeat with the opposite limbs.[22] See Figure 11.

Figure 11
Back: Extension

THINK PREVENTION

Hopefully, you are one of the lucky people who does not spend half of your sporting life in rehab. The exercises we have described above can also be used preventatively. Let's say you only play tennis during the summer months. After a winter of not playing, springtime may be a good time to start some forearm stretching and strengthening exercises so that your elbow will be in tip-top shape when you resume playing.

Keep in mind the importance of individualizing your rehabilitation program. Learn to recognize when it is safe to return to action. Try your best to avoid reinjury, and listen carefully to your body cues. Remember, prevention is the best medicine.

ENDNOTES

1. O'Connor, F. G., Sobel, J. R., & Nirschl, R. P. Five-step treatment for overuse injuries. *The Physician and Sportsmedicine*, October 1992, 20 (10), 128–142.

2. Stamford, B. Giving injuries the cold treatment. *The Physician and Sportsmedicine*, March 1996, 24 (3), 99–100.

3. White, J. Olympic insights. *The Physician and Sportsmedicine*, 1996, 24 (7), 111–114.

4. Levin, S. Early mobilization speeds recovery. *The Physician and Sportsmedicine*, August 1993, 21 (8), 70–74.

5. Torburn, L. Basic protocols of rehabilitation for the ankle, knee, hip, and shoulder. *Primary Care: Orthopedics*, June 1996, 23 (2), 389–403.

6. Connolly, J. F. Exercises to help you recover from a sprained ankle. *Consultant*, August 1966, 36, 1644–646.

   Torburn, L. Basic protocols of rehabilitation for the ankle, knee, hip, and shoulder. *Primary Care: Orthopedics*, June 1996, 23 (2), 389–403.

7. Connolly, J. F. Exercises to help you recover from a sprained ankle. *Consultant*, August 1966, 36, 1644–1646.

   Connolly, J. F. Acute Ankle sprains: Getting and keeping patients back up on their feet. *Consultant*. August 1966, 36, 1631–1643.

8. Case, W. S. Recovering from ankle sprains. *The Physician and Sportsmedicine*, November 1993, 21 (11), 43–44.

9. Connolly, J. F. Exercises to help you recover from a sprained ankle. *Consultant*, August 1966, 36, 1644–1646.

10. White, J. Olympic insights. *The Physician and Sportsmedicine*, 1996, 24 (7), 111–114.

11. Rizzo, T. D., Jr. Getting a leg up on anterior knee pain. *The Physician and Sportsmedicine*, October 1991, 19 (10), 147–148.

12. Hunter, L. Y. Women's athletics: The orthopedic surgeon's viewpoint. *Clinics in Sports Medicine*, October, 1984, 3 (4), 809–827.

13. Torburn, L. Basic protocols of rehabilitation for ankle, knee, hip, and shoulder. *Primary Care*, June 1996, 23 (2), 389–403.

14. Rizzo, T. D., Jr. Getting a leg up on anterior knee pain. *The Physician and Sportsmedicine*, October 1991, 19 (10), 147–148.

15. Torburn, L. Basic protocols of rehabilitation for ankle, knee, hip, and shoulder. *Primary Care*, June 1996, 23 (2), 389–403.

16. Rizzo, T. D., Jr. Recovering from shoulder pain. *The Physician and Sportsmedicine*, October 1992, 20 (10), 195–196.

17. Torburn, L. Basic protocols of rehabilitation for ankle, knee, hip, and shoulder. *Primary Care*, June 1996, 23 (2), 389–403.

    Rizzo, T. D., Jr. Recovering from shoulder pain. *The Physician and Sportsmedicine*, October 1992, 20 (10), 195–196.

18. Torburn, L. Basic protocols of rehabilitation for ankle, knee, hip, and shoulder. *Primary Care*, June 1996, 23 (2), 389–403.

19. Case, W. S. Acing tennis elbow. *The Physician and Sportsmedicine*, July 1993, 21 (7), 21–22.

    Patient Notes. Tennis elbow. *Postgraduate Medicine*, February 1995, 97 (2), 168.

20. Case, W. S. Acing tennis elbow. *The Physician and Sportsmedicine*, July 1993, 21 (7), 21–22.

21. White, J. Olympic insights. *The Physician and Sportsmedicine*, 1996, 24 (7), 111–114.

22. Rizzo, T. D. Getting your back in shape. *The Physician and Sportsmedicine*, February 1993, 21 (2), 177–178.

18

Beware of the Danger Zones

D O N N A I . M E L T Z E R , M . D .

THE FEMALE ATHLETE TRIAD

The Audition.   Picture these scenarios in your mind: A dozen or so young ballet dancers are anxiously waiting for the results of their first auditions. But only a couple of these eight- and nine-year-old girls will walk away with smiles, while the remainder will be very disappointed. Next, envision the group of ballet students who were chosen. They are now in their late teens, and are practicing at the barre as the artistic director of a ballet company looks them over from head to toe. Not only is the emphasis on grace and technique, but on thinness as well. Every dancer standing there nervously knows the essentials of a successful ballet body: long slender legs, a tiny waist, and a fairly flat chest.

Unfortunately, by this time, many of these young women will have adopted unhealthy lifestyles to achieve that long, lean, and leggy look. Some will have skipped meals, some may have purged themselves, and others will simply be obsessed with weight. These eating disorder symptoms may be accompanied by menstrual cycle irregularities and osteoporosis.

Defining the Triad.   When exercise, weight loss, and poor nutrition are taken to an extreme, some women and girls are at risk of developing the **female athlete triad**. Although the problem has been around for some time, the term "female athlete triad" has only recently received some well-deserved attention. The complete triad consists of an eating disorder, amenorrhea (absence of menstrual periods), and osteoporosis (low bone mass). In this chapter, we describe each of these conditions and how they are related.

How Common Is the Triad?   At this time, no one knows exactly how many women are affected by the female athlete triad.[1] We can, however, make some educated guesses about the prevalence of amenorrhea and even take a stab at estimating the frequency of disordered patterns of eating. As mentioned in Chapter 11, the reported prevalence of amenorrhea in young female athletes is anywhere from 3.4 percent to 66 percent. In contrast, only 2 to 5 percent of the general female population has amenorrhea.[2] Also disturbing are the reports that somewhere between 15 and 62 percent of female athletes exhibit disordered eating patterns.[3] The wide range in these figures stems from the fact that diverse populations of athletes have been studied. For example, the aspiring Olympic gymnast may feel pressure to maintain a specific body type and weight that is usually in stark contrast to that of the elite swimmer or bodybuilder. Also, researchers have utilized slightly different definitions of amenorrhea and eating disorders in their investigations.

Who's at Risk?   All female athletes are conceivably in danger of developing the triad. Although the exact prevalence of the complete triad is not known, those participating in endurance, highly competitive, and appearance-based sports seem to be at highest risk. Distance running, gymnastics, and ballet dancing are sports where a lean physique and low body fat are considered an advantage.[4] It may be the young woman who's striving to be the fastest marathoner, the gymnast looking for perfect tens, the dancer dreaming of being a prima ballerina, or maybe you. One explanation of the triad is that an athlete who is driven to excel in her sport or pressured to fit a certain body image maintains an unrealistically low body weight, resulting in abnormal menstrual periods, which in turn lead to premature bone loss.[5]

An Early Start. Females of all ages are now being encouraged to exercise and participate in sports. While youth is a time of rapid growth and development, it is also a time when social and emotional stressors may expose an individual to abnormal eating patterns. An obsession with thinness seems to have become pervasive in our culture. We need to get a better handle on this body fat fixation to make sure that it is not inadvertently transmitted from parent to child, from teacher to student, from coach to athlete, or from athlete to athlete.

I'm Too Old for the Triad . . . Not So! Adolescents and young athletes run a high risk of developing the complete triad, but you may be interested to know that adults are not immune, especially if they compete at an elite level.[6] We should be on the alert for any signs of the triad—not just in our daughters, but in our friends, colleagues, and ourselves as well.

Disordered Eating

In 1990, Patti Catalano was the first American woman to break 2:30 in the New York City Marathon. In 1980, she ran 48 races and produced 13 American or world records. Patti Catalano was also bulimic. She beat the problem in 1986 after years of secret bingeing and purging, and calls her recovery the "greatest race" of her life.[7]

Disordered patterns of eating are more common than many people realize, especially when they are viewed as a cluster of abnormal eating behaviors with poor nutritional practices at one end of the spectrum and **anorexia** and **bulimia** at the other extreme.[8] In simple terms, anorexia is a loss or lack of appetite. On the other hand, bulimia is characterized by binge eating. Anorexia nervosa and bulimia nervosa are medically defined syndromes, each with specific diagnostic criteria (see below). It is, however, not unusual for an affected individual to fluctuate between anorexia and bulimia. In fact, between 40 percent and 48 percent of anorexic patients have coexisting bulimia.[9]

Anorexia nervosa. Individuals suffering from anorexia nervosa starve themselves and may also develop rigid and intensive exercise programs to burn calories and lose weight. Anorexics possess a disturbed image of their body weight or shape, and have an intense fear of gaining weight or of becoming fat, even though they may be grossly underweight.[10] Paradoxically, this morbid preoccupation with weight gain often intensifies with further weight loss.

Bulimia or Binge Eating. Women with bulimia have recurrent episodes of binge eating: the consumption of huge amounts of food in short periods of time. Some (the purging type) will force themselves to vomit or will misuse laxatives, diuretics ("water pills"), or other medications. Unlike anorexics, bulimics do not see themselves with such a markedly distorted body image. Quite often, a female with bulimia is of normal or slightly above normal weight. Bulimics who do not engage in purging via vomiting or laxatives (the non-purging type) will often use other inappropriate behaviors such as fasting or excessive exercise to prevent weight gain.

Disordered Eating: Warning Signals

- Eating less at mealtime
- Obsession with food, calories, and weight
- "Closet" eating (not eating with others)
- Habit of visiting the bathroom immediately after mealtime
- Out-of-control eating binges

TABLE 18.1

....

Diagnostic Criteria for Anorexia Nervosa

- Refusal to maintain body weight at or above a minimally normal weight for age and height.
- Intense fear of becoming fat or gaining weight, even though underweight.
- Disturbed body image, or denial of the seriousness of the current body weight.
- Amenorrhea in postmenarchal females.

Restricting Type: Does not engage in binge eating or purging. Weight loss is accomplished primarily through dieting, fasting, or excessive exercise.

Binge Eating/Purging Type: Regularly engages in binge eating or purging behavior (or both). This includes self-induced vomiting and/or misuse of laxatives or diuretics.

....

Adapted from the *Diagnostic and Statistical Manual of Mental Disorders* (4th ed.).

Making an Exact Diagnosis.   Twenty-five years ago, the definition of anorexia was heavily weighted toward the physical symptoms of the syndrome. More recently, the importance of the psychological characteristics of the illness is being recognized. Diagnostic criteria for anorexia nervosa and bulimia nervosa were updated in the revised 1994 edition of the Diagnostic and Statistical Manual of Mental Disorders (DSM-IV).[11] (See Tables 18.1 and 18.2.) While some affected individuals may not fit these definitions to a tee, abnormal eating patterns should not be overlooked in any case. Making the earliest possible diagnosis of the problem correlates fairly well with a better chance of a successful cure.

Not for Young Women Only. Although it is primarily a disorder of young women, there are no age limits or gender requirements when it comes to anorexia or bulimia. Ninety-five percent of anorexic and 90 percent of bulimic cases occur in girls and women.[12] This higher female-to-male ratio may change as the public becomes better versed in identifying the symptoms of eating disorders and as we screen more carefully for signs of the illness.

Anorexic and bulimic behaviors usually develop in late adolescence or the early twenties, but can occur in the young and the elderly as well. Although one of the earliest

TABLE 18.2

Diagnostic Criteria for Bulimia Nervosa

- Recurrent, out-of-control episodes of binge eating, typically with large amounts of food ingested.
- Recurrent inappropriate compensatory behavior to prevent weight gain (purging or nonpurging).
- Binge eating and inappropriate compensatory behaviors occur, on average, at least twice per week for 3 months.

There are two subtypes: Purging and Nonpurging types

Purging Type: Regularly engages in self-induced vomiting or misuse of laxatives, enemas, or diuretics.

Nonpurging Type: Does not purge, but compensates inappropriately by fasting or by excessive exercise.

Adapted from the *Diagnostic and Statistical Manual of Mental Disorders* (4th ed.).

signals of anorexia nervosa is excessive physical activity, people have wondered whether striving to achieve athleticism precipitates an eating disorder or vice versa. However, we should not forget that an individual does not need to be considered athletic to develop anorexia or bulimia.

Psychological Profile of the "Typical" Anorexic. The typical individual with anorexia nervosa is an adolescent female who is a high achiever.[13] She is a perfectionist and a good student who independently completes her chores and homework. Over time, she develops a preoccupation with weight and begins to restrict her caloric intake. She begins to make excuses for her weight being below normal while maintaining food rituals and excessive exercise programs. Sometimes, the anorexic will resort to using diet pills, laxatives, and other methods to purge herself, especially if she feels guilty about bingeing. She continues to lose weight and feels good as long as the bathroom scale reflects a loss. She remains in a world of denial, fearful of becoming fat. Signs of depression frequently coexist with eating disorders. Eventually, her grades slide as the physical symptoms of her ever increasing obsession with dieting and thinness set in.

The Physical Signs. Aside from striking thinness and wasting, anorexics often have abnormal vital signs: low body temperatures, bradycardia (low heart rates), and low blood pressure.[14] They may have a prominent growth of lanugo, a fine, downy hair that covers the body. Those who have engaged in self-induced vomiting may have damaged tooth enamel (from repeated contact with stomach acid) and scars on the backs of their hands (caused by repeatedly scraping the hand against the front teeth while trying to induce a gag).[15]

The physical changes seen in puberty may be delayed in those with anorexia. In fact, 30 percent of anorexic women may not menstruate until their twenties, even when treatment is initiated.[15] While women may suffer from amenorrhea caused by lowered LH and FSH levels, anorexic males may have fluctuating levels of testosterone and lower sperm counts.

A Private Disorder. Anorexia and bulimia are often kept hidden. Parents, partners, or roommates of those who suffer from disordered eating often do not know what's going on. If confronted, the anorexic or bulimic will often be in a complete state of denial. She may also be convincing enough to fool those closest to her.

You don't have to be an elite athlete to master keeping an eating problem a secret. That's because the symptoms of these disorders aren't always obvious, especially in the early stages. Very few women will openly admit that they have a distorted body image or even recognize that they are preoccupied with food and exercise. This is all part of the disease process.

The Athletic Connection. A 1990 survey reporting that 64 percent of women athletes had some experience with an eating disorder supports the widespread nature of this problem.[16] Although more typically encountered in females and more prevalent in athletes than nonathletes, eating disorders are not limited to females. Contrary to popular belief, males, especially those involved in certain weight-conscious sports (such as wrestling), are not immune to eating disorders. Moreover, fitness buffs and athletes participating in all sports are vulnerable, especially as they rise though the ranks to stardom.

What We Can Do. Athletes are a special breed. You may know women who are perfectionists, competitive, driven, and athletic. These are the same personality traits that can be found in persons with eating disorders. If there is the least bit of concern, parents, coaches, and friends may want to ask the athlete about the use of diet pills, laxatives, or diuretics. A gentler approach may be to have regular open discussions about body image, self-esteem, and life stressors. Inquiries should be made about purging and levels of physical activity. Prolonged fasting and/or bingeing are other signs that a problem exists. Remember, the athlete is not likely to discuss these behaviors with others, even those close to her. Everyone's index of suspicion must remain high.

Treatment. Treatment begins with a thorough history and physical exam. Sometimes, individuals with anorexia nervosa may need to be hospitalized, especially if their vital signs are unstable or if they are suicidal. Whether treatment is initiated in an outpatient setting or within the hospital, it requires teamwork. Medical personnel must work in concert with nutritionists and counselors. Individual, family, and group counseling sessions are often helpful. Antidepressants may also be prescribed for individuals with anorexia or bulimia. Since anorexia nervosa and bulimia nervosa are often chronic disorders, therapy may need to be ongoing.

Menstrual Disorders

The athlete with a nutritional problem may go on to develop a menstrual disorder, the second aspect of the triad. She may go months or even years without having a period. To briefly review, if a girl reaches the age of 16 or 17 without ever having menses, she can be diagnosed with primary amenorrhea provided she has developed secondary sex characteristics such as breast development and pubic hair.

A woman who has already menstruated and then goes three to six consecutive cycles without a period has secondary amenorrhea. (Some authorities define secondary amenorrhea as less than six to nine periods annually.)[17] For a full discussion of menstrual cycle disorders, see Chapter 11. Please note that some menstrual abnormalities can occur in the absence of an eating disorder. Our focus in this chapter will be on secondary amenorrhea.

Body Fat and Menses. We used to believe that body fat was the critical factor regulating menstruation. Frisch's "critical fat" hypothesis (discussed in Chapter 11) speculated that menarche and menstrual cycles were related to an individual's percentage of body fat. In other words, a woman needed 17 percent body fat in order for menarche to occur and if she developed amenorrhea, she would need 22 percent body fat for normal menses to be resumed.[18] Although we don't fully understand the entire scheme of events yet, a woman's percentage of body fat, in and of itself, probably does not cause the menstrual cycle changes.[19] We also do not know what the long term consequences are for women who have chronically very low estrogen levels.

Osteoporosis

"Osteoporosis is a nasty disease," says research physiologist Barbara Drinkwater, Ph.D., who has done pioneering work on osteoporosis.[20] For those who suffer from it, it is more than just a nasty disease. It can be frightening and devastating to both athletes and nonathletes.

Osteoporosis, which makes up the third part of the triad, is defined by early bone loss or inadequate bone formation, resulting in low bone mass. Previously felt to be a disease of elderly women, it's now known that many young athletes may have bones that can't be distinguished from those of 60-year-old women. Unfortunately, the exact incidence of osteoporosis among female athletes is not known.[21]

A Silent Disease.   Osteoporosis is often called a silent disease. In the early stages, there are no symptoms. Suspicions may not be raised until a person develops a bone fracture. At the fortieth annual meeting of the American College of Sports Medicine, Drinkwater noted that women who resumed normal periods after having amenorrhea had a 6 percent increase in bone density over 14 months.[22] The bad news was that the bone density growth did not continue. Four years later, these women still had bone densities that were below normal. It is disturbing to think that once bone is lost, it may never be fully regained.

The Effects of Estrogen and Exercise.   A significant risk factor for osteoporosis among healthy, active women is estrogen deficiency, which may be a result of delayed menarche, amenorrhea, oligomenorrhea, or premature menopause.[23] Exercise-associated amenorrhea is the most common type of amenorrhea in athletes and is not limited to any one sport.[24] Training intensity, body fat, and nutrition are other factors that play a role in athletic amenorrhea.

Some of this may be confusing since you have been told that women who engage in regular, moderate exercise may lower their risk of osteoporosis. The key word here is *moderate*. Long, intense workouts may be associated with lower estrogen levels, which in turn may speed up bone loss. Our concern here is that some studies have demonstrated an increased risk of fractures among some athletes with menstrual irregularity. Many young amenorrheic athletes are losing bone at a time in their lives when they should be storing it.

Curbing the Triad

Prevention and early awareness of the female athlete triad are the best ways to reduce its incidence. In the last few decades, increased interest in sports has led many of us to become highly competitive, if not elite athletes, while some of us keep our participation at the recreational level. In addition, there is societal pressure to look good and have a perfect body. For some, this image means having very little body fat. Taken to extremes, this could develop into an unhealthy lifestyle. Women need to understand that very low body fat is not the key to optimal athletic performance.

The management of athletes with eating disorders should be individualized. For those who have poor nutritional habits, it may just be a matter of explaining the importance of good nutrition while focusing on the food pyramid. (For a thorough discussion, see Chapter 10.) Athletes with anorexia or bulimia require help from physicians, trainers, parents, nutritionists, and other professionals.

If an athlete develops amenorrhea, she may be able to lower the risk of acquiring the complete triad. Sometimes, by simply improving nutrition, an athlete may resume normal menstruation. If she is willing and able to decrease her activity by 10 to 20 percent and gain some weight, her periods may spontaneously return to normal.[25]

Unfortunately, reducing a training schedule is not always a realistic option for competitive athletes. For those athletes, prescribing hormone replacement is controversial, but may be considered. Prescribing estrogen and progesterone might not increase bone mass, but it may prevent further bone loss. We know this works for post-menopausal women, but it is too early to tell if it will be effective for younger athletes with amenorrhea. Alternatively, birth control pills (whether or not the athlete is sexually active) are another option. Birth control pills are also presumed to preserve the integrity of bone.[25] Dr. Mona Shangold, who directs a sports gynecology center, feels that hormone replacement therapy should be prescribed for any woman who has the female athlete triad.[26] She reasons that athletes diagnosed with the triad are estrogen deficient and therefore require hormone replacement. For a complete discussion of the pros and cons of hormone replacement therapy, see Chapter 11.

Athletes of all ages should realize that while there are many benefits to sports and exercise, there may be a downside if taken to extremes. If the pressure to excel results in unhealthy consequences, athletes' future health is at risk and the benefits of exercise may be lost. Healthy priorities need to be reestablished and myths dispelled so that women do not suffer the effects of the triad.

THE STEROID DILEMMA

A Race Cut Short

Competitive bike racer Cindy Olivarri's life changed dramatically when the International Olympic Committee announced that the 1984 Games would, for the first time, feature women's cycling events. Olivarri had been racing competitively since 1979 and made the team in the Olympic trials. Shortly thereafter she learned that she had tested positive for steroids and would have to relinquish her opportunity to compete in the Olympics.

Nearly a decade later, she admits: "I knew it was cheating. I'd been tested before and never gotten caught."[27]

Anabolic steroids have been used by athletes for decades. Weight lifters who used steroids strived for power and the ability to lift more, swimmers and runners aimed for better performances, and bodybuilders hoped to increase their lean body mass. So prevalent was the use of steroids that the International Olympic Committee placed a ban on the use of anabolic steroids at the 1976 Games in Montreal.

Youth and Steroids

Steroid use among adolescents is of special concern. A survey of over 900 high school students in 1988 found an overall male and female user rate of 3 percent.[28] In 1991, over 12,000 high school students were surveyed by the Centers for Disease Control. This pool revealed that approximately 4 percent of males and 1.2 percent of females were using anabolic steroids.[29] That same year, a survey of seventh-grade students between the ages of 12 and 15 revealed an even higher percentage of steroid users: 4.7 percent of the boys and 3.2 percent of the girls.[30] Much higher rates have been documented in college and elite athletes.[31] It is especially worrisome to think that the actual prevalence of anabolic steroid use among adolescents may be significantly higher than the figures quoted in these surveys. There is bound to be underreporting of steroid abuse because individuals often deny drug use for fear of being caught and punished.

A Natural Hormone

Anabolic steroids are derivatives of the natural male sex hormone, testosterone, which is the counterpart of estrogen, the predominant female hormone. Both males and females have varying amounts of these two hormones. The ratio of the hormones helps to determine sex. Males have principally testosterone, while females are estrogen dominant. You may recall from Chapter 2 that testosterone enhances the development of male secondary sexual characteristics and increases skeletal muscle mass at the time of puberty.

Athletes and Anabolic Steroids

The results of several surveys report that athletes use anabolic steroids in the belief that these drugs increase strength and improve athletic performance, in addition to preventing sports injuries and promoting rapid healing.[32] Others have noted that anabolic steroids help to decrease recovery time between workouts.[33] Still others believe that using steroids helps them to maintain a winning edge over their competitors.

Studies evaluating the effects of anabolic steroids have been controversial: Some support an increase in muscle size and strength, while others have been unable to confirm these findings. Gains in strength have been more consistently observed in the following two circumstances.[34] Athletes who had strength-trained prior to using anabolic steroids were more likely to show an increase in strength as long as they continued to train. Also, athletes using steroids who ingested high-protein, high-calorie diets were more likely to show a positive gain in strength. No matter what the scientific literature states, we know that anabolic steroids remain popular among athletes because athletes *believe* them to improve performance.

Shopping for Steroids. While anabolic steroids are occasionally prescribed by physicians to treat certain medical disorders, their use by athletes is quite controversial. Consequently, the black market supplies most of the anabolic steroids used by athletes.[35] In one study of elite power lifters, 73 percent of steroid users identified the black market as their primary supplier of steroids, followed by physician or pharmacist (20 percent) and mail order (7 percent).[36] The safety and sterility of smuggled drugs can never be assured, which should prompt some health care concerns.

The United States Drug Enforcement Agency (DEA) is responsible for regulating controlled substances like anabolic steroids.[37] The Anabolic Steroids Act of 1990 made it a federal crime, punishable by up to five years in prison, to possess or sell anabolic steroids for nonmedical purposes. This prompted some people to seek other performance-enhancing drugs that were not as tightly regulated as the anabolic steroids. Such products are often sold as "dietary supplements" and therefore fall under a different jurisdiction that does not require their manufacturers to submit proof of safety to the Food and Drug Administration (FDA).

The bottom line is that using anabolic steroids or steroid alternatives without supervision by a legitimate health care professional is risky business. Performance-enhancing dietary substances may also not produce the desired effects and may be dangerous to a person's health.

Stacking, Cycling, and Pyramiding. In order to maximize some of the effects of anabolic steroids, many athletes use more than one drug simultaneously; this is referred to as the **stacking** principle.[38] Stacking is also used to minimize adverse side effects that would result from taking a larger dose of just one steroid. Another pattern of use is **cycling**, which is taking an anabolic steroid for a specific interval of time, such as 4 to 18 weeks, and then stopping to clear the drug from the system.[39] Still another technique, **pyramiding**, implies starting out with a low dose of anabolic steroid, increasing it over time, and then tapering down to nothing. These different patterns may also be used to help minimize an athlete's chances of being detected as a user of anabolic steroids.

The Downside.   As with Cindy Olivarri, athletes are willing to risk their careers in an attempt to achieve ultimate performance. In doing so, they also take substantial health risks.

There is a long list of side effects associated with anabolic steroid usage. When steroids are taken in large doses, men and boys can develop acne, enlargement of breast tissue, and reduction in the size of their testes. Women and girls who use steroids may develop masculine traits such as deepening of the voice, breast shrinkage, male pattern baldness, and facial hair growth. They may also experience menstrual irregularities. Both sexes risk liver problems and negative changes in their cholesterol levels. Some of these effects take years to develop. Some are reversible, but others are not. Women who take anabolic steroids should realize that masculinizing traits may not be reversible. Clearly, some of the proven dangers outweigh potential benefits.

SUDDEN DEATH

Unhappy Endings

Since the death of the original marathoner in Ancient Greece, we have heard tragic stories of athletes, young and old, dying without warning. In 1988, "Pistol Pete" Maravich collapsed and died suddenly during a pickup basketball game. In 1995, 28-year-old Olympic gold medalist skater Sergei Grinkov suffered a sudden fatal heart attack while training at an ice rink in Lake Placid, New York. A common aspect of these stories is that they seem to happen mostly to men. We have not heard much about women athletes suffering sudden death. Assuming that women are as active as men, the next question to pose is whether sudden deaths in women are simply underreported and not publicized—or does the female sex imply some sort of cardiovascular protection?

In the medical literature, sudden death is defined as an unexpected death that occurs instantaneously and without evidence of trauma. When this tragedy occurs in athletes who appear healthy, it is paradoxical. Athletes are supposed to be fit and protected from such events.

Tracking the Causes

In young athletes, the cause of sudden death is often an undiagnosed congenital heart problem. Among athletes over age 30 who die suddenly, a heart attack caused by coronary artery disease is the most common reason.[40] In some cases, risk factors for coronary artery disease have been identified retrospectively. Other victims of sudden death due to heart disease have maintained high levels of athleticism without symptoms or risk factors.

The Number-One Killer.   Coronary heart disease (CHD) is the number-one killer of

American women. Studies now demonstrate that one in nine women between the ages of 45 and 64 years old has heart disease. After the age of 65 years, one in three women will be affected by heart disease.[41]

People with CHD do not always present with classic symptoms. For example, a woman suffering from a heart attack may not always experience chest pain with exertion. Instead, her symptoms may be shortness of breath or fatigue, or intermittent chest pressure with or without exercise. Compared to men, women with chest pain are more likely to delay seeking medical attention and are also less likely to attribute their symptoms to heart disease.

There is now evidence that heart disease in women, once diagnosed, has been treated less aggressively than in our male partners. Heart disease in women has generated a lot of interest and exciting research is currently ongoing.

Examining Your Risk

You may begin to wonder what your risk is for sudden death. There is no medical evidence that even strenuous physical activity is harmful to an individual with a healthy heart.[42] We do, however, know that sudden death in athletes can occur because of underlying coronary artery disease. Unfortunately, there is very limited information available on sudden cardiac death in female athletes.

It may seem that sudden deaths are more prevalent in athletic males than females—but this may be because women's participation in sports differs from men's. It may also be that some women are protected from cardiovascular disease. (Certainly, heart disease is uncommon in premenopausal women.) The perceived differences in sudden death may also be due to errors in reporting or evaluating exercise-related sudden death in women. We cannot infer that sudden death does not occur in women just because the media has not publicized the issue.

The Warning Signs. Exercising adults should be aware of warning signs for cardiac disease. Not everyone has chest pains prior to suffering a heart attack. For some, the warning signs are lightheadedness, nausea, or unusual shortness of breath during exertion. Sergei Grinkov's widow and training partner reported that he never complained of chest pain or any other symptoms of heart disease. The only foreshadowing of the impending tragedy was that the skater's father died in his fifties from a sudden heart attack.[43]

Runner and author Jim Fixx's sudden death while exercising stunned millions of people in 1984. Fixx had been a heavy smoker in the past and also had a strong family history of heart disease. Not surprising, his autopsy revealed severe heart disease and evidence of a prior heart attack.

Should fear of dying stop you from exercising? Absolutely not, provided you don't have any of the symptoms of heart disease. If you are about to embark on an exercise routine and have any health concerns, speak to your physician. Make sure that your health care provider is sensitive and aware of the fact that risk factors and symptoms of disease may differ between sexes. Exercisers have a lower risk of sudden death compared to nonathletes—or at least that is the data that has been compiled on men. Until gender-specific exercise guidelines become available, listen to your body cues, talk with your physician, and stay tuned for future developments in women's health care.

SAFETY ON THE STREETS

In April 1989, the young female investment banker who was brutally attacked one evening while running in Central Park captured national attention. While there are no statistics demonstrating how many runners are attacked, we know that someone becomes a victim of a violent crime every 17 seconds. More than one adult woman is raped in the United States every minute.[44]

With such chilling numbers, women athletes need to take special precautions to ensure their safety. Nancy Biele, former president of the National Coalition Against Sexual Assault, states: "Something irks me about giving safety tips to women when we ought to look at how to stop men from raping women."[45] While recognizing that eliminating rape should be society's goal, she suggests the following tips provided by the Road Runner's Club of America (RRCA):

- Carry identification.
- Don't wear jewelry.
- Run with a partner.
- Carry enough money to make a phone call.
- Run in familiar areas, but alter your route.
- Always stay alert.
- Ignore verbal harassment.

Many runners like to run to music, but for safety's sake, it's recommended that you leave the headsets at home. With music blasting in your ears, you may be unaware of approaching individuals or vehicles. If you run at dusk or before dawn, wear clothing that is reflective. Dress to look confident, but not vulnerable.

Mace, a self-defense spray that burns the eyes, is advocated by the RRCA for female runners.[45] It comes in a small canister that you should have in hand and be prepared to use. However, in some cities and states, carrying mace is illegal. For more information, check with your local authorities. Alternatively, you may consider carrying a whistle or screech alarm.

Keep in mind that these safety tips are not just for female runners. Women need to be careful at all times. Whether you are walking to the parking lot at the mall or entering an elevator at work, be aware of your surroundings and any nearby individuals. If possible, avoid being alone in unpopulated areas and buildings. There is much to be said about women's intuition. Follow your intuition—it's better to be safe than sorry.

Make Yourself Visible

In the spring of 1997, 57-year-old triathlon champion Judy Flannery was hit by an automobile while on a bicycle training ride. This mother of five did not take up running until she was 38 years old, but in the last decade had won four world and six national titles in the triathlon.

Risk is inherent in nearly all sports, even those such as walking, in which the dangers appear to be slight. While much attention has been paid in recent years to the design and fashioning of safety gear and clothing, accidents do happen. If you exercise outdoors near traffic, make sure that motorists can see you. Wear light, reflective clothing. Wear or attach blinking lights to your bike. If possible, try to avoid exercising at dusk. Make use of protective safety equipment. Be aware of the elements. Obey all traffic rules. Exercise defensively. Use your head, be a smart exerciser, and rely on common sense at all times.

If you heed this advice, the safety tips will eventually become second nature. Not only will you feel more comfortable, but you may avert disaster. Remember, exercising should be safe and healthful.

1. Skolnick, A. A. "Female athlete triad" risk for women. *JAMA*, August 25, 1993, 270 (8), 921–923.

2. Nattiv, A., Lynch, L. The female athlete triad: Managing an acute risk to long-term health. *The Physician and Sportsmedicine*, January 1994, 22 (1), 60–68.

3. Beim, G., & Stone, D. A. Issues in the female athlete. *Orthopedic Clinics of North America*, July 1995, 26 (3), 443–451.

4. Nattiv, A., Lynch, L. The female athlete triad: Managing an acute risk to long-term health. *The Physician and Sportsmedicine*, January 1994, 22 (1), 60–68.

5. Nattiv, A., Agostini, R., Drinkwater, B., & Yeager, K. K. The female athlete triad: The inter-relatedness of disordered eating, amenorrhea, and osteoporosis. *Clinics in Sports Medicine*, l994, 13(2), 405–418.

6. Skolnick, A. A. "Female athlete triad" risk for women. *JAMA*, August 25, 1993, 270 (8), 921–923.

7. Williams, K. Deadly dieting: eating disorders among women can devastate more than athletic performances. *Women's Sports and Fitness*, 1991, 13 (8), 22.

8. Nattiv, A., Lynch, L. The female athlete triad: Managing an acute risk to long-term health. *The Physician and Sportsmedicine*, January 1994, 22 (1), 60–68.

9. Ware, M., Lyles, W. B. Anorexia Nervosa: Assessment. *Family Practice Recertification*, 1989, 11 (5), 26.

10. Hobbs, W. L., Johnson, C. A. Anorexia Nervosa: An Overview. *American Family Physician*, 1996, 54 (4), 1273.

11. American Psychiatric Association. *Diagnostic and statistical manual of mental disorders*. 4th ed. Washington, D.C.: American Psychiatric Association, 1994, 539–45.

12. Yanovski, S. Z. Bulimia Nervosa: The role of the family physician. *American Family Physician*, 1991, 44 (4), 1231–1238.

Ware, M., Lyles, W. B. Anorexia Nervosa: Assessment. *Family Practice Recertification*, 1989, 11 (5), 26.

13. Hobbs, W. L., Johnson, C. A. Anorexia Nervosa: An Overview. *American Family Physician*, 1996, 54 (4), 1273.

14. Ware, M., Lyles, W. B. Anorexia Nervosa: Assessment. *Family Practice Recertification*, 1989, 11 (5), 26.

15. Giannini, A. J., Newman, M., Gold, M. Anorexia and bulimia. *American Family Physician*, 1990, 41 (4), 1169.

16. Williams, K. Deadly dieting: eating disorders among women can devastate more than athletic performances. *Women's Sports and Fitness*, 1991, 13 (8), 22.

17. Smith, A. D. The female athlete triad: causes, diagnosis, and treatment. *The Physician and Sportsmedicine*, July 1996, 24–30, 67–73.

White, C. M., Hergenroeder, A. C. Amenorrhea, osteopenia, and the female athlete. *Pediatric Clinics of North America*, 1990, 37 (5), 1125–1138.

18. Putukian, M. The female triad. *Clinics in Sports Medicine*, 1994, 78 (2), 345–355.

19. Nattiv, A., Lynch, L. The female athlete triad: Managing an acute risk to long-term health. *The Physician and Sportsmedicine*, January 1994, 22 (1), 60–68.

20. Skolnick, A. A. "Female athlete triad" risk for women. *JAMA*, August 25, 1993, 270 (8), 921–923.

21. Smith, A. D. The female athlete triad: causes, diagnosis, and treatment. *The Physician and Sportsmedicine*, July 1996, 24–30, 67–73.

22. Skolnick, A. A. "Female athlete triad" risk for women. *JAMA*, August 25, 1993, 270 (8), 921–923.

23. Dalsky, G. P. Guidelines for diagnosing osteoporosis. *The Physician and Sportsmedicine*, 1996, 24 (7), 96–100.

24. Putukian, M. The female triad. *Clinics in Sports Medicine*, 1994, 78 (2), 345–355.

25. Otis, C. L. Exercise-associated amenorrhea. *Clinics in Sports Medicine*, 1992, 11 (2), 351–361.

26. Smith, A. D. The female athlete triad: causes, diagnosis, and treatment. *The Physician and Sportsmedicine*, July 1996, 24–30, 67–73.

27. Pear, M. J. Steroid roulette: taking male hormones is risky business for women. *Women's Sports and Fitness*, 1992, 14 (7), 18–19.

28. Ghaphery, N. A. Performance enhancing drugs. *Orthopedic Clinics of North America*, 1995, 26 (3), 433–443.

29. DuRant, R. H., Escibedi, L. G., Heath, G. W. Anabolic-steroid use, strength training, and multiple drug use among adolescents in the United States. *Pediatrics*, 1995, 96 (1), 23–28.

30. Radakovich, J., Broderick, P., Garfield, P. Rates of anabolic steroid use among students in junior high school. *Journal of the American Board of Family Practice*, 1993, 6, 341–345.

31. Pope, H. G., Katz, D. L., Champoux, R. Anabolic-androgenic steroid use

among 1,010 college men. *The Physician and Sportsmedicine*, 1988, 16 (7), 75.

32. Ghaphery, N. A. Performance enhancing drugs. *Orthopedic Clinics of North America*, 1995, 26 (3), 433–443.

33. Windsor, D. E., Dumitru, D. Anabolic steroid use by athletes. *Postgraduate Medicine*, 1988, 84 (4), 37.

34. Johnson, M. D. Anabolic steroid use in adolescent athletes. *Pediatric Clinics of North America*, 1990, 37 (5), 1111.

    Windsor, D. E., Dumitru, D. Anabolic steroid use by athletes. *Postgraduate Medicine*, 1988, 84 (4), 37.

35. Buckley, W. E., et al., Estimated prevalence of anabolic steroid use among male high school seniors. *JAMA*, 1988, 260 (23), 3441.

36. Yesalis, C. E., Herrick, R. T., et al. Self-reported use of anabolic-androgenic steroids by elite power lifters. *The Physician and Sportsmedicine*, 1988, 16 (12), 91.

37. Monroe, J. Steroid substitutes. *Current Health*, 1996, 22 (8), 13.

38. Windsor, D. E., Dumitru, D. Anabolic steroid use by athletes. *Postgraduate Medicine*, 1988, 84 (4), 37.

    Johnson, M. D. Anabolic steroid use in adolescent athletes. *Pediatric Clinics of North America*, 1990, 37 (5), 1111.

39. Ghaphery, N. A. Performance enhancing drugs. *Orthopedic Clinics of North America*, 1995, 26 (3), 433–443.

40. Van Camp, S. P. Sudden death. *Clinics in Sports Medicine*, 1992, 11 (2), 273–288.

41. Hennekens, C. H., Judelson, D. R., Wenger, N. K. Coronary disease: The leading killer. *Patient Care*, 1996, 30 (13), 116.

42. Van Camp, S. Exercise-related sudden death: risks and causes (part 1 of 2). *The Physician and Sportsmedicine*, 1988, 16 (5), 97.

43. Fackelmann, K. Flaws of the heart: sudden death in athletes is often caused by cardiac defects. *Science News*, 1996, 150 (5), 76.

44. Miller, L., McKenzie, R., Dobler, M. Street smarts: to ensure their safety, women need to run strong and smart. *Runner's World*, 1993, 28 (6), 58.

45. Shroyer, J. Becoming streetwise: guidelines for female runners. *The Physician and Sportsmedicine*, 1990, 18 (2), 121–125.

Conclusion

You've reached the finale and we expect that by now you are fit and approaching peak performance. You are an active woman who knows fact from fiction. With this in mind, we hope you enjoy reading the exercise myths below:

EXERCISE MYTHS

Myth: Women should exercise differently than men.
Reality: The differences between men and women account for some of the differences in our training and fitness needs. Appreciating these distinctions may enable you to reach peak performance and lower your risk of injury. And don't forget—many of our physical differences are assets, not liabilities.

Myth: If you're fit, you don't have to do stretching exercises.
Reality: Even if you exercise on a regular basis, stretching can help to prevent injury and alleviate muscle soreness. It may even enhance your performance.

Myth: Exercise increases your appetite.
Reality: Moderate exercise may suppress your hunger, but vigorous activitiy may actually stimulate your appetite without resulting in weight gain.

Myth: Women with back problems should not exercise.
Reality: Not usually true. Although back problems may preclude exercising immediately, professionals now encourage you to restart, slowly and carefully, as soon as possible. Blame for a chronic bad back is, in many cases, now being placed upon lack of exercise.

Myth: You can be fit if you exercise only ten minutes per day.

Reality: The latest recommendations suggest that you should exercise moderately for at least 30 minutes on most if not all days of the week. Beginners probably require a different strategy with shorter periods of activity.

Myth: The more you exercise, the fitter and healthier you'll become.

Reality: That sounds logical, but it's not necessarily true. Remember overuse injuries and the female athletic triad.

Myth: The best time to exercise is in the afternoon.

Reality: The best time is a convenient time that enables you to stick with a routine. *Tip:* Try to avoid vigorous exercise immediately after a heavy meal.

Myth: The more out of shape you are, the longer it takes to see results from exercising.

Reality: Sedentary people who start to exercise see more dramatic and faster changes in fitness levels than those who are already exercising. It makes sense: Any improvement from a base of zero is going to be impressive.

Myth: Excessive sweating indicates that you're out of shape.

Reality: As you get into better shape, the body cools itself through perspiration more efficiently. *Tip:* no matter how fit you are, it's still important to drink plenty of water. Drink before, during, and after exercise to avoid dehydration.

Myth: Weight lifting creates large muscles in women and it's only for young girls.

Reality: While a woman's muscles may increase in tone and size, they will not develop the same muscle bulk as a man's because women do not have the same amount of testosterone as men do. It's particularly important as we age to do some type of weight-bearing activity to maintain bone and muscle strength and mobility.

Myth: Exercise is always fun.

Reality: People sometimes are misled by those promoting exercise. Not every single minute of every workout is going to be fun—although many of them will be. It's work, beneficial, and even glorious at times, but it's still work! Keep it up.

Glossary

abduction—a movement away from the vertical midline of the body; for example, when you move your leg straight out to the side.

acetylcholine—a chemical substance released at the nerve junction, which acts as a messenger and excites the muscle fiber, thereby initiating the process of contraction.

actin filaments—one of the main protein molecules contained within each muscle fiber.

adduction—a movement back toward the vertical midline of the body, for example, when you bring your legs together.

adenosine diphosphate (ADP)—the molecule that results from the breakdown of adenosine triphosphate (ATP).

adenosine triphosphate (ATP)—a molecule (composed of adenosine and three phosphate radicals) which releases energy when it breaks down.

ADP—see adenosine diphosphate.

aerobic capacity—the efficiency with which oxygen is transported throughout the body.

aerobic exercise—any sustained, moderately strenuous activity where the oxygen demand of the muscles is met by the heart and lungs.

agonistic muscles—the muscles that assist in a movement (contraction) but are not the primary movers.

alendronate sodium—a nonhormonal medication used to increase bone density and reduce the risk of osteoporotic fractures; marketed as *Fosamax*.

alpine skiing—downhill skiing.

amenorrhea—the absence of menses during reproductive years. See primary and second amenorrhea.

amino acids—the approximately 23 building blocks that make up proteins.

anabolic steroids—synthetic male hormones taken by people to enhance athletic performance and body composition.

anaerobic exercise—high-intensity activity where oxygen demand is greater than can be supplied by the heart and lungs.

androgenic—literally means "male producing." An androgenic hormone produces masculine body changes.

anemia—see iron-deficiency anemia.

anorexia—loss of normal appetite.

anorexia nervosa—an eating disorder that is characterized by a distorted body image and an obsessive preoccupation with body weight.

anovulatory—a menstrual cycle disturbance where ovulation has not occurred.

antagonistic muscles—the muscles that cause the opposite movement from that which is currently occurring.

arthrogram—a special X-ray film demonstrating a joint cavity after injection of dye.

arthroscope—an instrument used to examine the interior of a joint cavity.

articulation—the union between two or more bones, between two or more cartilages, or between cartilage and bone.

aspartates—the salts of aspartic acid, a non-essential amino acid.

ATP—see adenosine triphosate.

attribution theory—a psychological view of the factors that tend to result in a particular outcome. For example, females are more likely to say they performed well because they were lucky.

ballistic movements—movements that are initiated by a vigorous muscular contraction and completed by momentum (generated by that vigorous contraction). They are usually jerky, rapid, and bouncy.

ballistic stretching—bounce stretching; no longer considered safe or beneficial.

basal metabolic rate (BMR)—energy expenditure, expressed as the basic number of calories needed to maintain life at rest.

ß-endorphin—a chemical released by the brain that influences perceptions of pain and pleasure. See "endorphins."

Bill of Rights for Young Athletes—basic entitlements of young athletes enumerated by the American Alliance for Health, Physical Education, Recreation, and Dance.

BMI—see body mass index.

BMR—see basal metabolic rate.

body composition—the term used to describe the amount of fat relative to the amount of nonfat tissue in the body.

body image—the way in which each person sees her or his physical self.

body mass index (BMI)—measure of relative fatness. It is a ratio of weight to height (kg/m^2).

bone densitometer—technology used to measure the mineral content of bone. The dual energy X-ray absorptiometer (DEXA) is most commonly used.

bulimia—an eating disorder characterized by binge eating followed by purging.

calorie—the unit used to measure food energy.

carbohydrate (carbo) loading—a combination of diet and training prior to a long endurance competition.

carbohydrates—one of the six nutrients found in food. They consist of starches and sugars and are a major source of the body's energy.

cardiac output—the amount of blood pumped out by the heart in one minute.

cardiorespiratory endurance—the ability of lungs, heart, and blood vessels to deliver adequate amounts of oxygen to meet the demands of prolonged physical activity.

carnitine—a vitamin-like molecule found in meat and dairy products and in small amounts in grains, fruits, and vegetables.

catastrophe theory—the hypothesis that if a person is overly aroused, performance will deteriorate dramatically (catastrophically).

central nervous system (CNS)—the brain and spinal cord.

cholesterol—a waxy lipid substance that is manufactured by the body and is also found in the animal foods we eat.

chromium picolinate—a product which has been advertised as being able to increase lean body mass and delay fatigue (but has not always been shown to do so).

circumduction—when a movement segment as a whole describes a circle or a cone, for example, when you rotate your wrist or head in a circular motion.

CNS—see central nervous system.

collateral ligaments—the medial and lateral collateral ligaments support the knee on both sides.

complete proteins—proteins that contain all of the essential amino acids. They come only from animal sources.

concentric contractions—occur when the muscle actually shortens, as the back muscles do when you lift a weight from the floor.

concussion—a blow to the head that causes the brain to hit against the skull.

contractility—the ability of a muscle to shorten whenever it's used.

contraction—the process whereby a muscle moves its site of insertion closer to its site of origin and, in doing so, moves the bones to which it is attached.

cooldown (or warming down)—a strategy to diminish the exercise workload slowly thereby allowing for a gradual lowering of the pulse rate.

coronary heart disease (CHD)—also known as cardiovascular disease. A disorder arising from the failure of the coronary arteries to supply sufficient blood and oxygen to the heart muscle.

corpus albicans—the term for the graffian follicle approximately eight to ten days after ovulation. If there is no pregnancy, the follicle becomes white (albicans).

corpus luteum—Latin for body and yellow, respectively. The term for the graffian follicle after ovulation when it is producing the hormones necessary for sustaining a pregnancy.

cross training—a method of exercising whereby a mix of activities over a week's period are performed in order to exercise a greater number of muscles and joints than would be exercised with just one activity.

cruciate ligaments—the ACL (anterior cruciate ligament) and the PCL (posterior cruciate ligament) of the knee prevent forward and backward rocking of the knee.

cycling—taking anabolic steroids for a period of time, followed by temporarily discontinuing, then beginning a new period of use.

decompression sickness—(or the "bends") symptoms caused by not allowing enough time to equilibrate when ascending from a deep sea dive.

dehydration—the condition that results from not replacing water lost through sweating or excretion.

DEXA—dual-energy X-ray absorptiometer; a device used to measure bone mineral density.

dietary fiber—the indigestible components of the plant food we eat. Dietary fiber can be divided into two main categories: those that are soluble in water and those that are not.

duathlons—competitions that are usually a combination of biking and running events.

duration—the length of time of a workout.

dysmenorrhea (painful menstruation)—cramping just before or during menses.

eating disorder—an array of abnormal eating behaviors.

eccentric muscle contraction—the lengthening of muscle fibers during a contraction. It occurs when there is a gradual release of a contraction whereby the rate and range of movement is checked, moderated, or controlled.

echocardiogram stress test—computerized monitoring of heart size, motion, and function to diagnose suspected cardiovascular disease.

elasticity—a property of a muscle that allows it to be stretched.

endorphins—peptides produced by the brain that are released into the bloodstream during and after strenuous physical activity. See ß-endorphin; also exercise high.

endurance—see cardiorespiratory or muscular endurance.

episiotomy—an incision made in the perineum (the area between the vagina and the rectum) to enlarge the birth opening during delivery.

essential amino acids—the eight to ten amino acids that cannot be manufactured by the body and must be obtained from food.

essential fatty acids—the fatty acids that cannot be manufactured by the body and must be ingested.

estrogen replacement therapy (ERT)—administration of estrogen as treatment before and after menopause. See HRT.

estrogenic—pertaining to the female hormones.

eumenorrhea—a normal menstrual cycle, which is commonly defined by the presence of more or less regular menstrual bleeding every 23 to 35 days.

excitability—the property of muscle that allows it to respond to a stimulus from the nervous system.

exercise—planned, structured, and repetitive bodily movement engaged in to improve or maintain one or more components of physical fitness.

exercise addiction—the commitment to large amounts of exercise despite serious harm to one's physical self or other aspects of one's life.

exercise-associated amenorrhea—loss of menses associated with participation in intense physical activity.

exercise "high"—the good feeling that many individuals obtain after and sometimes during vigorous exercise. See ß-endorphin, endorphins.

exercise pyramid—A schematic representation of exercise goals. Level one activities should be engaged in every day by most people. Level two requires higher levels of fitness and should be done three to five times a week if possible. Level three activities are especially vigorous and should be engaged in when and if one is able.

extensibility—the property of a muscle that allows it to return to its normal resting length after having been stretched.

extension—a movement in which the bones move farther apart. It is usually the return movement from flexion. Straightening your fingers to open your hand (extension) after you've made a fist (flexion) is an example.

fartlek training—a technique where bursts of speed are added to the slower, steadier, continuous aerobic workout. Between these fast segments, the activity is continued at a relaxed pace until regular breathing returns.

fast-twitch muscle fibers—a type of muscle fiber that responds rapidly to stimulation.

fat-soluble vitamins—vitamins A, D, E, and K.

fats—one of the nutrients found in food.

fatty acids—any of several organic acids that make up lipids; found in both plant and animal foods.

fear of success—focusing on the negative aspects of succeeding.

female athlete triad—a recently coined phrase to describe a syndrome consisting of an eating disorder, amenorrhea, and osteoporosis.

femur—the thigh bone.

ferning—the branching pattern of the cervical mucus during ovulation as viewed under a microscope.

fetal bradycardia—an abnormally low heart rate in the unborn fetus.

fetal tachycardia—an abnormally high heart rate in the unborn fetus.

fiber—see dietary fiber.

fitness—taken together, the five components of cardiorespiratory endurance, muscular endurance, muscular strength, flexibility, and body composition.

fitness walking—walking at a brisk rate of four to five miles an hour for 30 to 45 minutes.

fixators—the muscles that steady or stabilize a part of the body so that prime movers and agonists will contract more effectively in a desired movement.

fixed load—weight training in which the resistance, repetitions, sets, and rest remain the same throughout the workout.

flat bones—bones like the ribs, pelvic bones, and knee caps, which are relatively thin but provide protection.

flexibility—ability to bend a joint through a range of motion.

flexion—a movement that brings bones closer together (decreases the angle at the joint).

flow—performing with total concentration and enjoyment.

follicle stimulating hormone (FSH)—a hormone released by the pituitary gland that stimulates the ovaries.

Food Guide Pyramid—a schematic representation of the Dietary Guidelines that also serves as a guide for daily food choices.

Fosamax—see alendronate sodium.

free weights—bars with weight plates on each end. Dumbbells have short bars and barbells have long bars. Used in weight training.

frequency—the number of days per week that one exercises.

FSH—see Follicle Stimulating Hormone.

gelatin—derived from collagen. It contains approximately 25 percent of the nonessential amino acid glycine.

general warm-up—a total body exercise such as brisk walking or jogging in place prior to beginning an activity.

glucose—a carbohydrate. It is the fuel burned by cells to generate energy.

glycogen—chains of glucose that have been stored in the liver or muscles.

GnRH—see Gonadotropin Releasing Hormone.

golfer's elbow—(medial epicondylitis) injury to the common tendon origin of the forearm flexors causing pain on the inner forearm muscles and inner part of the elbow.

Gonadotropin Releasing Hormone (GnRH)—the hormone released by the hypothalamus that stimulates the pituitary gland to secrete gonadotropins (FSH, LH).

heart rate—the number of times the heart beats in one minute; often measured by putting a finger on one of the arteries in either the wrist or neck and counting for one minute.

heart rate monitor—a device used to measure heart rate.

heat illness—hot weather problems, ranging from muscle cramps to elevated body temperature, associated with changes in mental function.

herbal supplements—single or combinations of various herbs used typically as self-prescribed medications.

herniated disc—injury to the spine; also known as a slipped disc.

hill training—running up and down hills as part of an aerobic training regimen.

hitting the wall—the expression often used by runners to describe the physiological condition that occurs when muscle glycogen is depleted and blood sugar declines.

hormone replacement therapy (HRT)—the use of estrogen and progesterone supplementation, most often in postmenopausal women. HRT that uses estrogen without a progestin is referred to as estrogen replacement therapy (ERT).

hypertrophy—an enlargement or increase in size. With muscle hypertrophy, the muscle fibers enlarge but do not increase in number.

hypoestrogenic—the condition of low estrogen levels.

hypoglycemia—the condition that results when glycogen is depleted and blood sugar declines.

iceberg profile—a pattern of psychological traits that is typical of elite athletes. These athletes tend to be below average in tension, depression, anger, fatigue, and confusion, but higher than normal in vigor.

iliotibial band—the long and strong ligament running from the hip to the side of the thigh.

impingement syndrome—when various tendons repeatedly get compressed against bony structures, causing chronic pain.

impostor syndrome—the generally misguided self-perception that an individual is fooling others into believing that he or she is successful.

improvement conditioning stage—the time in a training regimen that follows the initial conditioning stage. It can last 12 to 20 weeks, during which progress is rapid.

initial conditioning stage—the initial segment, about four to six weeks, of a training regimen.

intensity—the rate or degree of vigor with which an exercise is performed.

interval training—also known as speed training; a series of short, measured distances performed at a race pace or faster (approximately 90 percent of maximum heart rate), alternated with rest periods.

inverted U—a hypothesis suggesting that a moderate amount of psychological arousal produces the highest level of performance.

inward rotation—when the front side of a bone is turned inward toward the midline of the body; for example, when you stand pigeon-toed (toes pointing inward).

iron deficiency—a medical condition reflecting insufficient iron stores.

iron-deficiency anemia—the most common type of anemia, caused by inadequate iron intake, inadequate iron absorption, and/or accelerated iron loss.

irregular bones—bones uniquely designed to suit specific assignments, such as the vertebrae and the bones of the jaw.

isometric contraction—a muscle contraction in which no movement occurs.

isotonic contraction—motion of the bone in the direction of the contraction, with a concomitant shortening of the muscle.

jogger's nipples—abrasions of the nipples of either female or male runners.

joint—the union between two or more bones, between two or more cartilages, or between cartilage and bone.

Kegel exercises—exercises designed to improve vaginal tone that may help to correct some forms of urinary incontinence and enhance sexual satisfaction; also called pelvic floor exercises.

kinesthetic sense—the self-awareness of muscular movement and body position.

last—the foot-shaped form around which a shoe is constructed.

LH—see Luteinizing Hormone.

lipids—any of the fatty acids found in the blood, such as triglycerides (fats and oils), phospholipids (lecithin), and sterols (cholesterol).

long, slow distances (LSD)—relaxed, comfortably paced workouts performed at about 75 percent of maximum heart rate.

longitudinal muscles—long straplike muscles whose fibers lie parallel to their long axis, allowing for the largest range of movement.

lumbar lordosis—commonly used to refer to abnormal or exaggerated curvature of the lower part of the spine; medically refers also to the natural curvature of the lower spine.

luteal phase—the time in the menstrual cycle after ovulation has occurred when the uterus is being prepared for implantation of a fertilized egg.

luteal phase disturbances—menstrual cycle problems occurring when either the hormone level (specifically progesterone) or the normal length of the luteal phase (approximately 14 days) are not as expected.

luteal phase suppression—a shortening of the luteal phase (less than ten days from ovulation to the start of menstrual flow) accompanied by decreased levels of progesterone.

luteinizing hormone (LH)—a hormone released by the pituitary that acts on the ovaries and uterus in females and the testes in males.

macro minerals—minerals such as calcium, magnesium, potassium, phosphorus, and sodium, which are needed in relatively large amounts by our bodies.

matrix—the bone's inner composition. The matrix is about one-third organic substances (chiefly collagen) and two-thirds inorganic salts.

max HR—see **maximal heart rate**.

maximal heart rate (max HR)—the greatest number of beats per minute at which the heart is capable of functioning. An easy approximation of that rate is achieved by subtracting one's age from 220.

maximal oxygen consumption (VO_2max)—the point at which oxygen consumption does not rise despite increased exercise intensity; the highest rate at which oxygen can be taken in and utilized during exercise.

menarche—the first menstrual period.

meniscus—the cushion of cartilage that helps to stabilize a joint and aid in gliding motions.

menses—the menstrual (blood) flow.

menstrual cycle—women's reproductive cycle including: the follicular phase, ovulation, the luteal phase, and menses.

menstruation—the part of the menstrual cycle when women bleed (because the uterine lining has been sloughed off).

mental imaging—actively visualizing excellent performance.

metabolism—the sum of all the chemical processes that go on in the body.

METS—metabolic equivalents; units for measuring physical exertion; one MET is the energy expended in a minute by somebody resting quietly.

minerals—a class of nutrients that help to regulate body functions, aid in growth and maintenance of tissues, and serve as catalysts for the release of energy.

mittelschmerz—a German term for abdominal pain, usually related to ovulation, that occurs in the middle of the monthly menstrual cycle. The actual mechanism is not clearly understood.

mixte—bike frame with a diagonal top tube.

motor neuron—the type of nerve that provides the impetus for movement.

motor unit—a single motor neuron together with all of the muscle fibers that its branches supply.

movers—muscles that are directly responsible for performing a movement.

muscle specificity—the concept that each bodily movement or activity uses a specific set of muscles; engaging in one sport may not improve performance in another.

muscular endurance—the muscle's ability to perform without fatiguing over a set period of time.

muscular strength—the amount of force that a muscle (or muscle group) is capable of exerting.

myosin filaments—one of the main protein molecules contained within each muscle fiber.

myotonia—the tonic spasm of a muscle; buildup of tension and energy in nerves and muscles, especially as a result of sexual arousal.

neurogenic urinary incontinence—inability to control urination due to disorders affecting the nervous system, such as Parkinson's disease and diabetes mellitus.

nordic skiing—cross-country skiing.

NSAIDs—abbreviation for "nonsteroidal anti-inflammatory drugs," which are medications used to reduce inflammation and pain; see NSAID appendix.

nuclear stress test—a method for evaluating the heart when the body is engaging in physical activity. A nuclear camera is used to capture an image of the heart during exercise; thallium or technetium-99m (Cardiolite) are the most commonly used radioactive tracers.

oligomenorrhea (infrequent periods)—when a woman has menstrual cycles at intervals ranging from 36 days to six months.

osteocytes—the living bone cells located inside the hard matrix.

osteoporosis—insufficient bone mineral content, resulting in fragile bones that are vulnerable to breakage.

outward rotation—a movement of the front side of a bone away from the midline of the body; for example, when a ballerina stands with her legs and feet "turned out."

over-training—"too many" hours spent in repetitive movements which often lead to "microtraumatic" injuries.

ovulation—the rupture of the ovarian wall by the graffian follicle, so that the released egg can travel through the fallopian tube.

oxygen debt—when physical exertion calls for larger quantities of oxygen than the body can provide, exercise must stop.

oxygen deficit—the short transition period when circulatory and respiratory adjustments lag behind the need for oxygen.

patella—the knee cap.

patella alta—a knee cap that sits high in the groove of the thigh.

patellofemoral syndrome—a group of disorders that cause pain, inflammation, or instability of the knee.

pelvic floor exercisers—devices used to strengthen the vaginal muscles; designed to correct some forms of urinary incontinence and improve sexual satisfaction.

pelvic floor exercises—see Kegel exercises.

perceived level of exertion—an estimate of how hard one is working. A scale to interpret individual ratings of perceived levels of exertion was devised by Gunnar Borg; versions of this are commonly posted in gyms, health clubs, and other places where people exercise.

Perception of Success Questionnaire—a paper-and-pencil self test which is designed to measure an individual's motivation to do well in athletic activities.

pessary—a rubber or silicone device inserted into the vagina to help support the bladder and thereby decrease urinary incontinence.

physical activity—any bodily movement produced by skeletal muscles that results in energy expenditure.

physical fitness—those attributes that relate to a person's ability to perform physical activity. These include cardiovascular endurance, muscular strength and endurance, flexibility, and body composition.

plantar fascia—a connective tissue structure that stretches from the ball of the foot to the toes. It provides support for the arch of the foot.

PMS—see premenstrual syndrome.

PNF—see **proprioceptive neuromuscular facilitation** techniques.

power—the ability to move objects in the shortest time possible. Power is a combination of strength and speed.

premenstrual syndrome (PMS)—a group of symptoms, both behavioral and physical, that occur in the second half of the menstrual cycle and often interfere with work and personal relationships.

primary amenorrhea—absence of onset of menses in a woman over 16 or 17 years of age.

prime movers—the one or two muscles of greatest importance involved in executing a particular movement.

pronate—to rotate the front surface down or back; for example; to turn the forearm so the palm faces downward or backward. For the foot, it involves inward and downward rotation of the arch.

proprioceptive neuromuscular facilitation techniques (PNF)—alternating contractions and stretches while another person holds the individual being stretched in a particular position; a variation of passive stretching.

proprioceptors—sensory nerve terminals that respond to movement and send signals to the central nervous system.

puberty—the age at which reproductive organs become mature.

pubescence—the period of time and concomitant physiological changes leading to puberty.

pubic symphysis—the site where the pubic (hip) bones join in the front of the body.

pyramiding—taking a low dose of anabolic steriods and gradually increasing the dose and then tapering off.

Q angle—(quadriceps angle); the angle formed when a line drawn from the hip to the kneecap is intersected with a line from the tibia to the kneecap.

race walking—a method of very fast walking where one foot stays on the ground at all times, and the knee of the supporting leg is straight.

RDA—see Recommended Dietary Allowance.

Recommended Dietary Allowance (RDA)—the term used by the National Academy of Sciences to describe the body's daily need for specific nutrients.

repetitions—a term used in weight training and elsewhere to refer to the number of continuous times an exercise is performed.

RICE—an acronym for the four key steps of rehabilitation: rest, ice, compression, and elevation.

rotation—a movement in the horizontal plane about a vertical axis; for example, when saying "no" with one's head.

rotator cuff muscles—the major stabilizing muscles of the shoulder.

sacroiliac joint—the junction of the lower part of the spine (sacrum) with the hip bone.

saturated fats—lipids derived mainly from animal sources such as meats, egg yolks, and dairy products.

secondary amenorrhea—absence of menses, usually for greater than six months, in an individual who has previously menstruated.

sensory neurons—nerves that transmit impulses from muscles, tendons, skin, visceral, and sense organs, to the central nervous system.

set—in weight training, a series of repetitions. For example, a weight may be lifted for three sets of ten repetitions each.

shin splint—inflammation causing pain over the front part of the lower leg.

short arc extensions—exercise of the lower leg that involves placing a rolled towel under a slightly bent knee and straightening the lower leg out.

skeletal muscles—the muscles that are involved in bodily movements.

slow-twitch muscle fiber—a type of muscle fiber that responds slowly but also fatigues slowly. They are the key fibers in endurance activities.

smooth muscles—the muscles found in blood vessels and the walls of visceral organs.

spinbarkeit—the increase in elasticity of cervical mucus as the level of estrogen increases.

spondylolysis—a fracture of part of the spine that is not displaced or slipped out of place.

Sports Inventory for Pain—a paper and pencil test that rates self-perceived tolerance for pain.

sports—physical activities that usually have structured rules and involve competition.

sprain—an injury to the ligaments that support joints.

stacking—taking more than one drug at a time. A pattern of anabolic sterioid use to help minimize adverse side effects.

stand-over height—the distance from the ground to your crotch when you straddle the crossbar of a bicycle.

static stretching—a method of stretching in which a position is assumed and held for approximately 15 to 30 seconds until a mild tension (not pain) in the muscle is felt. This is followed by relaxation of the muscle.

steady state—in exercise, it refers to the condition where the amounts of oxygen inhaled and delivered to the muscles are adequate to allow for continued muscular activity.

strain—an injury to muscle-tendon units.

stress test—any of several medically monitored procedures to assess cardiovascular fitness. Typically a person exercises on a treadmill or stationary bicycle while pulse, blood pressure, and heart activity (as assessed by an electrocardiogram) are measured.

stroke volume—the amount of blood pumped by the heart with each beat.

subluxation—incomplete dislocation of a joint.

sudden death—an unexpected death that occurs without being precipitated by illness or trauma.

Sun Protection Factor (SPF)—indicates how much longer it will take to tan or burn with a sunscreen than without it.

supinate—to rotate the front surface upward or forward. For example, to turn the forearm so the palm faces up or front. For the foot, it involves an upward rotation of the arch.

symbolic annihilation—women's activities that are not brought to public view; it is as if they never happened.

target heart rate (THR)—the heart rate selected as a goal during exercise. When it is set and reached, between 60 to 90 percent of the maximum heart rate, peak cardiovascular benefit is derived.

task-specific warm-up—preparing to exercise by engaging in low intensity levels of the activity in order to ease into it.

telemark—a form of downhill skiing with cross-country type equipment.

tennis elbow (lateral epicondylitis)—injury to the tendon origin of the extensor muscles, causing localized pain on the outside aspect of the elbow and the forearm muscles.

tibia (shin)—the lower front leg bone.

Title IX—the 1972 Federal Education amendments, which state that no person in the United States shall be subjected to discrimination in educational programs or activities that receive federal financial assistance.

tonus (muscle tone)—the capacity to maintain a state of steady, partial contraction.

trace minerals—the minerals, such as iron, zinc, and copper, that our bodies need in minute amounts.

training intensity/training zone—the area between 60 and 90 percent of maximum heart rate during aerobic exercise that provides for the development of aerobic fitness.

triangular or fan-shaped muscles—relatively flat muscles with fibers radiating from a narrow attachment at one end to a broad attachment at the other.

triathlon—a single competition usually consisting of running, biking, and swimming.

triglycerides—lipids consisting of a molecule of glycerol and three fatty acids. Triglycerides make up about 95 percent of the lipids in foods and in our body.

unsaturated fats—lipids that are generally liquid at room temperature. They are derived primarily from plant sources such as corn, soybean, and peanut. Unsaturated fats are further divided into monounsaturated and polyunsaturated, depending on their chemical structure.

urinary stress incontinence—leakage of urine associated with exercise, coughing, sneezing, laughing, and so on.

urinary urge incontinence—an uncontrollable urination that is not activity-related but may be due to infections, tumors, nervous system disorders, or side-effects of certain medications.

vaginal perineometer—a biofeedback device used to monitor the effectiveness of pelvic floor exercises.

vaginitis—infection or inflammation of the vagina.

valsalva maneuver—exhaling against a closed glottis (i.e., holding your breath and bearing down).

variable load—a term used in weight training to refer to the changing of resistance and repetitions for each set.

vasocongestion—the increased blood flow to and enlargement of the genitals, breasts, and other body tissues related to sexual arousal.

vegetarian diet—a diet that does not include meat. Vegetarian diets may vary considerably.

vitamins—a category of food nutrient that promotes specific chemical reactions within our cells.

VO$_2$max—see maximal oxygen consumption.

warm-up—preparations for exercise, which allow the body to ease into activity.

water-insoluble fiber—the dietary fiber that remains essentially unchanged during digestion.

water-soluble fiber—the type of dietary fiber that becomes gel-like and is fermented by bacteria in the colon.

water-soluble vitamins—the 8 B-vitamins and vitamin C, which do not require fat for absorption.

weight machine—exercise machine to help build strength and fitness.

weight training—a form of resistance exercise whereby a muscle is placed under a heavy load, slowly contracted, and then relaxed. Typically, a given number of repetitions is performed (one set) and each set is repeated, usually three times in one session.

zones of optimal performance—the theory that each individual functions best at his or her own personal level of emotional arousal.

Appendix

NON-STEROIDAL ANTI-INFLAMMATORY DRUGS

Non-steroidal anti-inflammatory drugs (NSAIDs) are regularly prescribed in the treatment of sports injuries. There are a large number of NSAIDs currently available. Some are available by prescription only, while others may be purchased over the counter (OTC). Several pharmaceutical companies are currently marketing OTC versions of their prescription drugs.

NSAIDs have analgesic (pain relief), anti-inflammatory, and antipyretic (fever-reducing) properties. They may be prescribed for acute, as well as chronic, medical problems. Athletes should be careful not to use NSAIDs to mask pain so they can partake in physical activities that might actually worsen the problem that caused the initial pain.

Some NSAIDs are better analgesics, whereas others are better anti-inflammatory agents. Clinical experience has shown us that when an individual fails to get pain relief and/or a reduction in inflammation with one NSAID, another NSAID may prove to be more effective. NSAIDs belong to different chemical classes and come in a variety of doses and dosage schedules. (See Table 1.)

If you are taking NSAIDs, you should be aware of some of the side effects and drug interactions. The most common side-effects are gastrointestinal symptoms, such as heartburn, indigestion, nausea, and ulcer formation. NSAIDs may interact with other medications such as blood thinners, water pills, and blood pressure pills.

If you have any medical problems, speak with your health care provider before self-prescribing any NSAID that can be bought OTC. If you develop any unusual symptoms while taking an NSAID, even during short-term use, be sure to contact your physician or pharmacist.

TABLE 1

....

Dosing information for NSAIDs

Generic Name	Trade Name	Usual Adult Dosage
Aspirin	Ecotrin, Extended Release* (or other brands)	325+mg every 4 hours
Diclofenac sodium	Voltaren	25, 50, or 75 mg every 12 hours
Diflunisal	Dolobid	250–500 mg every 8 to 12 hours
Etodolac	Lodine	200–400 mg every 6 to 8 hours
Fenoprofen	Nalfon	300–600 mg every 6 hours
Flurbiprofen	Ansaid	100 mg every 8 to 12 hours
Ibuprofen	Motrin	400–600 mg every 6 hours
	Motrin IB*, Advil*, Nuprin*	200–400 mg every 4 to 6 hours
Indomethacin	Indocin	25–50 mg every 8 hours
Ketoprofen	Orudis	25–50 mg every 6 to 8 hours
	Orudis KT*	12.5–25 mg every 4 to 6 hours
	Actron*	12.5–25 mg every 4 to 6 hours
Ketorolac tromethamine	Toradol	10 mg every 6 hours (not to exceed 5 days of usage)
Meclofenamate	Meclomen	100 mg every 6 to 8 hours
Mefenamic acid	Ponstel	250 mg every 6 hours
Nabumetone	Relafen	500–1,000 mg every 12 to 24 hours
Naproxen	Naprosyn	250–500 mg every 6 to 8 hours
Naproxen sodium	Anaprox	275 mg every 6 to 8 hours
	Anaprox DS	550 mg every 12 hours
	Aleve*	200 mg every 8 to 12 hours
Oxaprozin	Daypro	600–1,200 mg daily
Phenylbutazone	Butazolidan	100 mg every 6 hours
Piroxicam	Feldene	10–20 mg daily
Sulindac	Clinoril	150–200 mg every 12 hours
Tolmetin sodium	Tolectin	200–600 mg every 8 hours

....

*Available over the counter

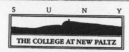

WOMEN AND EXERCISE

Little scientific information is available about women's participation in physical activity. We are seeking to better understand our exercise involvement and to gather information which might help us improve our physical pursuits.

This survey is being conducted under guidelines established by The College at New Paltz, State University of New York Institutional Review Board. By participating, you will help the survey administrators find answers to important questions; however, your involvement is strictly voluntary. Please remember that you may choose not to answer any questions which you find objectionable.

This questionnaire should take about 15 - 30 minutes to complete.
When you have finished, please fold and return this form to the designated box or mail to us in the enclosed prepaid envelope. Thank you in advance for your contribution!

– Susan L. Puretz, Ed.D., Adelaide Haas, Ph.D., Donna Meltzer, M.D.

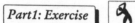

Part1: Exercise

1. What do you do when you exercise? (Please circle all that apply)

1. Aerobics	2. Backpack	3. Badminton
4. Bike	5. Bowl	6. Canoe
7. Cross-Country Ski	8. Dance	9. Down-Hill Ski
13. Mountain/Rock Climb	14. Run	15. Soccer
16. Softball	17. Swim	18. Tennis
19. Volleyball	20. Walk	21. Weight/machines
22. Triathalon (any cross-training competition)	23. Other (Please specify up to four:)	

_____
_____
_____

2. Which of the above, if any, do you consider your major source(s) of exercise?

_____

3. Do you compete in any of the above?   1. Yes 2. No

☞   If yes, which one(s) _____

4. Do you make a distinction between your sports activity(s) and the things you do for exercise?
                                                          1. Yes 2. No
Explain _____

5. Do you view your regular exercise primarily as a physical preparation for your sports activities?
                                                          1. Yes 2. No
Explain _____

6. Where do you regularly exercise?

     1. Private health club   2. YMCA/YWCA   3. At a track   4. At home
     If other, please specify up to four
     _____   _____   _____

7. Generally, how frequently do you exercise?

1. 1 day a week	4. 4 days a week	7. every day
2. 2 days a week	5. 5 days a week	8. other _____
3. 3 days a week	6. 6 days a week	

8. On the average, how long are your exercise sessions?
   1. About 15 minutes   2. About a half hour   3. About an hour   4. More than one hour

9. In general, would you judge your overall exercise to be:
   1. Mild   2. Moderate   3. Intense

10. How long have you exercised regularly?
    1. Less than 6 months   2. 6-12 months   3. 1-5 Years   4. More than 5 years
    5. Other _____

11. How old were you when you started exercising regularly?
    1. Under 12   2. In my teens   3. In my twenties   4. In my thirties
    5. In my forties   6. Other _____

12. Why did you start engaging in regular exercise? (Please rank order those responses applicable to you where 1=most important reason)

    ____ weight control   ____ tension reducer   ____ health goals
    ____ to look better   ____ competition   ____ social
    ____ pleasure   ____ parents started me as a child
    ____ other _____

13. Why do you engage in regular exercise now? (Please rank order those responses applicable to you where 1=*most important reason*)

    ____ weight control   ____ tension reducer   ____ health goals
    ____ to look better   ____ competition   ____ social
    ____ pleasure   ____ parents started me as a child
    ____ other _____

14. Have you ever stopped exercising for periods of time due to an injury?
    1. Yes   How long _____ Why _____
    2. No

15. Have you ever stopped exercising for periods of time for reasons other than injury?
    1. Yes   How long _____ Why _____
    2. No

16. Do you have any limitations to your exercise schedule? (Please rank order those responses applicable to you where 1=*most important reason*)

    ___ Time   ___ Age   ___ Injury
    ___ Illness   ___ Medical Advice   ___ Money
    ___ Other   Explain _____

17. What benefits have you experienced that you attribute to exercise?
    _____
    _____

18. What problems have you had that you attribute to exercise?
    _____
    _____

19. Have these problems been solved?

    1. Yes   2. No   Explain _____

20. What level of athlete are you?

    1. Hobbyist
    2. Competitor in local competitions
    3. Competitor in state competitions
    4. World class
    5. Other _____

Part 2: Nutrition & Habits

☞ 21. Do you have a special diet?   1. Yes 2. No
      If yes, please describe _____

22. Do you restrict the intake of certain foods?   1. Yes 2. No
☞   If yes, p lease describe _____

23. Do you take vitamin supplements?   1. Yes 2. No
☞   If yes, what vitamins do you take? _____
      How often do you take these vitamins? _____

24. Do you use any prescription, over-the-counter, or other drugs/medications?
           1. Yes 2. No
☞   If yes, which ones/explain _____

25 Do you smoke?   1. Yes 2. No
☞   If yes, how much do you smoke? _____

26. Do you drink caffeine?   1. Yes 2. No
☞   If yes, what form, & how much? _____

27. Do you drink alcohol?   1. Yes 2. No
☞   If yes, what form, & how much? _____

28. How much sleep do you ordinarily get? _____

29. Do you think any of the behaviors you noted in this section *help* your physical performance?
      1. Yes   2. No   Explain _____

30. Do you think any of the behaviors you noted in this section *hinder* your physical performance?
      1. Yes   2. No   Explain _____

Part 3: Personal Information

31. Age _____

32. Occupation _____

33. Education _____

34. Where do you live?   1. Rural or country area
                2. Small village or town
                3. Small city
                4. Large city or metropolitan area

35. In what state or country do you currently live? _____

36. Marital Status _____

37. Do you have children?   1. Yes   2. No
☞   If yes, what are your children's ages? _____

38. Did you continue exercising while you were pregnant?
           1. Yes   2. No   3. Not applicable
      Explain _____

39. Did you continue exercising while nursing a baby?
           1. Yes   2. No   3. Not applicable
      Explain _____

40. Did/does having children influence your exercise patterns?

                                                1. Yes   2. No   3. Not applicable

    Explain _____

41. Rate your current level of physical fitness: 1.Poor   2. Fair   3.Good   4.Excellent

42. Rate your current level of health: 1.Poor   2. Fair   3.Good   4.Excellent

43. Do you currently have menstrual periods?   1. Yes 2. No

44. Are you pre-puberty (too young to have menstrual periods)?   1. Yes 2. No

45. Are you menopausal or post-menopausal?   1. Yes 2. No

  ☞   If yes, did/do you take hormone replacement therapy?

                                 1. Yes   2. No   3. Not applicable

    Explain _____

46. Are/were you aware of physical discomfort during your period?

                            1. Yes   2. No Explain _____

47. Are/were you aware of physical discomfort immediately prior to your period?

                            1. Yes   2. No Explain _____

48. Do/did you have premenstrual psychological tension?

                            1. Yes   2. No Explain _____

49. Did you ever stop menstruating as a result of your participation in exercise/sports?

                            1. Yes   2. No

  ☞   If yes, how long did you stop menstruating _____
         Was the situation corrected?   1. Yes   2. No
         How was the situation corrected?_____

50. Is your performance affected by your menstrual cycle?

                            1. Yes   2. No Explain _____

  ☞   If yes, at what point in your cycle (Circle all that apply)
                  1. Before period   2. During period   3. After period
    Explain_____

51. Do you have objective evidence to support this?

                            1. Yes   2. No Explain _____

52. What type of birth control do you currently use? (Circle all that apply)

       1. Pills   2. Rhythm   3. IUD
       4. Norplant   5. Diaphragm   6. Condom
       7. I am sterilized   8. My partner is   9. I am
                            sterilized   postmenopausal
       10. I am not heterosexually active
       11. I am heterosexually active but do not use any birth control
       12. Other _____

53. Have you experienced problems with exercise or sports activities which you believe are unique to women?

                            1. Yes   2. No Explain _____

54. Are you satisfied with the exercise clothing, equipment, and facilities that are available to women?

                            1. Yes   2. No Explain _____

Please use the attached page to make any additional comments that you feel important to your overall exercise history.

Again, thank you very much for your participation.

Index

A

Abdominals
    exercises for, 80
    lower back injuries and, 79
    weight training exercises for, 99
Abduction, 43
Acetylcholine, 45–46
Achilles tendon, 41
    stretches for, 76–77
Actin filaments, 39–40
Addiction to exercise, 16–17, 93
Adduction, 43
Adenosine diphosphate (ADP), 40
Adenosine triphosate (ATP), 40
    breakdown of, 46
Adipose tissue, 237
Adrenaline, cooldowns and, 77
Aerobics, 7, 8
    cross-training activities, 106
    high-impact aerobics, 81
    low-impact aerobics, 81
    older athletes and, 365
    pregnancy and, 313
    stress incontinence and, 373
Affordability of activity, 107
Afterglow, 14
Age
    bone and, 35
    eating disorders and, 424–425
    and exercise, 5
    for menarche, 270–271
Aging process, 342–362
Agonists, 44–45
Alcohol and bone density, 11, 351
Alendronate sodium tablets, 352–353
Allen, Mark, 72
Allergies to herbal supplements, 262
Alpha-adrenergic drugs, 378
Altitude training, 126–127
Amenorrhea, 17, 282
    bone health and, 289–290
    caloric drain and, 287–288
    emotional factors, 288
    exercise-associated amenorrhea, 282, 285–289

intensity of exercise and, 285–287
    primary amenorrhea, 280–281
        treatment of, 293
    problems associated with, 289–290
    profiles of exercising women and, 284
    reproductive protection, 288
    secondary amenorrhea, 281
    stress and, 288–289
    treatment of, 292–293
American College of Obstetricians and
        Gynecologists (ACOG), 312
American College of Sports Medicine, 1–2,
      12
    "Guidelines" of, 14
    METs, tables of, 69
    overload principle and, 70
    training guidelines, 89
    weight training exercises, 100
American Council on Exercise, 80
American Dietetic Association, 230, 261
American Heart Association, 220
    VO$_2$max data, 359
American National Standards Institute
      (ANSI), 172
American Society for Clinical Nutrition,
      230
American Women's Track and Field:
    A History (Tricard), 124
Amino acids, 220
    in energy bars, 262
    supplements, 233
Anabolic steroids. *See* Steroids
Anabolic Steroids Act of 1990, 431
Anatomy, 34–43
Androgenic hormones, 24
Anemia. *See* Iron-deficiency anemia
Ankles
    injuries, 406
    rehabilitation of, 413–414
Anorexia nervosa, 93, 423
    age and, 424–425
diagnostic criteria, 424–425
    osteoporosis and, 350–351
    physical signs of, 425–426
    psychological profile, 425
    treatment of, 427
Antagonists, 45
Anterior cruciate ligament (ACL), 401–402

Anti-prostaglandin medication, 277
Anxiety and competition, 151–152
Appalachian Trail, 135, 366, 367
Aqua jogging, 6
Are We Winning Yet (Nelson), 159
Arginine, 233
Arms
    extensions, 75
    horse riding, arm lifts for, 141
    length of, 30–31
    weight training exercises for, 99
Arnsdorf, L., 373
Arthritis, 11
Arthrograms, 404
Arthroscopes, 404
Articulation of joints, 36
Aspartates, 233
Aspirin, 262, 277
Assessment
    cardiorespiratory endurance
        assessment, 57–58
    of physical fitness, 57
Astronauts, weight training and, 96
Attribution theory, 149

B

Baby carriers, 324–325
Backpacking, 135–138
    fitness for, 136
    foods for, 263–264
    injuries, 136–138
Backs. *See also* Lower back
    athletic backs, 398–399
    flexibility test, 355
    injuries to, 396–399
    pregnancy and, 305–306
    rehabilitation of, 418–419
    slipped disks, 397–398
    stretches, 75–76
    weight training exercises for, 98, 99
    young athletes, injuries in, 397
Backward leg stretch, 141
Backwards walking/running, 134
Badminton, 6
    pregnancy and, 314
Balance in exercise, 93
Baldwin, Dan, 202–203
Ball and saddle joints, 37

Gerbner, George, 162
Giardia lamblia, 138
Gillett, Patricia, 366
Gilligan, Carol, 149
Ginseng, 262
Gjerdingen, Dwenda, 316
Gliding joints, 37
Glossary, 440–454
Gloves
    for bicycling, 171, 191
    ski gloves, 181
Glucose, 220, 222
    chromium picolinate and, 233–234
    energy and, 237
    in sports drinks, 259–260
Gluteus maximus, 42–43
Glycine, 234
Goals
    for child competitors, 331–333
    for competition, 150–151
    performance, improvement of, 94
    realistic goals, 17
Goggles for swimming, 184–185
Goldberg, Barry, 337
Golf, 6
    back problems, 398–399
    equipment, 200–201
Golfer's elbow, 400
Gonadotropin releasing hormone (GnRH), 273
    caloric drain and, 288
Gorp, 263
Graf, Steffi, 162
Grains, 221
Greek sports, 3
Greendale, G. A., 11
Grilo, C. M., 66
Grimwood, Tamara, 88
Grinkov, Sergei, 432, 433
Grove City College v. Bell, 160
Growth periods, 23
Guthrie, S. R., 359
Gymnastics. *See also* Female athlete triad
    children, 327
        competition by, 333
    injuries in, 154
    pregnancy and, 314
    pondylolysis, 398

H

Haas, Adelaide, 1–21, 90, 146–164, 341–370, 351, 371–391
Hall, Evelyn, 157
Hammill, Dorothy, 162
Hamstrings
    flexibility test, 355
    stretch, 76
Harding, Tonya, 147
Hartford Female Seminary, 4
Harvard School of Public Health, 14
Hats and caps
    ski hats, 181
    swim caps, 184
Hawaiian Ironman Triathlon, 130–131
Head injuries, 393
Headsets for music, 214
Health and fitness clubs, 209
    cleanliness of, 211
    cost of, 211
    daycare at, 325
    equipment in, 210
    etiquette of, 211
    guidelines for selecting, 210–311
    staff rating, 210
Health as motivation, 9
Health spas, 212
Heart. *See also* Coronary heart disease (CHD)
    aerobic conditioning and, 340
    aging and, 344–350
    cardiac output, 50
    improving condition of, 349–350
    overweight and, 56
    pregnancy, heart in, 302
    warning signs for, 345–349
Heart Action Step test, 345–346
Heart rate, 50–51. *See also* Pregnancy; Target heart rate (THR)
    and gender, 26
    monitors, 68–69, 215, 347–348
    response to exercise, 51
Heat illness, 28–29, 257
Heel spurs, 406
Heel-toe roll, 113
Height, 23
Helmets
    bicycling helmets, 172–173

for children, 325
    head injuries and, 393, 394
    for horse riding, 143
Hemoglobin, 38
Henie, Sonja, 162
Herbal supplements, 262–263
Heredity
    depression and, 30
    stature and, 23
Herniated disks, 398–399
High-density lipoprotein (HDL), 11
    child athletes and, 338
    moderate exercise and, 70
High–impact aerobics, 81
Hiking, 6. *See also* Backpacking
    foods for, 263
Hinge joints, 37
Hip stretches, 76
Hip-to-shoulder ratio, 27
Home exercise equipment, 203–209
    cross-country ski machines, 207–208
    rowing machines, 208–209
    stair machines, 203–204
    stationary bikes, 206–207
    treadmills, 204–206
Home stress test, 345–346
Home videos, 212–213
Honey, 234
Honig, Daniel, 131
Hormone replacement therapy, 352
    urinary incontinence and, 377–378
Hormones, sexuality and, 387–388
Horner, Matina, 150
Horse riding
    exercises for, 140–143
    fitness for, 139
    head injuries, protection from, 143
    mental conditioning for, 142–143
    pregnancy and, 314
    Ride and Tie, 138–139
    tacking up the horse, 139–140
    warm-ups for, 139
Hot tubs, 363
Housework, 1, 2
How to Shit in the Woods (Meyer), 383
Hudson, Jackie, 155
Hybrid bikes, 189–190

Hyperandrogenism, 291
Hyperprolactinemia, 291
Hypertension, 362
Hypoestrogenism, 282, 291
Hypoglycemia, 249, 255
Hypothalamus
    amenorrhea and, 282, 285
    tests for function of, 291
Hypothyroidism, 291

I

Ibuprofen, 277
Iceberg profile, 146
Icing injuries, 412
Ideal diet, 228
Iliotibial band syndrome, 404
Imipramine, 378
Immovable joints, 36
Impingement syndrome, 395–396
Impostor syndrome, 149
In a Different Voice (Gilligan), 149
Inch, Sally, 372
Incontinence. See Urinary incontinence
Infants
    exercise programs for, 326–327
    gender and, 22–23
Injuries. See also Pain; Rehabilitation
    ankle injuries, 406
    avoidance of, 108
    back injuries, 396–399
    backpacking injuries, 136–138
    to breasts, 394–395
    chest injuries, 394–395
    child competitors, 333
    diabetic athletes, 364
    elbow injuries, 399–400
    to genital area, 400–401
    gymnastic injuries, 154
    head injuries, 393
    horse riding injuries, 143
    knee injuries, 401–404
    lower leg injuries, 405
    mental states and, 154
    neck injuries, 394
    older athletes, 360–364
    overexercising, 92–93, 147
    plantar fasciitis, 406–407
    from race walking, 119

RICE therapy, 411–413
shoulder injuries, 395–396
In-line skates, 198
Inner thigh stretches, 76
Insoluble fiber, 228
Insulin, soluble fiber and, 228
Intensity of exercise, 14, 66–69, 91
    amenorrhea and, 285–287
    classification of activities by, 238
    fuel use and, 241
    for older athletes, 365
    survey on, 91
    warm-up, intensity of, 72
Interval training, 94–95
    for running, 94–95, 124
Inverted U hypothesis, 152
Inward rotation, 44
Iodine, 224
Iron, 224
    misconceptions about, 231
    recommended daily allowance (RDA)
        for, 264
    tips for boosting intake, 265
Iron-deficiency anemia, 231, 264
    menstrual cycle and, 264–265
    prevention of, 265
Irregular bones, 36
Isoleucine, 233
Isometric contraction, 46
Isotonic contraction, 46

J

Jackson, Susan, 153
Jealousy, 388
Jennings, Lynn, 868
Jet skiing, 6
    pregnancy and, 314
Jewish Community Centers, 212
Jogger's nipples, 167–168
Jogging. See Running/jogging
Joints, 35, 36
    flexibility, 48
    overweight and, 56
    types of, 36, 37
Jones, Kathy Myers, 80
Jones, Kim, 260
The Jones Guide to Fitness and Health in
    New York (Jones), 80

Joyner, Florence Griffith, 162
Joyner-Kersee, Jackie, 162
Jumping rope, 81

K

Karvonen Method, 68
Kayaking, wetsuits for, 215
Kegel, Arnold, 376–377, 378
Kegel exercises, 376–377
    orgasm and, 387
Kerrigan, Nancy, 147
Kinesiology, 43–49
    defined, 34
Kinesthetic sense, 42
King, Billie Jean, 22, 162
Kishton, J. M., 334
Knees
    flexibility test, 355
    iliotibial band syndrome, 404
    injuries to, 401–404
    patellofemoral syndrome, 403
    rehabilitation of, 414–415
    sprains, 402
    treatment of injuries, 404
Korbut, Olga, 162
Kramer, Arthur, 13
Kushi, Lawrence, 366
Kutner, Lawrence, 330

L

Lactic acid, 40
LaLanne, Jack, 209
Lasts in shoes, 175
Lateral collateral ligament, 402
Lateral epicondylitis, 399–400
Lecithin, 222
Lee, I-Min, 14
Legs
    back pain and length of, 398
    flexibility test, 355
    lower leg injuries, 405
    weight training exercises for, 98
Legumes, 221
Leisure-time activity, 2
Leon, Arthur, 14, 15
Leucine, 233
Leukotrienes, 261
LeUnes, A., 158

energy needs and, 238
maximal oxygen consumption
(VO$_2$max), 51–52
running/jogging, use during, 240

P

Paffenbarger, Ralph, 14
Pain
    dealing with, 157–158
    endorphins and, 157
    feminist perspective on, 158–159
    sports inventory for, 157–158
Pantothenic acid, 224, 230
Parabolic skis, 194
Parasites, 138
Parkinson's disease, 372
Park Nicollet Medical Foundation, 14
Partners
    for exercise, 19
    Ride and Tie, 138–139
    sex and, 388–389
    for weight training, 102
Patella, 402
    dislocation of, 403–404
Patellofemoral syndrome, 403
Pelvic waist turns, 142
Pelvis, pregnancy and, 304
Performance, improvement of, 93–96
Perineometer, 379
Perreault, Bonnie, 140–143
Personal fitness profile, 67
Personal stereos, 214
Personal trainers, 79–80
    certification of, 80
    selection of, 80
    terminating relationship with, 80–81
Pessary, 379
Phelps, Almira, 4
Phidippides, 77
Phinney, Connie Carpenter, 418
Phosphate salts, 234
Phospholipids, 222
Phosphorus, 224
Physical activity, defined, 2
Physical fitness
    activities for development, 54
    assessment of, 57
    defined, 2, 53, 55

focus on, 7–8
overload principle, 66–70
profile of, 64, 67
The Physician and Sportsmedicine, 136–137
*The Physiological Effects of Wheat Germ Oil
    on Humans* (Cureton), 234
Pipes, Thomas, 155
Pippig, Uta, 87, 282
Piston rowing machines, 208
Pituitary function, 291
Pivot joints, 37
Places to exercise, 17–18
Plantar fasciitis, 406–407
Playgrounds, 327–328
PNF (proprioceptive neuromuscular facili-
    tation techniques), 74
Polartec, 178
Polyunsaturated fats, 223
Posterior (PCL) cruciate ligament, 402
Postpartum exercise, 316–319
Posture
    with cross-country ski machines, 207
    lower back and, 78
    pregnancy and, 206
    for stair machines, 204
    walking posture, 113
Potassium, 224
    misconceptions about, 231
    side effects, 232
Power, strength and, 56
PowerBar, 261
PR*Bar, 261
Pregnancy
    back problems, 305–306
    balance changes, 304–305
    birth weight and, 311
    blood pressure and, 302–303
    body changes and, 301–306
    body temperature and, 309
    contraindications to exercise,
        315–316
    dehydration and, 315
    fetal health and exercise, 308–310
    guides for pregnant athletes, 312–316
    heart rate
        fetal heart rate, 309–310
        maternal heart rate, 302
    iron deficiency in, 231

labor and exercise, 311–312
nighttime suggestions, 307
pelvis during, 304
postpartum exercise, 316–319
posture and, 206
problems with exercise and, 307–311
recommendations for exercise, 310
stress incontinence and, 372
warning signs, 309
weight gain, 303–304
Premature labor, 308
Premenstrual syndrome (PMS), 275
    help for, 277
Prentice, W. E, 60–62
Preschoolers, exercising with, 325
Press, Gwynn, 324
Primary amenorrhea, 280–281
    treatment of, 293
Prime movers, 44–45
Priority, exercise as, 18
Progestin Challenge test, 291
Pronators, 175
Proprioceptors, 42
Prostaglandins, 261
Proteins, 220
    growth and, 235–236
    increased protein diet, 261
    muscles and, 40
    sources of, 221
    supplements, 233
Prudden, Bonnie, 341, 345–346
Psychological barriers, 17
Psychological support for exercise, 17
Puberty, 23, 269–270
    muscle strength and, 25
Pubic symphysis, 304
Puretz, Susan, 34–52, 53–85, 86–110, 90,
        111–145, 351
Push-ups, 60
Pyramiding steroids, 431

Q

Q angle, 27
    patellofemoral syndrome, 403
Quads stretch, 76
Quality of life, 366
Quedenfeld, Ted, 336
Quinine, 262

Swimming, 6. *See also* Triathlons
  body fat and, 31
  breast size and, 28
  caps, 184
  children, instruction of, 330
  cross-training activities, 106
  fartlek training, 95
  goggles, 184–185
  hyperandrogenism and, 282
  impingement syndrome, 395–396
  interval training, 94–95
  menarche and, 271
  menstrual dysfunction, 280
  pregnancy and, 313
Swimsuits, 181–184
  body image and, 182–183
  for surfing, 181–184
  vaginitis and, 183–184
Swoopes, Sheryl, 162
Symbolic annihilation, 162
Synchilla, 178

T

Target heart rate (THR), 67–68
  aging and, 342–344
  perceived exertion, 69
Target training zone, 66
Task-specific warm-ups, 71–72
Tastes in exercise, 81
Teenagers, 329
  steroid use, 430
Telemark equipment, 193
Tendons, 41
Tennis, 6
  clothing for, 179
  equipment, 198–200
  grips on rackets, 199
  pregnancy and, 314
  rackets, 198–200
  shoes for, 197
  size of rackets, 199–200
Tennis elbow, 399–400
Terry, Georgena, 189
Terry Precision Cycling for Women, 189
Testosterone
  cholesterol and, 223
  steroids from, 430
Therma Fleece, 178

Thermax, 180
Thiamine, 224, 230
Thigh stretches, 76
Thirst, 248
Thromoxanes, 261
Thru-hiking, 135, 366
Tibia, 401
Tibialis posterior muscle, 39
Time for exercise, 17
Title IX, Education Amendment Act of
      1972, 8–9, 159–160, 392–393
Toenail loss, backpacking, 137
Tonus of muscle, 39
Top performers
  basketball players, 155
  long-distance runners, 155
  older athletes, 366–367
  training by, 86–88
  volleyball players, 156
Touring bikes, 189
Trace minerals, 225
Trail mix, 263
Trainers. *See* Personal trainers
Training. *See also* Weight training
  carbohydrates and, 242
  conflicting guidelines, 90–91
  fartlek training, 95
  fats and, 241–242
  foods and, 240–249
  intensity of, 66
  interpreting recommendations, 91–92
  interval training, 94–95
  quantity of, 89–91
  race walking, 118–120
  speed training, 95–96
  top performers, training by, 86–88
Trapezius, 39
  coordination of, 44
  as fixator, 45
Travel suggestions, 82
Treadmills, 204–206
  belts and decks for, 205
  display, 206
  speed and incline on, 205–206
Treasure, Darren C., 331, 332
Trends in exercise, 81
Triangular muscle, 39
Triathlons, 130–135

cross training for, 104, 131
overexercise injuries, 105
tips for, 131, 134
training schedule for, 13
Tricard, Louise Mead, 123, 124, 125, 129
Tricep stretch, 75
Trichomonas, 183–184
Triglycerides, 222
  soluble fiber and, 228
Troy Female Seminary, 4
Trunk stretch, 75–76
Truscott, Jamie, 328

U

Ultramarathons, 128–130
Unsaturated fats, 222–223
Upper back stretches, 75
Urge incontinence, 371–372
Urinary incontinence. *See also* Stress
      incontinence
  biofeedback techniques, 379
  drug therapy, 378
  during exercise, 380–381
  mechanical support, 379
  professional help, 377–378
  surgery for, 379–380
  types of, 371–372
Urinary tract infection (UTI), 400
U.S. Drug Enforcement Agency (DEA), 431
Uterine cancer, 12
Uznis, Mary Ann, 356

V

Vacation suggestions, 82
Vagina
  cancer of, 12
  injuries to, 400–401
Vaginal cones, 379
Vaginal perineometer, 379
Vaginitis, 183–184
Valine, 233
Valsalva maneuver, 313, 363
Van Nostrand, J. F., 361
Vassar College, 4
Vecsey, George, 162
Vegetable oils, 223
Vegetables, proteins in, 221
Vegetarian diet, 261